THE LANCET

Treating Individuals

From randomised trials to personalised medicine

For Elsevier:

Commissioning Editor: Alison Taylor
Development Editor: Kim Benson
Production Manager: Susan Stuart
Typesetting and production: Helius
Design: Patricia Stubberfield
Cover design: Kneath Associates

THE LANCET
Treating Individuals

From randomised trials to personalised medicine

Edited by: Peter M. Rothwell MBChB MD PhD FRCP
Professor of Clinical Neurology, University of Oxford, Oxford, UK

Foreword by: Richard Horton Editor, *The Lancet*

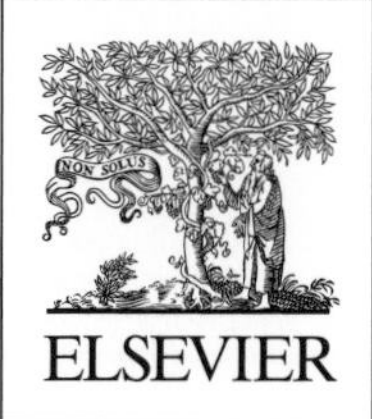

EDINBURGH • LONDON • NEW YORK • OXFORD • PHILADELPHIA • ST LOUIS • SYDNEY • TORONTO • 2007

THE LANCET

An imprint of Elsevier Limited

First published 2007

ISBN: 978-0-08-044739-1

British Library Cataloguing in Publication Data
A catalogue record for this book is available from the British Library.

Library of Congress Cataloging in Publication Data
A catalog record for this book is available from the Library of Congress.

Note
Knowledge and best practice in this field are constantly changing. As new research and experience broaden our knowledge, changes in practice, treatment and drug therapy may become necessary or appropriate. Readers are advised to check the most current information provided (i) on procedures featured or (ii) by the manufacturer of each product to be administered, to verify the recommended dose or formula, the method and duration of administration, and contraindications. It is the responsibility of the practitioner, relying on their own experience and knowledge of the patient, to make diagnoses, to determine dosages and the best treatment for each individual patient, and to take all appropriate safety precautions. To the fullest extent of the law, neither the Publisher nor the Editor or Authors assumes any liability for any injury and/or damage to persons or property arising out or related to any use of the material contained in this book. *The Publisher*

Printed in Spain

Contents

Contributors vii

Preface ix

Foreword, *Richard Horton, Editor, The Lancet* xiii

Section 1: Reliable determination of the overall effects of treatments **1**

1 Reliable assessment of the effects of treatments on mortality and major morbidity 3
Rory Collins and Stephen MacMahon

2 The lethal consequences of failing to make full use of all relevant evidence about the effects of medical treatments: the importance of systematic reviews 37
Iain Chalmers

Section 2: Is the trial relevant to this patient? **59**

3 Assessment of the external validity of randomised controlled trials 61
Peter M. Rothwell

4 Applying results to treatment decisions in primary care 83
Paul Glasziou and David Mant

5 The older patient 97
John Grimley Evans

6 Applying results to treatment decisions in complex clinical situations 111
Louis R. Caplan

7 External validity of pharmaceutical trials in neuropathic pain 121
C. Peter N. Watson

8 External validity of pharmaceutical trials in asthma and chronic obstructive pulmonary disease 131
Justin Travers, Suzanne Marsh, Philippa Shirtcliffe and Richard Beasley

Section 3: Is the overall trial result sufficiently relevant to this patient? **137**

9 When should we expect clinically important differences in response to treatment? 139
Peter M. Rothwell

10 Genes and the individual response to treatment 151
Urs A. Meyer

11 Reliable estimation and interpretation of the effects of treatment in subgroups 169
Peter M. Rothwell

12 Can meta-analysis help target interventions at individuals most likely to benefit? 183
Simon G. Thompson and Julian P. T. Higgins

13 Use of risk models to predict the likely effects of treatment in individuals 195
Peter M. Rothwell

14 Evaluating the performance of prognostic models 213
Douglas G. Altman and Patrick Royston

15 Are *n*-of-1 trials of any practical value to clinicians and researchers? 231
Graeme J. Hankey

Section 4: Targeting of treatment in routine practice 245

16 Primary prevention of cardiovascular disease: the absolute-risk-based approach 247
Rod Jackson

17 Antithrombotic therapy to prevent stroke in patients with atrial fibrillation 265
Robert G.Hart

18 Reperfusion therapies in acute cardiovascular and cerebrovascular syndromes 279
David M. Kent

19 Choice of agent in treatment of epilepsy 297
Sanjay M. Sisodiya

20 Pharmacogenomic targeting of treatment for cancer 307
Sharon Marsh and Howard L. McLeod

Index 319

Contributors

Douglas G. Altman DSc
Director, Centre for Statistics in Medicine, University of Oxford, Oxford, UK

Richard Beasley MD FRCP DSc
Medical Research Institute of New Zealand, Wellington, New Zealand; University of Southampton, UK

Louis R. Caplan MD
Professor of Neurology, Harvard Medical School; Chief, Cerebrovascular Diseases, Beth Israel Deaconess Medical Center, Boston, MA, USA

Sir Iain Chalmers DSc
Editor, *James Lind Library*, The James Lind Initiative, Oxford, UK

Rory Collins FMedSci FRCP
Professor, Clinical Trial Service Unit (CTSU), Oxford University, Oxford, UK

Paul Glasziou MBBS FRACGP PhD
Professor of Evidence-Based Medicine, Centre for Evidence-Based Medicine, Department of Primary Health Care, University of Oxford, Oxford, UK

Sir John Grimley Evans MD FRCP FFPH FMedSci
Professor Emeritus of Clinical Geratology, University of Oxford, Green College, Oxford, UK

Graeme J. Hankey MD FRCP FRACP
Consultant Neurologist and Head of Stroke Unit, Royal Perth Hospital, Western Australia; Clinical Professor, School of Medicine & Pharmacology, University of Western Australia

Robert G. Hart MD
Professor of Medicine (Neurology), University of Texas Health Science Center, San Antonio, TX, USA

Julian P. T. Higgins BA PhD
MRC Biostatistics Unit, Cambridge, UK

Rod Jackson MBChB PhD FAFPHM
Professor of Epidemiology, and Head of Section of Epidemiology and Biostatistics, Auckland, New Zealand

David M. Kent MD MS
Institute of Clinical Research and Health Policy Studies, Tufts–New England Medical Center, Boston, MA, USA

Howard L. McLeod PharmD
UNC Institute for Pharmacogenetics and Individualized Therapy, University of North Carolina, Chapel Hill, NC, USA

Contributors

Stephen MacMahon DSc PhD FACC FCSANE
The George Institute for International Health, University of Sydney, Sydney, NSW, Australia

David Mant MA FRCGP FRCP
Professor of General Practice, Department of Primary Health Care, University of Oxford, Oxford, UK

Sharon Marsh PhD
Washington University School of Medicine, Division of Oncology, St Louis, MO, USA

Suzanne Marsh MBChB MRCP
Medical Research Institute of New Zealand, Wellington, New Zealand

Urs A. Meyer MD
Professor of Pharmacology, Division of Pharmacology/Neurobiology, Biozentrum, University of Basel, Basel, Switzerland

Peter M. Rothwell MBChB MD PhD FRCP
Professor of Clinical Neurology, University of Oxford; Stroke Prevention Research Unit, University Department of Clinical Neurology, John Radcliffe Hospital, Oxford, UK

Patrick Royston BA MSc DSc
Statistical Methodology and Cancer Groups, MRC Clinical Trials Unit, London, UK

Philippa Shirtcliffe MBChB FRACP
Medical Research Institute of New Zealand, Wellington, New Zealand

Sanjay M. Sisodiya MA PhD FRCP
Reader in Neurology, Institute of Neurology, University College London, London; Honorary Consultant Neurologist, National Hospital for Neurology and Neurosurgery, Queen Square, London; National Society for Epilepsy, Chalfont St. Peter, UK

Simon G. Thompson MA DSc
MRC Biostatistics Unit, Cambridge, UK

Justin Travers MBChB FRACP
Medical Research Institute of New Zealand, Wellington, New Zealand

C. Peter N. Watson MD FRCPC
Assistant Professor, University of Toronto, Toronto, Ontario, Canada

Preface

All of us would hope and expect that if we required medical or surgical treatment we would receive the intervention that was most likely to be of benefit to us in our own particular situation. We might well also assume that doctors would have developed methods of predicting as precisely as possible which interventions would be most appropriate for which individuals.

Indeed, a huge amount of effort has gone into popularising and doing randomised trials and systematic reviews of medical interventions over the last 50 years, and the first section of this book considers in detail how and why they should be done and reminds us of the harm to patients that will result if we proceed without them in future. However, in stark contrast, there has been remarkably little research into how best to use the results of trials and reviews to ensure that as many individual patients as possible receive the most appropriate treatment in routine clinical practice. In fact, there is evidence of widespread underuse of potentially effective treatments, due at least in part to concerns on the part of clinicians about the relevance of some trials and reviews to their clinical practice and/or to decisions about treatment of individual patients.

This book focuses on the two key questions that are most frequently asked by clinicians about applying the results of randomised controlled trials and systematic reviews to decisions about their individual patients. Is the evidence relevant to my clinical practice? How can I judge whether the probability of benefit from treatment in my current patient is likely to differ substantially from the average probability of benefit reported in the relevant trial or systematic review?

There is evidence that many trials are not relevant to routine clinical practice (i.e. they are not externally valid), particularly some of those funded or performed by the pharmaceutical industry, and that funding agencies, journals and licensing authorities need to place greater emphasis on external validity. The second section of the book considers the determinants of external validity in general and with specific reference to primary care, the treatment of older patients, and the management of complex disorders, and illustrates the extent of the problem by systematically assessing the external validity of trials of treatments for chronic neuropathic pain and for asthma and chronic obstructive pulmonary disease.

The last two sections of the book consider the different approaches to predicting the likely effects of treatments in subgroups and individuals. This issue of the 'individualisation' of treatment decisions is the most controversial. The crux of the debate centres on the extent to which it is possible to use data from randomised controlled trials and systematic reviews to reliably inform the targeting of treatments (see panel I). Some observers argue that when large randomised controlled trials and systematic reviews are done, the effects of most medical interventions are shown to be relatively modest, and that very large pragmatic trials with broad entry criteria are therefore necessary to have the statistical power even to quantify these modest overall effects reliably. Others argue, however, that the measured effects of treatment are often so modest precisely because the trials are performed in such heterogeneous populations of patients, and that stratification into less heterogeneous clinical subgroups or risk groups is

Preface

Panel I: A selection of quotes that summarise the apparently contradictory points of view that are commonly expressed on how best to inform treatment decisions about individual patients

On the one hand ...

Anyone who believes that anything can be suited to everyone is a great fool, because medicine is practised not on mankind in general, but on every individual in particular. (Henri de Monville, 1320)

If it were not for the great variability between individuals, medicine might as well be a science, not an art. (William Osler, 1892)

In my indictment of the statistician, I would argue that he may tend to be a trifle too scornful of the clinical judgement, the clinical impression. (Austin Bradford Hill, 1952)

Far better an approximate answer to the right question, which is often vague, than an exact answer to the wrong question, which can always be made precise. (John W Tukey, 1962)

The paradox of the clinical trial is that it is the best way to assess whether an intervention works but arguably the worst way to assess who will benefit from it. (David Mant, 1999)

On the other hand ...

...it would be unfortunate if desire for the perfect (i.e. knowledge of exactly who will benefit from treatment) were to become the enemy of the possible (i.e. knowledge of the direction and approximate size of the effects of treatment of wide categories of patient). (Salim Yusuf, Rory Collins and Richard Peto, 1984)

It is right for each physician to want to know about the behaviour to be expected from the intervention or therapy applied to his individual patient ... it is not right, however, for a physician to expect to know this. (John W. Tukey, 1986)

One should look for treatment-covariate interactions, but ... one should look very cautiously in the spirit of exploratory data analysis rather than that of formal hypothesis testing. (David Byar, 1985)

Subgroup analysis kills people. (Richard Peto, 1995)

necessary. The third section of the book reviews the different potential approaches to exploring the likely extent of differences in the probability of benefit from treatment between subgroups and individuals, and the final section reviews six areas of clinical practice where some progress towards evidence-based personalised medicine has been made.

The book expands on the *Treating Individuals* series of articles published in *The Lancet* in 2005, which attempted to address these same issues, and brings together the thoughts of a much larger group of highly experienced clinicians, trialists and statisticians. With the exception of the Editor, contributors have not generally seen or commented on other chapters and the writing of the book was not preceded by any consensus meeting. Consequently, the views expressed are sometimes inconsistent, or even contradictory, which reflects the core purpose of the book – to present (unedited) the different perspectives of clinicians, trialists and statisticians on what is perhaps the main challenge still facing evidence-based medicine – how best to inform the treatment of individuals.

Peter M. Rothwell

Foreword

How good are doctors at treating individual patients? The word 'treatment' can be interpreted in several different ways. If we mean the overall management of patients—the way in which doctors take a history, complete a physical examination, and the style with which they conduct the interaction with the patient—then we are defining a set of behaviours that are largely about respect, compassion and trust. Common sense, many would say. Who needs a book about common sense?

But 'treatment' in the context of *Treating Individuals* means applying the results of research evidence—ideally, but not exclusively, from randomised trials or systematic reviews of randomised trials—to the individual patient. This interpretation of 'treatment' is certainly not resolved by appealing to common sense. This book might be worth reading after all.

Two concepts dominate. First, reliability: how consistently good are the data, whatever their provenance, in terms of inherent quality (otherwise known as internal validity)? Second, relevance: how appropriate are those data to the problem the patient presents (sometimes called external validity)? Reliability and relevance are the only two questions that should matter to the physician considering how to use data to inform his or her decision-making.

There are many examples where the rigorous application of these two principles would have prevented a great deal of misunderstanding and harm. Some years ago, observational studies suggested that the short-acting calcium-channel blocker nifedipine was associated with an increased risk of myocardial infarction. Concern soon spread to the entire class of these drugs. A frenzy ensued. Considerable professional and public fear was generated. It took almost a decade for the issue to be settled experimentally. Readers (and editors) of superficially startling preliminary research jumped to quick conclusions, forgot the essential concepts of reliability and relevance (both low in this particular instance), and fostered a largely unproductive era of scepticism about a valuable class of drug.

By contrast, the cautious analysis and interpretation of non-randomised data can be usefully instructive for treating individuals. In a before-and-after study, the UK's national teenage pregnancy strategy after 1999 was subjected to the kind of scrutiny few health policies receive. Although not conclusive, this non-experimental comparison has suggested a tantalising reversal of a previously rising trend in teenage pregnancies. The investigation carried moderate reliability and moderate relevance. Not conclusive, to be sure, but certainly informative.

The obsessive ambition to secure reliable and relevant information for public and patient alike can sometimes seem astonishingly irrational. Who would think of using randomisation to evaluate a country's entire health-system reform? Crazy. Yet that is what the Mexican Ministry of Health sought to do when it introduced far-reaching reforms in 2001. The question facing the ministry was how effective their reforms were likely to be for individuals. They had hopes—even policies—but few data. They needed information that was reliable and relevant. They turned to an experimental evaluation. It is hard to imagine a western nation of over 100 million people taking such a bold (and scientific) step.

Foreword

A sterile debate stains the question about evidence for treatment—what counts: observational or randomised studies? Instead of pitting one set of methods (and communities: epidemiologists versus trialists and systematic reviewers) against another, a better approach might be to encourage a more critical attitude to the whole question of decision-making about treatments. Evidence-based medicine has constructed an impressive foundation for the appraisal and application of research into practice. Despite its success, there are still those who raise questions about the claims of evidence-based medicine. Some say it is creating doctors 'conditioned to function like a well-programmed computer framework'.[1]

Peter Rothwell helps us to move beyond these old ideological obstacles. He has assembled an extraordinary family of writers to lead readers through a compelling array of issues that are literally matters of life and death for patients. *The Lancet* has good reason to thank him and his contributors for expanding the reach and depth of their original *Lancet* series. They have taken a good idea and, impossibly, made it better.

Richard Horton, Editor, The Lancet

References

1 Groopman J. *How Doctors Think*. Boston, MA: Houghton Mifflin, 2007.

Section 1

Reliable determination of the overall effects of treatments

1

Reliable assessment of the effects of treatments on mortality and major morbidity

Rory Collins and Stephen MacMahon

Introduction

This chapter is intended principally for basic scientists and practising clinicians who want to know why some types of evidence about the effects of treatment on survival, and on other major aspects of chronic disease outcome, are much more reliable than others. Although there are a few striking examples of treatments for serious disease which really do work extremely well, most claims for big improvements turn out to be evanescent. Unrealistic expectations about the chances of discovering large treatment effects could misleadingly suggest that evidence from small randomised trials or from non-randomised studies will suffice. By contrast, the reliable assessment of any more moderate effects of treatment on major outcomes – which are usually all that can realistically be expected from most treatments for most common serious conditions – requires studies that guarantee both strict control of bias (which, in general, requires proper randomisation and appropriate analysis, with no unduly data-dependent emphasis on specific parts of the overall evidence) and strict control of random error (which, in general, requires large numbers of deaths or of some other relevant outcome). Past failures to produce such evidence, and to interpret it appropriately, have already led to many premature deaths and much unnecessary suffering.

Some treatments for the chronic diseases of middle age have been found to produce large effects on death and disability. For example, it is obvious that prompt treatment of diabetic coma or cardiac arrest saves lives. But, given the heterogeneity of any particular condition (as indicated by the different survival durations of apparently similar patients) and the variety of different mechanisms that can lead to death or disability (only one of which may be appreciably influenced by any one treatment), hopes of large effects of treatment on major outcomes have often been unrealistically high.[1, 2] Some such expectations might derive from extrapolation of the effects of treatment on 'surrogate' outcomes. For example, cardiac arrhythmias are associated with a poor prognosis, and antiarrhythmic drugs can markedly reduce their frequency. However, various antiarrhythmic regimens have been found to increase, rather than decrease, mortality.[3, 4] Many other treatments have large effects on one part of a disease process – for example, zidovudine on viral titre in early human immunodeficiency virus (HIV) infection, and radiotherapy on local recurrence in breast cancer – but uncertainty remains as to whether their routine use produces a favourable balance of benefits and risks for major clinical outcomes.[5–7] In general, if such uncertainty exists about a treatment, any effects on mortality or major morbidity are likely to be either negligibly small or of only moderate size.[2] As will be discussed, support for this conclusion comes from the modest effects typically suggested by the aggregated results (i.e. meta-analyses or systematic overviews) of all relevant clinical trials of any particular therapy for a chronic disease;[2, 8] and, in certain special cases, by the modest strength of the relationship in observational studies between disease risk and a risk factor that treatment can modify (e.g. blood pressure[9] or cholesterol[10]).

In many circumstances, even moderate improvements in survival or in major morbidity would still be regarded as worthwhile by patients and their doctors (provided, of course, that any benefits are not substantially offset by some serious adverse effects). Clearly, however, if such treatment effects are to be reliably detected or reliably refuted, then any errors in their assessment need to be much smaller than the difference between a moderate but worthwhile effect and an effect that is too small to be of any material importance. Systematic errors (i.e. biases) in the assessment of treatment can be produced by differences in factors other than the treatment under investigation (panel 1.1). Observational studies, in which outcome is compared between individuals who received the treatment of interest and those who did not, can be subject to large systematic errors.[11]

Instead, the guaranteed avoidance of material biases typically requires the proper randomised allocation of treatment and appropriate statistical analysis, with no unduly data-dependent emphasis on specific subsets of the overall evidence[2] (panel 1.2). Random errors in the assessment of treatment effects relate to the impact of the play of chance on outcome among those exposed or not exposed to the treatment of interest (see panel 1.1). These errors are determined by the number of deaths or other relevant outcomes in the study, and their size can be quantified (e.g. in terms of a confidence interval that indicates the range of effects statistically compatible with the observed result). The only way to guarantee small random errors is to study large numbers of outcomes by doing large individual studies and large meta-analyses[2] (see panel 1.2). It is not much use, however, having very small random errors if there could be moderate biases, so even the large size of some observational studies cannot guarantee reliable assessment of moderate treatment effects.[12]

Clinical trials and observational studies have provided much of the available evidence about the effects on death and major non-fatal outcomes (e.g. heart attacks, strokes,

Panel 1.1: Main sources of error in epidemiological studies of the effects of treatment

Systematic errors

- Biases due to the differences in outcome caused by factors other than the treatment being investigated
- Frequent problem in the interpretation of observational studies
- Can cause either overestimation or underestimation of treatment effects
- Difficult to determine the size or direction of bias

Random errors

- Impact of chance on comparisons of outcome between those who did and did not receive the treatment
- Frequent problem in the interpretation of clinical trials
- Can prevent real effects of treatment being detected or their size being estimated reliably
- Easily quantified

Panel 1.2: **Requirements for reliable assessment of moderate treatment effects: simultaneous avoidance of moderate systematic errors and moderate random errors**

Avoidance of moderate systematic errors

- Proper randomisation (non-randomised methods may cause moderate or large biases)
- Analysis by allocated treatment (including all randomised patients: intention-to-treat analysis)
- Chief emphasis on overall results (without undue data-dependent emphasis on particular subgroups)
- Meta-analyses of all relevant studies (without undue data-dependent emphasis on particular studies)

Avoidance of moderate random errors

- Large numbers of major outcomes in any new studies (with streamlined study methods to facilitate recruitment)
- Meta-analyses of all relevant studies (yielding the largest possible numbers of deaths and other major outcomes)

cancers) of different treatments for disease. But not all such epidemiological evidence is reliable, and the consequences of this may be substantial: for example, ineffective or dangerous treatments might continue to be used, or effective and safe treatments might not be used appropriately widely. The first part of this chapter is concerned with the reliable demonstration of any moderate effects of treatment on mortality and major morbidity, which requires the simultaneous avoidance of moderate biases and moderate random errors. This requirement determines the need for appropriately large, properly randomised, trials. As will be discussed, non-randomised observational studies, and unduly small randomised trials or meta-analyses, are all much inferior as sources of evidence about such moderate, although potentially important, effects of treatment. In the second part of this chapter, the ways in which observational studies can be useful for the assessment of treatment effects are discussed; in particular, for the detection of large effects on rare outcomes, and for helping to generalise the results of randomised trials to different circumstances.[11]

Clinical trials: minimising both systematic and random errors

Avoidance of moderate systematic errors

Proper randomisation

The fundamental reason for random allocation of treatment in clinical trials is to maximise the likelihood that each type of patient will have been allocated in similar proportions to the different treatment strategies being investigated.[12] In a properly randomised trial, the decision to enter a patient is made irreversibly in ignorance of which trial treatments that patient will be allocated. Foreknowledge of the next treatment allocation could affect the decision to enter the patient, and those allocated one treatment might then differ systematically from those allocated another.[13] For example, in a study comparing amniotomy (rupture of membranes) versus oxytocin for induction of labour that was described as randomised, allocation was actually based on whether the woman's date of birth was odd or even. Foreknowledge of this led to women with an 'unripe' cervix being far less likely to be recruited if they were to have been allocated amniotomy (i.e. had an odd date of birth; table 1.1).[14] Similarly, in the Captopril Prevention Project (CAPPP) trial,[15] envelopes containing the antihypertensive treatment allocation could be opened before patients were irreversibly entered in the study, and – presumably as a consequence – there were highly significant differences in pre-entry blood pressure (and other characteristics) between the treatment groups, which might have introduced bias.[16]

Studies in which treatment has not been properly allocated at random do not necessarily provide misleading evidence about the effects of treatment.[17, 18] For example, in the Salk polio vaccine studies of the 1950s,[19] the halving in poliomyelitis cases observed in the large non-randomised comparison between those children who had been vaccinated and those who had not was confirmed by the large randomised trial of vaccine versus placebo (table 1.2). But, since non-random methods introduce the potential for moderate biases, non-randomised studies cannot be guaranteed to provide appropriately unbiased assessments when the real effects of treatment are of moderate size.[13, 20] So, for example, the mortality reduction observed in the aggregate of all available

Cervical 'ripeness'	Amniotomy: odd dates of birth (n = 110)	Oxytocin: even dates of birth (n = 113)
Least	7	28
Intermediate	58	56
Most	45	29

Comparison of the distribution between treatment groups of cervical ripeness before treatment allocation: $\chi^2 = 16.1$ ($p < 0.0005$).

***Table* 1.1: Imbalance in patients' characteristics between treatment groups due to foreknowledge of treatment allocation: trial of amniotomy or oxytocin for induction of labour[14]**

Type of study	Poliomyelitis cases/total (rate per 100 000)		Odds ratio (95% CI)
	Vaccine	Control	
Non-randomised	60/231 902 (26)	391/725 173 (54)	0.55 (0.44–0.68)
Randomised*	57/200 745 (28)	142/201 229 (71)	0.43 (0.32–0.56)

*Excludes 8484 vaccine-allocated and 8577 placebo-allocated non-compliant children with data on outcome not fully available.

***Table* 1.2: Confirmation by randomised trial of observed effect in non-randomised trial: Salk vaccine for poliomyelitis[19]**

randomised trials of oral anticoagulants for acute myocardial infarction was found to be only about a third as large as the highly significant 30–40% mortality reduction observed in the non-randomised concurrently-controlled studies (which mainly used alternate allocation).[21] Hence, the biases inherent in non-randomised studies can be at least as big as any moderate effects of treatment on mortality and major morbidity that might exist (and it can be difficult to predict their direction).

Intention-to-treat analysis

Even in a properly randomised trial, bias can be inadvertently introduced by the post-randomisation exclusion of certain patients (e.g. those who are non-compliant with the study treatment), especially if the prognosis of those excluded from one treatment group differs from that of those excluded from another. This point is illustrated by the Coronary Drug Project randomised trial of cholesterol-lowering therapy: patients who took at least 80% of their allocated clofibrate had substantially lower 5-year mortality than those who did not (15.0% versus 24.6%, respectively; $p = 0.0001$), but there was an even more striking difference in outcome between good and poor compliers in the placebo group (15.1% versus 28.3%, respectively; $p < 0.00001$).[22] The primary statistical analysis of any trial should, therefore, compare outcome among all those originally allocated one treatment (even though some of them may not have actually received it) versus outcome among all those allocated the other treatment – that is, an intention-to-treat analysis of the impact of a general policy of using the treatment. This is not to say that additional analyses may not also be of value: for example, in describing the frequency of some very specific side-effect, it may be preferable to describe its incidence only among those who actually received the treatment because strictly randomised comparisons might not be needed to assess extreme relative risks.[1]

Since there is bound to be some non-compliance with the allocated treatments in clinical trials, intention-to-treat analyses will tend to underestimate the effects produced by full compliance with the study treatments. But, rather than using potentially biased 'on treatment' comparisons among only those who were compliant, more appropriate allowance can be made by applying an approximate estimate of the level of compliance to the estimate of the treatment effect provided by the intention-to-treat comparison.[23] For example, in a meta-analysis of the randomised trials of prolonged use of aspirin and other antiplatelet agents among patients with occlusive vascular disease, the average compliance 1 year after treatment allocation seemed to have been no more than 80%.[24] Application of this estimate of compliance to the proportional reduction of about 30% in non-fatal heart attacks and strokes estimated from intention-to-treat analyses of these trials suggests that full compliance with antiplatelet therapy produces reductions in risk of about 35–40%.

Problems produced by data-dependent emphasis

Apparent differences between the therapeutic effects in different subgroups of study participants can often be produced just by the play of chance and, in particular subgroups, chance can mimic or obscure moderate treatment effects. For example, in the large Second International Study of Infarct Survival (ISIS-2) randomised trial of the emergency treatment of heart attacks, the 1-month survival advantage produced by aspirin was particularly clear (804 vascular deaths among 8587 patients allocated aspirin versus 1016 among 8600 allocated placebo-control; proportional reduction of 23% (standard deviation (SD) 4); $p < 0.000001$).[25] To illustrate the unreliability of subgroup analyses, these overall results were subdivided by the patients' astrological birth signs into 12 subgroups. In some subgroups the results for aspirin were about average, but in others they were, by chance, slightly better or slightly worse than average. Taking the subgroups with the least promising results, which happened to be Libra or Gemini, no fewer deaths were observed with aspirin than with placebo (table 1.3). Clearly, it would be unwise to conclude from such an analysis that patients born under the astrological birth signs of Libra or Gemini are unlikely to benefit from aspirin. Yet, similar conclusions based on 'exploratory' data-derived subgroup analyses that are no more reliable than these are often reported and may be accepted, with inappropriate effects on practice. For example, despite the highly significant survival advantage observed overall in the large Gruppo Italiano per lo Studio della Streptochinasi nell'Infarto Miocardico (GISSI) randomised trial, it was suggested that fibrinolytic therapy might not save lives among patients who had had a previous heart attack (based on 157 deaths among such patients allocated streptokinase versus 147 among those allocated control).[26] By contrast, subsequent trials have shown unequivocally that the benefits of fibrinolytic therapy are similar among those with and without a history of prior infarction.[27] In another example of the impact of unduly selective emphasis on small subgroups in particular trials, the use of aspirin after transient ischaemic attacks was, until recently, approved in the USA for men but not for women.[28] This has turned out to have been a lethal error, resulting in many women being denied a life-saving treatment that produces about the same benefits for women as for men.[24]

Similarly, when several studies have all addressed much the same therapeutic question, choice of only a few of them for emphasis could be a source of serious bias, as chance fluctuations for or against treatment might affect this choice. To avoid such bias, it is often appropriate to base inference chiefly on a meta-analysis of all of the results from all randomised trials that have addressed the particular question (or, at least, on an unbiased subset of the relevant trials).[7, 29] Such meta-analyses will also minimise random errors in the assessment of treatment effects, because far more patients (and, most importantly, more events) are typically included in a meta-analysis than in any individual trial that contributes to it. The separate trials might well be heterogeneous, but this merely argues for careful interpretation of the results of any meta-analysis (rather than arguing against any such analyses)[30] since, without meta-analyses, moderate biases and

Astrological birth sign	Vascular death by 1 month		*p*
	Aspirin	Placebo	
Libra or Gemini	150 (11.1%)	147 (10.2%)	0.5
All other signs	654 (9.0%)	869 (12.1%)	< 0.0001
Any birth sign	804 (9.4%)	1016 (11.8%)	< 0.0001

***Table* 1.3: Unreliability of 'data-dependent' subgroup analyses: ISIS-2 trial of aspirin among over 17 000 patients with suspected acute myocardial infarction[25]**

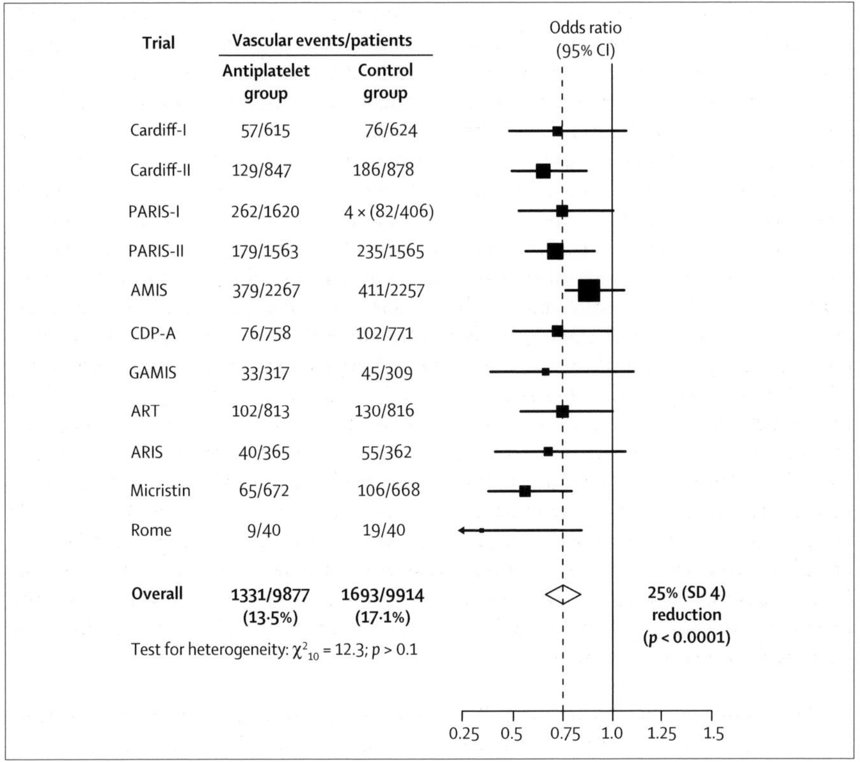

Figure 1.1: **Clear demonstration of worthwhile benefits in meta-analysis of available trial data, by contrast with failure of individual trials to provide convincing evidence. (Reproduced from Collins and MacMahon,[1] copyright 2001, with permission from Elsevier.)**

random errors often cannot both be avoided reliably. For example, meta-analysis of the relevant randomised trials showed clearly that prolonged antiplatelet therapy after myocardial infarction reduces the risk of major vascular events (i.e. death, recurrent infarction, stroke) by about a quarter (figure 1.1).[24] These findings have led to the appropriately widespread use of such treatment (in particular, low-dose aspirin), and the prevention of tens of thousands of deaths and disabling events each year worldwide. By contrast, selective emphasis on the trial with the least promising result[31] could lead to the dangerously misleading conclusion that antiplatelet therapy is not beneficial for such patients.[32] Similarly, the inference drawn from a subgroup of one trial that the beneficial effects of angiotensin-converting-enzyme inhibitors on mortality and hospital admission for heart failure are lost in the presence of aspirin[32] is not supported by a meta-analysis of all such trials in patients with ventricular dysfunction.[33]

Subgroups defined by post-randomisation characteristics

In general, any prognostic features that are to be used in analyses of treatment effects in randomised trials should be irreversibly recorded before the treatment is allocated.

For, if the recorded value of some feature is affected by the trial treatment allocation, then comparisons within subgroups that are defined by that factor might be biased. As an example, consider a study of mastectomy with axillary clearance versus lumpectomy alone for women with breast cancer. An unusually careful search of the axilla among those allocated axillary clearance could result in the discovery of tiny deposits of cancer cells that would otherwise have been overlooked. Hence, some of the women in the axillary clearance group who would otherwise have been classified as 'stage I' will be reclassified as 'stage II', biasing any comparisons with women in the lumpectomy-alone group for whom the staging was less careful.[34] Similarly, in randomised trials of treatment with 3-hydroxy-3-methylglutaryl-coenzyme A reductase inhibitors (statins) versus no such treatment, comparisons between the coronary disease rates seen among patients who achieved large cholesterol reductions and those who achieved small reductions[35] are potentially biased. For, groups of patients defined by the difference in post-randomisation cholesterol-lowering response to treatment cannot be guaranteed – and, indeed, are unlikely – to differ only randomly from each other (e.g. factors related to the apparent biochemical response might also be related to outcome). Hence, inferences drawn from such non-randomised comparisons of 'responders' versus 'non-responders' could be seriously misleading. Such potential for bias is also inherent in analyses of randomised trials that involve statistical 'adjustment' or stratification for post-randomisation levels of the risk factors altered by the study treatment (e.g. blood pressure with antihypertensive drugs[36, 37]) which may be interpreted falsely as providing reliable evidence that the observed risk reductions cannot be explained fully by the change in those risk factor levels alone (and, hence, that other factors must be relevant).

Avoidance of moderate random errors

Problems with false-negative results

It is still not sufficiently widely appreciated just how large clinical trials need to be to detect reliably the sort of moderate, but important, differences in major outcomes that might exist (especially if effects in different subgroups are to be assessed reliably).[1, 2] For example, between the late 1950s and the early 1980s, about two dozen randomised trials of intravenous fibrinolytic therapy for the emergency treatment of heart attacks were reported.[38] Each of those trials was too small – none involved even 1000 patients – to provide reliable evidence about any moderate effects of this treatment on mortality (figure 1.2), although several were large enough to show the large relative effects on bleeding. As a result, fibrinolytic therapy was generally regarded as both ineffective and dangerous, and thus inappropriate for routine coronary care. By contrast, during the mid-1980s, the GISSI-1[26] and ISIS-2[25] 'mega-trials' each involved more than 10 000 patients (and, most relevantly, more than 1000 deaths), and provided such definite evidence about the beneficial effects of fibrinolytic therapy that worldwide treatment patterns changed rapidly. Consequently, at least half a million patients per year are now given fibrinolytic treatment, avoiding at least 10 000 premature deaths annually. But, if GISSI-1 and ISIS-2 had been only a tenth as large (which would still have been larger than any of the previous trials), the observed reduction in mortality of about a quarter would not have been conventionally significant, and would therefore have had much less influence on medical practice. Indeed, the inadequate size of the earlier trials –

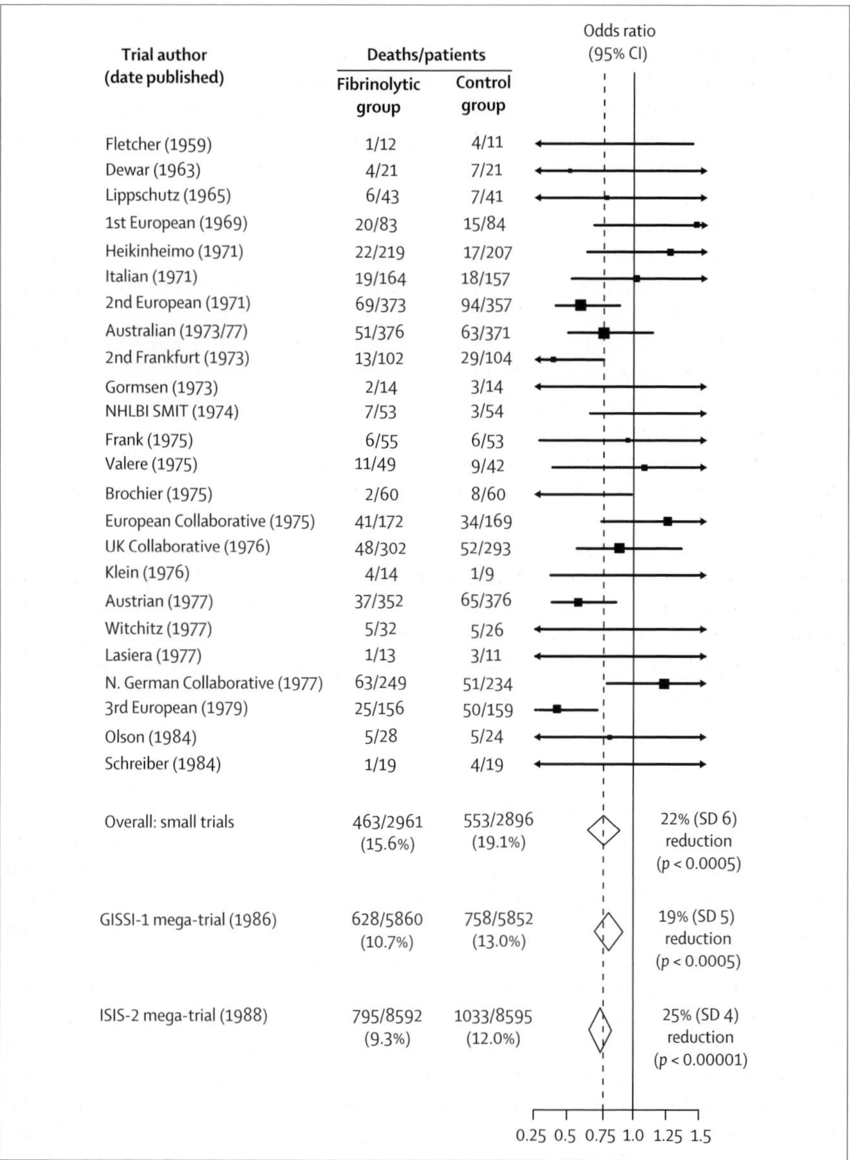

Figure **1.2: Clear demonstration of worthwhile benefits in mega-trials, by contrast with failure of previous much smaller trials. (Reproduced from Collins and MacMahon,[1] copyright 2001, with permission from Elsevier.)**

which delayed the convincing demonstration of the benefits of fibrinolytic therapy for more than two decades – can now be seen to have been the cause of some hundreds of thousands of unnecessary deaths.

1 Assessment of effects of treatments on mortality and morbidity

Problems with false-positive results

Small-scale evidence about the effects of treatment on major outcomes (whether from a single randomised trial or from a meta-analysis of trials) is often unreliable, and will frequently be found in retrospect to have been misleading. For example, a review of the small randomised trials of antiplatelet therapy in pregnancy suggested that such treatment reduced the incidence of pre-eclampsia by about three-quarters, and produced a much better outcome for the fetus (with less intrauterine growth retardation and fewer perinatal deaths).[39] By contrast, the effects in several subsequent, much larger, randomised trials[40, 41] were much less promising, indicating reductions of only about a sixth in pre-eclampsia and no apparent improvement in fetal outcome. Small-scale evidence from randomised trials can be misleading, not just about the size but even about the direction of the effects of treatment on major outcomes. For example, it was concluded from a small randomised trial among patients with heart failure that the inotropic agent vesnarinone more than halved the risk of death (13 vesnarinone versus 33 placebo deaths, $p = 0.002$).[42] By contrast, when the same regimen was studied in much larger numbers of the same type of patient, mortality was significantly increased (292 vesnarinone versus 242 placebo deaths, $p = 0.02$).[43] Similarly, although a meta-analysis of small trials had indicated that intravenous steroids reduced mortality following head injury, a large-scale randomised trial designed to confirm this hypothesis had to be stopped prematurely because mortality was significantly increased by this treatment.[44] Further examples of treatments for which extreme observations from initial small trials have not been confirmed by much larger randomised trials include calcium[45, 46] or vitamin[47, 48] supplementation for the prevention of pre-eclampsia,[45, 46] intravenous nitrates[49, 50] or magnesium[51, 52] for the emergency treatment of heart attacks, heparins[53, 54] or calcium antagonists[55, 56] for the emergency treatment of strokes, and vitamin E[57–60] or antibiotics[61–64] for the prevention of coronary disease.

There are several possible explanations for such discrepancies. One theoretical possibility is that the benefits of the treatment are confined to particular categories of patients that were selectively included in the small trials. Often this possibility can be investigated by separate analyses in these selected subgroups within the large randomised trials: for example, with antiplatelet therapy in pre-eclampsia, such analyses did not identify any particular category of woman in which the effects were as great as those reported in the small trials.[40] Similarly, when considering the disappointing results of a large trial of extracranial–intracranial bypass surgery for symptomatic carotid stenosis,[65] some neurosurgeons suggested that the findings might not be generally relevant because many of the patients thought to benefit from surgery had been excluded from the trial.[66] But, when those categories of patient were defined, it could be shown that the results within the trial among such patients were no more promising.[67] Another, perhaps more plausible, explanation for the failure of large trials to confirm reports of extreme results in selected small trials is that other small trials with unpromising results might be less likely to have been published because they were less remarkable[68] (e.g. for pre-eclampsia, at least as many women had been randomised in other small trials of antiplatelet therapy that had not had their pre-eclampsia results published[41]). Moreover, since large trials of a particular question are often done because the results of initial small trials (or small meta-analyses) are extremely promising, the 'hypothesis-generating' trial evidence might well provide an overestimate of the real effects of treatment (especially if those trials were stopped prematurely because of extreme results[69]), whereas the subsequent large trials would not.

Generalisation from clinical trials to clinical practice

Clinicians are used to dealing with individual patients, and might feel that the results of trials somehow deny that individuality. This is almost the opposite of the truth, as one of the main reasons for doing randomised trials is because patients are so different from one another that it is only when the effects of treatment on outcome are compared among sufficiently large groups of patients divided at random that the proportions of patients with good and bad prognoses allocated the different treatments can be relied on to be sufficiently similar. Moreover, the identification of those particular types of patient most likely to benefit from a treatment will often require even larger scale evidence from randomised trials, and even more careful interpretation, than is required to show an overall treatment effect reliably. panel 1.3 lists the three main remedies for this unavoidable conflict between the reliable subgroup-specific conclusions that doctors and their patients want, and the unreliable findings that subgroup analyses of clinical trials might offer.[2,70]

Basing inference on overall effects on particular outcomes

The first approach is to emphasise chiefly the overall results of a trial – or, better still, of a meta-analysis of all such trials – for particular outcomes as a guide to the qualitative results in various specific subgroups of patients, and to give less weight to the actual results in each separate subgroup.[1,2] This is clearly the right way to interpret the astrological subgroups in table 1.3, but it is also likely in many other circumstances to provide the best assessment of whether a treatment is effective in particular subgroups. For example, on the basis of adjusted analyses of large observational databases, it has been claimed that 1-month mortality is increased by fibrinolytic therapy in patients aged 75 years or older who present within 12 h with electrocardiographic changes indicative of acute myocardial infarction.[71,72] By contrast, a meta-analysis of the major randomised trials of fibrinolytic therapy has provided especially strong evidence of overall benefit,[73] with no significant difference between the mortality reductions seen among such patients at different ages: 27 (SD 3) fewer deaths per 1000 patients younger than 75 years compared with 34 (SD 16) fewer deaths per 1000 older patients.[26] Similarly, although patients with severe heart failure have tended to be excluded from previous trials of cholesterol-lowering therapy, the overwhelmingly strong evidence of benefit demonstrated by large randomised trials in a wide range of circumstances

Panel 1.3: Estimating the effects of treatment in particular types of patient

- Base inference on the overall effects observed on particular outcomes (without unduly selective emphasis on the results in each separate subgroup of patients)
- Give greater emphasis to results in prespecified, rather than retrospectively data-derived, subgroups (provided they involve sufficiently large numbers of outcomes)
- Consider subgroup analyses of mortality in the context of analyses of other relevant major outcomes (which might be more statistically stable)

(including among people with coronary heart disease, which is the most common cause of heart failure)[74] provides compelling evidence for the routine use of such treatment in heart failure (unless good evidence against such practices emerges from subsequent trials[75, 76]). Hence, when a treatment has been shown unequivocally to be beneficial overall, really good evidence should be required of lack of benefit in some particular subgroup (rather than merely lack of a clearly significant effect in that subgroup taken on its own) before it is considered safe to conclude that the treatment is not of value for such patients.

Because the effects of treatment on different outcomes may differ in terms of size or direction, estimates from trials of the separate effects on each outcome are likely to be more widely generalisable than would be an estimate of the combined effect on these outcomes. For example, the average reduction in diastolic blood pressure of 5–6 mmHg achieved in previous trials of antihypertensive therapy produced proportional risk reductions of about 40% for stroke and of about 15% for coronary heart disease, and each of these proportional effects seemed to be similar among different types of patient.[77] Hence, the relative frequency of strokes and of coronary events in different circumstances will influence both the proportional and absolute effects of blood-pressure lowering on the overall risk of vascular disease. Similarly, for endarterectomy in patients with symptomatic carotid-artery stenosis, the net effect on stroke risk is dependent on the balance in a particular population between the beneficial effects of surgery on ipsilateral stroke and the adverse effects of surgery on other strokes. Consequently, estimates from trials of the separate effects on each of these types of strokes would be expected to be more informative about the net effect on the risk of stroke in different situations[78] than would the overall effects on total stroke observed in any single population.[79]

Prespecification of analyses within particular subgroups

The second approach to determining effects in particular types of patient is to prespecify a limited number of subgroup analyses, provided there are good a priori reasons for anticipating that the effect of treatment might be different in different circumstances. Generally, such prespecified analyses should then be taken more seriously than other subgroup analyses, as long as they are based on sufficiently large numbers of events. For example, the benefits of fibrinolytic therapy for heart attacks were expected to be greater the earlier patients were treated, so some studies prespecified that the analyses should be subdivided by time from onset of symptoms to treatment. None of the individual studies of fibrinolytic therapy could show this clearly on its own, but a meta-analysis of the major trials included large enough numbers of patients to show that the benefit was indeed greatest for those treated earliest after the onset of acute myocardial infarction (although the mortality reduction was still substantial for those treated several hours after symptom onset).[25] In such circumstances, however, it may be unwise to prejudge the outcome of such an analysis by excluding patients in whom it is thought the benefits might be smaller or non-existent: for example, several statin trials excluded elderly patients, and so delayed the emergence of clear evidence of benefit in such patients.[80]

Interpretation of mortality analyses in the context of morbidity analyses

Finally, in considering the likely effects of treatment on the survival of particular patients, it might be useful to take account not only of the mortality data in specific subgroups but also of the data on some other relevant major outcomes (e.g. recurrence-free survival in cancer trials, or non-fatal as well as fatal myocardial infarction in heart disease trials). If the overall results for such outcomes are similar but much more highly significant than for mortality (due chiefly to the larger number of events, but perhaps also because effects on non-fatal outcomes emerge more rapidly), subgroup analyses of these major outcomes will be more stable. Hence, the results of these analyses may provide a better guide to the existence of any large differences between subgroups in the effects of treatment (particularly if such subgroup analyses were specified before results were available). For example, in the early 1990s, a collaborative meta-analysis of all relevant randomised trials of the oestrogen-receptor-blocking drug tamoxifen in women with early breast cancer showed clearly that tamoxifen reduces the risks of breast cancer recurrence and of death from breast cancer among postmenopausal women.[81] Far fewer data were available at the time for premenopausal women and, although there was a definite improvement in recurrence-free survival, there was no clear improvement in survival among such women considered on their own. As a consequence, tamoxifen was not used routinely for these younger women,[82] yet it has more recently been shown that prolonged treatment with tamoxifen produces substantial survival advantages not only for postmenopausal but also for premenopausal women.[83] In retrospect, therefore, the decision by many clinicians not to place sufficient emphasis on the overall findings for survival, supported by the age-specific benefits for recurrence, was mistaken.

Conclusions: the need for really large-scale randomised evidence

In a world in which moderate effects of treatment on mortality or major morbidity are generally more plausible than large effects, claims of striking effects from small-scale randomised trials, and from other sources (including observational studies[1]), will often prove evanescent. The assumption that both a moderate difference or no difference may be plausible, and that an extreme difference is much less so, has surprisingly strong consequences for the interpretation of evidence from trials. In particular, it implies that even highly significant (e.g. $2p = 0.001$) differences that are based on only relatively small numbers of events in selected studies may provide untrustworthy evidence of the existence of any real difference,[2,84] as was the case with the initial results for aspirin in pre-eclampsia,[39] vesnarinone in heart failure,[42] magnesium in heart attacks,[51] and heparin in stroke.[53] For this reason, recent claims based on small randomised trials of large effects (e.g. the healing of leg ulcers with oral aspirin,[85] the prevention of dementia with antihypertensive therapy,[86] vascular complications with antioxidant vitamins in end-stage renal disease[87]) should probably be treated with far greater caution – both by journal editors and by their readers – than is often, at present, customary. Moreover, when there is not good evidence of any effect on major outcomes, estimates of the 'number needed to treat' (NNT) to prevent such outcomes are of little or no value, and it is particularly inappropriate to fail to provide a clear indication of the range of uncertainties around such estimates[88] (e.g. with the claim that lowering blood pressure could prevent 19 cases of dementia per 1000 patients treated for 5 years,[86] when the results were also compatible with the prevention of no cases of dementia and, hence, with an infinite NNT).

As discussed below, observational studies may provide useful evidence about any large effects of treatment that do exist (e.g. rare, but serious, hazards), and about the risks of death and disability in particular types of patient that may help to generalise from clinical trials to clinical practice. But, only sufficiently large-scale evidence from randomised trials can reliably assess moderate effects of treatment on mortality and major morbidity – and past failures to produce such evidence, and to interpret it appropriately, have already led to many premature deaths and much unnecessary suffering.

Observational studies: non-randomised assessment of treatment

Important (but limited) role of observational studies

Observational studies and randomised trials can contribute complementary evidence about the effects of treatment on mortality and on major non-fatal outcomes. In particular, observational studies have an important role in the identification of large adverse effects of treatment on infrequent outcomes (i.e. rare, but serious, side-effects) that are not likely to be related to the indications for (or contraindications to) the treatment of interest.[11] Such studies can also provide useful information about the risks of death and disability in particular circumstances that can help to generalise from clinical trials to clinical practice. But, due to their inherent potential for moderate or large biases, observational studies have little role in the direct assessment of any moderate effects of treatment on major outcomes that might exist. Instead, sufficiently large-scale evidence from randomised trials is needed to assess such treatment effects appropriately reliably. Wider appreciation of the different strengths and weaknesses of these two types of epidemiological study should increase the likelihood that the most reliable evidence available informs decisions about the treatments that doctors use – and that patients receive – for the management of a wide range of life-threatening conditions.

Epidemiological studies of the effects of treatments on mortality and major non-fatal outcomes can take the form of either clinical trials or observational studies. The first part of this chapter dealt with clinical trials – in particular, those in which the treatment is assigned to patients at random. As discussed, randomisation minimises systematic errors (i.e. biases) in the estimates of treatment effects, allowing any moderate effects that exist to be detected unbiasedly in studies of appropriately large size.[1, 2] By contrast, observational studies – such as cohort studies and case–control studies – involve comparisons of outcome among patients who have been exposed to the treatment of interest, typically as part of their medical care, with outcome among others who were not exposed (or comparisons between those with different amounts of exposure).[11] The reasons why certain patients received a particular treatment while others did not are often difficult to account for fully, and, largely as a consequence, observational studies are more prone to bias than are randomised trials. The primary objective of the second part of this chapter is to distinguish between situations in which biases in observational studies could lead to misleading conclusions and those in which such studies could provide useful evidence about the effects of treatment.

Assessment of adverse effects of treatment

Observational studies can have an important role in the identification of large adverse effects of treatments, particularly on infrequent outcomes that are not likely to be related to the indications for, or contraindications to, the treatment of interest (panel 1.4). Perhaps one of the best illustrations of this is the detection of increased risks of abnormal fetal limb development after maternal use of thalidomide.[89] A decade later, observational studies also detected the many-fold increased risk of vaginal clear-cell adenocarcinoma among the daughters of women who used diethylstilboestrol.[90] Other, more recent, examples include the demonstration of a 20-fold increased risk of cardiac-valve abnormalities among patients taking the appetite-suppressant drugs fenfluramine, dexfenfluramine and phentermine[91] (table 1.4), and even larger increases in the risk of Stevens–Johnson syndrome and toxic epidermal necrolysis with antiepileptic therapy.[92] In each of these examples, the outcome was rare among unexposed individuals and the excess risk was large among exposed individuals, making it unlikely that systematic errors could reasonably account for the entire association.

On the other hand, as the disease of interest is rare in such circumstances, individual studies may well involve too few cases to detect, or quantify reliably, even large increases in risk. Hence, to minimise random error, combined analyses of the aggregated results (i.e. meta-analyses) of all relevant observational studies are being done with increasing frequency. For example, a meta-analysis found that more than 10 years of oestrogen replacement therapy unopposed by progestogen was associated with an almost ten-fold increase in the risk of endometrial cancer among postmenopausal women.[93] Such large effects are unlikely to be entirely the consequence of bias, but it is not so easy to exclude the possibility that biases might largely or wholly explain more modest increases in risk: for example, the 40% increased incidence of malignant melanoma seen among users of hormone replacement therapy in another meta-analysis of observational

***Panel 1.4:* Situations in which an observational study is more likely to provide reliable evidence about adverse effects of treatment**

- The outcome of interest is rare among individuals not exposed to the treatment
- The excess risk among individuals exposed to the treatment is large (e.g. a several-fold increase in risk)
- There are no obvious sources of bias likely to account for most, or all, of the observed association

	Any appetite suppressant (*n* = 233)*	Unexposed controls (*n* = 233)†	Odds ratio (95% CI)
Valve abnormalities	53 (23%)	3 (1%)	22.6 (7.1–114.2)

*163 on fenfluramine and phentermine, 31 on dexfenfluramine and phentermine, and 39 on dexfenfluramine alone. †Matched for sex, age, height, and body-mass index.

***Table 1.4:* Detection of large adverse effects of treatment in an observational study: cardiac-valve regurgitation with appetite-suppressant drugs[91]**

studies.[94] For, although these meta-analyses may help avoid the biases produced by unduly selective emphasis on particular parts of the available evidence (as with meta-analyses of randomised trials[1, 2]), the combination of observational evidence that is subject to other systematic errors might merely compound those biases – that is, produce more precise, but still biased, estimates of the effects of treatment.

Assessment of beneficial effects of treatment

Reliable evidence about beneficial effects of treatment on mortality and major morbidity can also emerge from observational studies when outcome among untreated patients is typically poor and a large proportion of patients derive benefit from the treatment. For example, the beneficial effects of penicillin on survival in patients with sepsis,[95] and of antihypertensive treatment on death and stroke in patients with malignant hypertension,[96] were demonstrated in simple case series. Another example is provided by oral rehydration therapy, which reduced mortality from about 30% to less than 5% when introduced during a cholera epidemic among Bangladeshi refugees.[97] But, as discussed in the first part of this chapter, outcome for many other common serious conditions is less predictable, and the most plausible expectation of benefit is that a treatment produces only moderate (although still potentially worthwhile) effects on serious outcomes. For the reliable assessment of these effects of treatment, observational studies have a much more limited part to play,[98] since the potential biases could obscure, inflate or even seem to reverse the real effects of treatment – and these biases cannot be quantified reliably. Despite these widely recognised limitations,[11] however, observational studies have been the basis for many claims of such treatment benefits: for example, a two-thirds lower risk of dementia[99] and a halving in fracture risk with statins,[100] a one-third lower risk of cancer with angiotensin-converting enzyme (ACE) inhibitors[101] and a one-third lower risk of coronary heart disease,[102] and a one-fifth lower risk of colorectal cancer[94] with hormone replacement therapy. Each of these claims (and many similar ones) has been refuted by the results of large-scale randomised trials, but new claims from observational studies of such benefits continue to be prominently published (e.g. improved muscle strength and physical function with ACE inhibitors,[103] reduced risk of sepsis with statins,[104] reduced risk of coronary disease with celecoxib compared with rofecoxib,[105] reduced risk of oral cancer with non-steroidal anti-inflammatory drugs[106]). Based on previous experience, it seems likely that most (if not all) of these claims of potentially important benefits of treatment will prove to be false – although, in the absence of randomised trials of sufficient size, it is impossible to determine reliably whether any of these reports is misleading.

Major sources of bias in observational studies

Confounding by factors associated with both treatment and outcome

Perhaps the most important potential source of bias in observational studies is confounding, whereby some factor is associated with the exposure of interest – but is not a direct consequence of it – and, independently, influences the risk of the outcome of interest (panel 1.5). Observational studies of the effects of exposure to treatment are particularly prone to confounding by indication (or by contraindication), with the development of a medical condition leading both to the use of the treatment (or its avoidance) and to the outcome of interest. This type of bias can produce misleading

Panel 1.5: **Major sources of bias in observational studies of treatment**

Confounding

A factor (such as pre-existing disease severity) is associated with the use (or avoidance) of the treatment and, independently, influences the risk of the outcome of interest. For example, 'confounding by indication (or contraindication)' may occur when the treatment tends to be provided more (or less) frequently to individuals with medical conditions associated with increased or decreased risks of the outcome of interest

Recall bias

The reliability of recall of treatment exposure differs between those who develop an adverse outcome and those who do not

Detection bias

The reliability of detection of adverse outcomes differs between those exposed to the treatment of interest and those not exposed

estimates, not just of the size but also of the direction of treatment effects, depending on the nature of the associations between the confounding factors and the outcome.

An example of misleading evidence about the size of a treatment effect is provided by a large observational study in which patients who received beta-blockers after myocardial infarction were about half as likely to die as those who did not receive such treatment (table 1.5).[107] By contrast, large-scale evidence from randomised trials has clearly shown that long-term beta-blocker use in patients with a history of myocardial infarction reduces the risk of death by only about a quarter[108] (as have trials in higher risk patients with congestive heart failure[109–111]). The patients who received beta-blockers in this observational study were significantly younger, and had a lower risk medical history, than those who did not receive these drugs. Statistical adjustments were made for these, and other, potential confounding factors that had been recorded, but such adjustments may well be incomplete due both to insufficient correction for

Study type	Deaths/patients		Risk ratio† (95% CI)
	Beta-blocker*	No beta-blocker*	
Observational study‡	~123/785 (16%)	~886/2952 (30%)	0.57 (0.47–0.69)
Randomised trials	827/10 452 (8%)	986/9860 (10%)	0.77 (0.70–0.85)

*Treatment recorded at baseline in the observational study and assigned at random in the trials. †Multivariate adjusted relative risk in the observational study, and stratified odds ratio in the meta-analysis of randomised trials. ‡Exact numbers in each treatment group of the observational study were not reported.

Table 1.5: **Different sizes of apparent effect in an observational study[107] and in randomised trials:[108] beta-blocker use and death after myocardial infarction**

factors that were recorded (because of random errors in their measurement[112]) and to lack of correction for differences in other relevant factors. Hence, it seems likely that the overestimation in this observational study of the survival advantage produced by beta-blocker therapy reflects some residual bias (due, perhaps, to a selective tendency for these drugs to be used less frequently in higher risk patients).

An example of misleading evidence about the direction of a treatment effect is provided by an observational study in which there was almost a two-fold greater risk of coronary events among patients receiving antihypertensive therapy than among those not receiving such treatment (table 1.6).[113] By contrast, randomised controlled trials (RCTs) have clearly demonstrated that antihypertensive treatment reduces the risks of coronary heart disease (as well as those of stroke).[114] Similarly, whereas a large observational study found nearly a doubling in the risk of major coronary events among those regularly taking aspirin,[115] RCTs have shown unequivocally that antiplatelet therapy reduces the risks of heart attacks by about a quarter.[116] These misleading findings from observational studies persisted after statistical adjustment for a variety of confounding factors and after restriction of analyses to individuals without a recorded history of cardiovascular disease. Once again it seems that uncontrolled residual bias remains the most likely explanation – probably, in these examples, due to an understandable tendency for the treatments to be used more frequently in higher risk patients. Fortunately, for both antihypertensive and antiplatelet therapy, the evidence from the randomised trials has chiefly influenced practice patterns, resulting in the appropriately widespread use of these treatments and the consequent prevention of many hundreds of thousands of premature deaths each year. By contrast, reliance on the evidence from the observational studies might have led to the inappropriate abandonment of these treatments (or, at the very least, to restriction of their use) and to much unnecessary suffering.

Observational studies can also provide misleading evidence about the effects of different drug doses. For example, retrospective observational analyses of outcome among participants in the North American Symptomatic Carotid Artery Endarterectomy Trial (NASCET) indicated that the risk of perioperative stroke among patients who

Study type	CHD events/patients		Risk ratio† (95% CI)
	Antihypertensive therapy*	No antihypertensive therapy*	
Observational study	50/839 (6%)	420/20 475 (2%)	1.8 (1.3–2.6)
Randomised trials	934/23 847 (4%)	1104/23 806 (5%)	0.84 (0.77–0.92)

CHD, coronary heart disease. *Treatment recorded at baseline in the observational study and assigned at random in the trials. †Multivariate adjusted relative risk in the observational study and stratified odds ratio in the meta-analysis of randomised trials.

***Table 1.6*: Different directions of apparent effect in an observational study[113] and in randomised trials:[114] antihypertensive therapy and coronary heart disease**

Study type	Stroke/patients		Risk ratio† (95% CI)
	Lower dose aspirin (< 650 mg/day)*	Higher dose aspirin (650–1300 mg/day)*	
Observational study	96/1391 (7%)	15/835 (2%)	2.3 (1.3–3.9)
Randomised trial	64/1417 (5%)	86/1432 (6%)	0.74 (0.53–1.03)

*Treatment recorded at baseline in the observational study and assigned at random in the randomised trial. †Univariate relative risk in the observational study and odds ratio in the randomised trial.

***Table 1.7*: Discordance between apparent effects of different drug doses in an observational study[117] and a randomised trial:[118] higher dose versus lower dose aspirin and stroke after carotid endarterectomy**

had been taking 650–1300 mg/day aspirin was less than half that among patients who had taken lower doses (table 1.7).[117] Subsequently, however, a randomised trial designed to test this hypothesis in patients undergoing carotid endarterectomy found a non-significantly higher stroke incidence with 650–1300 mg/day aspirin than with lower doses (as well as a marginally significant higher risk of the composite of stroke, myocardial infarction or death).[118] In this instance, reliance on the evidence from the observational study alone could have led to the inappropriate abandonment of lower dose regimens, which cause fewer side-effects and are better tolerated long term.

Bias due to differential recall of treatment exposure

Recall bias can be a problem in observational studies when there is a difference in the reliability of the data collected on treatment exposure between cases that have the disease of interest and controls that do not.[119] Although it is unlikely that recall bias could account for the many-fold increases in risk seen, for example, with limb abnormalities and thalidomide use,[89] it might well be responsible for more moderate differences in apparent risk. For example, an early case–control study of childhood cancer obtained data on maternal x-ray exposure through interviews with mothers, and observed that the risk of death from malignancy among the children of women who reported being exposed to abdominal x-rays was almost twice as great as that among the children of women who reported no such exposure.[120] To determine whether this association might, at least in part, reflect more complete recall of exposure by the mothers of affected children, a second study was done in which exposure was determined from prenatal medical records.[121] That study also found an increased risk of cancer among offspring of exposed women, but the relative risk was only half as large as in the first study. It has been suggested that such bias might be kept to a minimum by making comparisons between exposures reported by mothers of children with some particular birth defect and those reported by mothers of children with other anomalies.[122] That strategy would not, however, exclude entirely the possibility of differential recall between the mothers of children with different types of birth defect. Moreover, it might obscure a real effect of the treatment if exposure was associated with more than one type of congenital anomaly.

Bias due to differential detection of outcomes

Individuals receiving any treatment will tend to be seen by doctors or other health professionals more frequently than will others, and this may result in the earlier detection of a variety of outcomes. For example, although a highly significant increase of a quarter in the risk of breast cancer was seen among women taking hormonal contraceptives,[123] this finding could largely reflect the earlier detection of less advanced breast cancer among such women. For, much of the observed excess risk was due to an excess of localised tumours, without any clear increase in the risk of tumours that had spread beyond the breast. Another possible example of such detection bias is provided by studies of first-trimester exposure to the antifungal drug itraconazole. Congenital malformations were seen in 13% of children of exposed women in a retrospective study compared with only 3% in a prospective study,[124] perhaps reflecting the greater likelihood of including women who have affected babies in a retrospective study.

Efforts to control biases in observational studies

The effects of biases in observational studies are frequently underestimated in the interpretation of associations found between treatment and outcome. Even when statistical adjustment for measured confounding factors fails to reduce the size of such associations materially, this provides little reassurance that residual bias is not still a major cause of any observed associations. These difficulties are illustrated by an observational study of antihypertensive treatment in which a 60% higher risk of heart attacks was seen among patients receiving a calcium antagonist compared with those receiving other agents.[125] In that study, calcium antagonists seem to have been preferentially prescribed to higher risk patients (e.g. those with pre-existing coronary heart disease or other risk factors for cardiovascular disease), but the association between use of calcium antagonists and subsequent myocardial infarction remained conventionally significant after adjustment for measured confounders and after excluding those with a history of cardiovascular disease. Residual bias remains a plausible explanation for at least part of the observed excess risk, however, since the data collected on prognostic factors are unlikely to describe all of the factors that contributed to the tendency to prescribe calcium antagonists to higher risk patients. This could explain why the large excess risk reported in that observational study was not confirmed by a prospectively planned meta-analysis of all relevant randomised trials comparing the effects on heart attack incidence of calcium antagonists and diuretics or beta-blockers (relative risk (RR) 1.01; 95% CI 0.94–1.08).[126]

Various statistical methods have been proposed to deal with the problem of residual biases in observational studies of treatment. For example, instrumental variable estimation involves grouping patients according to their likelihood of receiving the treatment of interest based on observable factors (i.e. instrumental variables) that affect treatment use but – it is hoped – do not directly affect patients' outcomes.[127] Although this method has been described as mimicking randomisation, it depends entirely on the untestable assumption that the observed instrumental variables are not correlated with unobserved factors that directly affect outcome. Moreover, since the range of variation, between groups of patients, in the likelihood of receiving some particular treatment might be narrow (e.g. one such assessment of coronary artery catheterisation was based on its use in 20% versus 26% of patients[127]), any difference in outcome due to this differential use of the treatment would probably be very small (and, hence, difficult to assess even in a properly RCT).

Another method that has been proposed involves case-crossover (or case-series) analysis,[128, 129] in which outcomes are compared between periods before and after treatment exposure within the same individuals. But, although this may avoid biases resulting from differences between exposed and non-exposed patients, variations in the underlying disease state within individuals could still determine both the necessity for treatment and the likelihood of the outcome of interest occurring. For example, a case-crossover study reported a 60% higher risk of road-traffic accidents during periods of exposure to benzodiazepines.[130] At least in part, this could have been due to exacerbation of certain conditions that led both to an increased use of benzodiazepines and, independently, to an increased risk of accidents. Hence, these and other non-randomised methods[131] do not provide assurance that all sources of known and unknown bias are adequately controlled, and so cannot exclude the possibility that moderate biases have obscured or inflated any moderate effects, or have falsely indicated a treatment effect when none existed.

Potential for small random errors in observational studies

One advantage of observational studies is that it is often easier to study much larger numbers of patients – and, consequently, much larger numbers of deaths and other relevant outcomes – in such studies than it is in randomised trials. Observational studies can, therefore, provide estimates of treatment effects that are subject to relatively small random errors, allowing the reliable detection of some extreme, although rare, adverse effects of treatments. However, as discussed earlier, small random errors in large observational studies can also lead to the detection of more moderate differences in risk that are merely the result of bias, rather than the effect of treatment (i.e. more precise, but biased, estimates). For example, in meta-analyses of observational studies of hormone replacement therapy, women who had taken such treatment were seen to have significantly lower risks of coronary heart disease with oestrogen alone (RR 0.70; 95% CI 0.65–0.75) or with oestrogen plus progestin (RR 0.66; 95% CI 0.53–0.84),[132] lower risks of colorectal cancer (RR 0.8; 95% CI 0.7–0.9),[94] higher risks of breast cancer (RR increasing by 2.3% (95% CI 1.1–3.6) with each year of use)[133] and higher risks of malignant melanoma (RR 1.4; 95% CI 1.2–1.7).[94] But, there is evidence that women who take hormone replacement therapy may have better pretreatment coronary risk-factor profiles[134] and better access to preventive healthcare[135] than those who do not take such therapy, and several of the risk factors for coronary heart disease that differ between users and non-users of hormone replacement therapy (e.g. physical inactivity, obesity) are also risk factors for colon cancer.[136] On the other hand, women who take hormone replacement therapy (like those who take oral contraceptives[123]) may be more likely to have breast cancer and melanoma diagnosed at an earlier stage because of greater contact with doctors. As a consequence, the balance of any true benefits and risks of hormone replacement therapy cannot be determined reliably from observational studies. This has been clearly demonstrated by the results of the Women's Health Initiative, a large-scale trial of hormone replacement therapy, which failed to detect any reduction in the risk of coronary heart disease after several years of treatment with either oestrogen alone (RR 0.91; 95% CI 0.75–1.12)[137] or with oestrogen plus progestin

(RR 1.24; 95% CI 1.00–1.54).[138] Conversely, however, that trial did report an increase in the risk of breast cancer[139] and a reduction in the risk of colorectal cancer[140] among women assigned oestrogen plus progestin, but no such effects were apparent among women assigned oestrogen alone.[141]

Evidence from observational studies in the context of results from randomised trials

A more prominent role for observational studies in the assessment of treatment effects has been proposed in two reviews[142, 143] on the basis of examples in which there were considered to be no apparent differences between the results of observational studies and those of randomised trials. However, several of the examples included in those reviews involved estimates of treatment effects that were subject to large random errors. For example, separate meta-analyses of the observational studies and of the randomised trials comparing laparoscopic and open appendectomy were interpreted as having shown similar reductions in infection rates with laparoscopic procedures,[142] even though the 95% CI for the risk reduction in each type of study ranged from about 10% to about 70%. It has also been noted[144] that other examples in those reviews did not even involve observational studies of treatment, but instead misleadingly compared the effects found in randomised trials of treatment that alter risk factors (e.g. lowering blood cholesterol or blood pressure) with estimates from observational studies of the associations between risk-factor levels and disease risk.[143] Most pertinently, any similarity of the treatment effects estimated from observational studies and from randomised trials in any one particular circumstance provides little reassurance that observational studies will provide unbiased estimates of the effects of treatment in some other circumstance.

Furthermore, it makes little sense to continue to base inference on observational studies when their results have been reliably refuted by large-scale randomised trials. For example, it had previously been suggested by observational analyses that digoxin might increase mortality substantially.[145] By contrast, the large randomised trial conducted by the Digitalis Investigation Group (DIG) showed unequivocally that the addition of digoxin to current therapy reduces the risk of hospital admission for heart failure (RR 0.72; 95% CI 0.66–0.79) by about as much as do ACE inhibitors, with no apparent adverse effect on total mortality (1181 deaths in patients allocated digoxin and 1194 in patients allocated placebo; RR 0.99; 95% CI 0.91–1.07).[146] In the light of this evidence, the prominent reporting of subsequent claims from observational analyses that digoxin doubles the risk of death in just the sort of patients studied in the DIG trial is inappropriate.[147, 148]

Without clear confirmatory evidence from large-scale randomised trials or their meta-analyses, reports of moderate treatment effects from observational studies should not be interpreted as providing good evidence of either adverse or protective effects of these agents (and, contrary to other suggestions,[149, 150] the absence of evidence from randomised trials does not in itself provide sufficient justification for relying on observational data). In this regard, it is salutary to note the example provided by early reports from observational studies of moderately increased risks of breast cancer among hypertensive patients treated with reserpine.[151, 152] Those reports led to avoidance of one of the few effective antihypertensive agents available at that time, and only much later

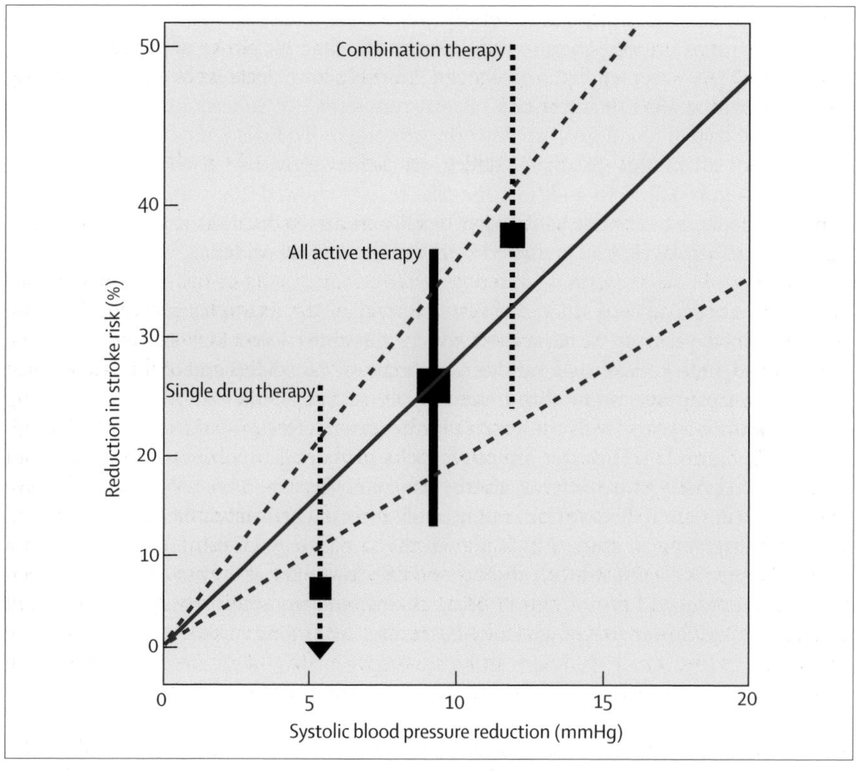

Figure 1.3: **Blood pressure lowering for the prevention of recurrent stroke among individuals with a history of ischaemic cerebrovascular disease: effects predicted from an observational study and observed in a randomised trial.[156–158] Predicted and observed effects of blood pressure lowering among patients with ischaemic stroke or TIA.[158] Predicted reductions in stroke risk and 95% CI for a given reduction in usual systolic blood pressure are indicated by the diagonal lines.[156] Observed effects of treatment on stroke risk and 95% CIs are indicated by vertical lines and boxes.[157] Box sizes are proportional to the number of strokes. All estimates of reductions in stroke risk are plotted on a logarithmic scale.**

was this association with breast cancer shown to be the likely result of bias.[153] A subsequent report from an observational study has suggested a moderately high risk of cancer among hypertensive patients treated with a calcium antagonist.[154] But, once again, no such excess of cancer has been reported from large-scale randomised trials of calcium antagonists.[155]

Use of observational studies to estimate potential effects of treatment

Prediction of the relative effects of treatment

When a treatment alters an established risk factor for disease, observational studies of the association between that risk factor and the disease may provide some indication of the potential effects of the treatment on disease risk. For example, an observational study of outcome among patients with a history of ischaemic stroke or transient ischaemic attack (TIA), observed that a prolonged 9 mmHg lower systolic blood pressure was associated with a 25–30% lower risk of recurrent stroke.[156] Subsequently, a large-scale randomised trial of blood-pressure lowering among individuals with a history of stroke showed that all of this predicted effect was achieved within 4 years of beginning treatment (figure 1.3).[157] In addition, the trial results showed that patients randomised to more intensive treatment with larger blood pressure reductions experienced larger reductions in stroke risk, as predicted by the observational evidence.[158]

Similarly, in observational studies of general populations, a prolonged 5 mmHg lower diastolic blood pressure is associated with a one-third lower risk of stroke among middle-aged individuals,[8] and randomised trials of blood-pressure lowering among hypertensive patients[77] show that much, or all, of this predicted long-term effect is achieved within 5 years (with similar relative treatment effects in a variety of subgroups of patients; figure 1.4). However, although such estimates from observational studies of the potential effects of treatments may be valuable, they could overestimate the actual effects of treatment if disease risk is only partly reversed (at least in the short term). For example, observational studies have shown that a prolonged 5 mmHg lower diastolic blood pressure is associated with about a one-fifth lower risk of coronary heart disease,[8] and that a prolonged 1 mmol/l lower blood cholesterol concentration is associated with about a one-half lower risk of coronary heart disease[9] among middle-aged individuals.

Subgroups of entry characteristics	No. of patients	% with events: Treatment	% with events: Control	Odds ratio (95% CI)	% reduction (SD)
DBP (mmHg)					
All < 110	35 139	1.3	2.2		39 (6)
Some > 110, all > 115	7669	4.6	6.5		32 (8)
Some or all > 115	4845	4.7	8.2		45 (9)
Age (years)					
Some or all < 60	12 483	4.6	7.0		34 (6)
All > 60	35 170	1.3	2.3		43 (6)
Prior stroke					
Most no	47 104	2.0	3.2		38 (5)
All yes	549	18.8	27.3		38 (16)
All patients	47 653	2.2	3.5		38 (4)

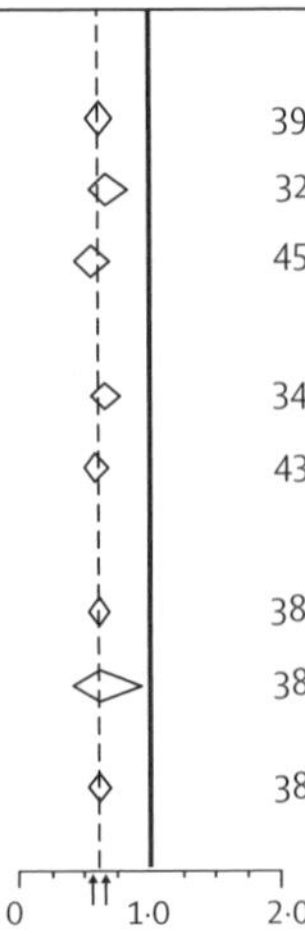

Figure 1.4: **Meta-analysis of RCTs of antihypertensive therapy:[77] achievement of full effects on stroke risk predicted from observational studies[8] for a 5–6 mmHg reduction in usual diastolic blood pressure. (Reproduced from Collins and MacMahon,[1] copyright 2001, with permission from Elsevier.)**

By contrast, randomised trials of treatments that reduce blood pressure[77,159] or cholesterol[74,160,161] suggest that only about a half or two-thirds of the long-term effects predicted from the observational studies are produced within about 5 years of altering these risk factors.

Treatments might also have independent effects on disease risk that offset or augment the benefits of altering a particular risk factor. For example, the reduction in coronary heart disease risk of about a quarter observed in randomised trials of ACE inhibitors[162–164] is nearly twice what would be predicted from observational studies[8] with the achieved 5 mmHg reduction in systolic blood pressure. Moreover, differences in outcome associated with some putative risk factors may not be causal. For example, many observational studies have found that greater consumption, and higher blood concentrations, of β-carotene are associated with a lower incidence of cancer. The first reviews of these findings stressed that such associations might merely reflect some type of confounding, and emphasised the need for large-scale randomised trials of the effects of long-term β-carotene supplementation on the incidence of cancer.[165,166] Even after more than 10 years of treatment in such trials, no clear evidence of benefit has emerged,[167] suggesting that the inverse associations in observational studies were indeed due largely, or wholly, to differences in other aspects of health-related behaviour, which determined differences in cancer risk between those with different β-carotene intakes. Numerous observational studies also showed that higher intakes of vitamin E were associated with reduced risks of coronary heart disease. However, while a few small-scale randomised trials suggested beneficial effects of vitamin E supplementation, large-scale, long-term trials demonstrated no worthwhile effects.[57–60] Similarly, blood concentrations of fibrinogen,[168] C-reactive protein[168] and homocysteine[169] seem to be strongly associated with the risk of vascular disease, but it remains unclear whether blood concentrations of these factors are raised largely as a consequence of underlying vascular disease (rather than being a cause of it) – in which case, lowering the concentrations of these factors would not be expected to produce any material reduction in risk. Without large-scale randomised trials of interventions that influence the levels of these factors it is difficult to know whether these associations are causal (and, even if they are, whether any effects on disease are reversible).

Prediction of the absolute effects of treatment

Another way in which observational studies may help to determine the potential effects of treatment is by providing more representative estimates of the absolute rates of death, and of other relevant outcomes, in particular circumstances in the absence of the treatment. For, although RCTs will usually provide the most reliable estimates of the relative effects of treatment on cause-specific outcomes,[1,2] restrictive inclusion criteria can result in the recruitment of patients at higher or lower than usual risk. In circumstances where the relative effects of treatment are similar across a wide range of disease risks (e.g. with blood-pressure lowering and stroke risk; see figure 1.3), the absolute effects of treatment will vary in approximate proportion to the background disease risks. So, for example, the likely absolute effects of antihypertensive treatment might be best estimated by applying the relative reductions in stroke and in coronary heart disease shown by the randomised trials[77] to the absolute rates of the same outcomes found in observational studies of specific populations. Hence, the absolute benefits of such treatment at the same levels of blood pressure would be expected to be much greater in populations with stroke and coronary disease rates that are very high (as in parts of eastern Europe and Russia,[170] or among patients with pre-existing vascular disease) than in those with much lower rates (as in parts of southern Europe,[170] or among patients without vascular disease or other important risk factors).

Conclusions: improving healthcare by the appropriate use of epidemiological evidence

Both randomised trials and observational studies can contribute important evidence about the effects of treatment on mortality and major non-fatal outcomes. The appropriate role for each type of evidence is determined primarily by the extent to which random error and bias can be guaranteed to be sufficiently small for the question posed to be answered reliably. Observational studies can often reduce random error substantially by involving very large numbers of individuals with a specific disease outcome, thereby providing useful evidence about any large effects of treatment on relatively uncommon outcomes (e.g. rare, but serious, side-effects). Such studies may also provide an indication of the eventual effects of a treatment that markedly alters levels of a risk factor, provided there is a causal relation with disease. But, due to their inherent potential for moderate or large biases, observational studies have little role in the direct assessment of any more moderate effects of treatment on major outcomes, which are generally all that can realistically be expected from most treatments for most common serious conditions. By contrast, random allocation of treatment minimises bias and, when random error is also reduced sufficiently by the study of appropriately large numbers of patients (whether in individual trials or meta-analyses), randomised trials can provide reliable evidence about moderate treatment effects.[1, 2]

Failure to recognise the limitations of observational studies in the assessment of moderate treatment effects may well have serious consequences, including both the use of ineffective treatments (e.g. β-carotene supplements for cancer prevention[167]) and the inappropriate abandonment, or insufficiently widespread use, of effective treatments (e.g. as occurred when concerns were raised about the safety of certain antihypertensive drugs[125, 154]). Despite this, it has been argued by some that observational studies can provide useful information when there are substantial barriers to conducting randomised trials, such as the requirement for an extremely large sample size or a very long period of follow-up (e.g. in assessing the effects of hormone replacement therapy on breast-cancer risks); when the conduct of randomised trials is hindered by the reluctance of patients or their doctors to participate (e.g. in assessing treatments for multiple sclerosis) or when there are considered to be other ethical, economic, regulatory or political obstacles.[149, 150] Difficulties in obtaining reliable evidence in randomised trials as a consequence of such obstacles are not, however, sufficient to justify the use of unreliable evidence from observational studies that may, due to the potential biases, be importantly misleading. Instead, greater efforts need to be made to remove or overcome any obstacles that inappropriately prevent the provision of reliable evidence from randomised trials of adequate size (as has been achieved for treatments of numerous vascular and neoplastic conditions).

It has also been argued that observational studies could provide more generalisable evidence about the effects of treatment because they involve populations of patients, or clinicians, that are more representative of particular practice settings than those involved in clinical trials.[149, 150] However, the inclusion of more representative participants does not prevent observational studies from producing biased estimates of any moderate treatment effects that might exist. Moreover, as has been discussed, careful consideration of the effects seen among the different types of patient included in randomised trials can often allow the results of clinical trials to be generalised widely. In particular, applying estimates derived from appropriately large randomised trials (or meta-analyses of trials) of the relative effects of a treatment on specific outcomes to the absolute risks of those outcomes observed in representative patient populations may well provide a broadly reliable guide to the balance of the absolute benefits and absolute risks conferred by the treatment in routine clinical practice.

In conclusion, observational studies and randomised trials provide complementary evidence about the effects of treatment on mortality and major morbidity. Wider appreciation of the different strengths and weaknesses of these two types of epidemiological study should increase the likelihood that the most reliable evidence available informs decisions about the treatments that doctors use – and that patients receive – for the management of a wide range of life-threatening conditions.

Acknowledgments

We thank Colin Baigent, Iain Chalmers, Richard Doll (deceased), Richard Peto, Anthony Rodgers and Peter Sandercock for comments and suggestions on previous drafts of this manuscript. This work was supported by awards from the National Health and Medical Research Council of Australia, The Medical Foundation of the University of Sydney, a British Heart Foundation personal chair (RC), and direct support from the UK Medical Research Council and Imperial Cancer Research Fund.

References

1 Collins R, MacMahon S. Reliable assessment of the effects of treatment on mortality and major morbidity, I: clinical trials. *Lancet* 2001; **357:** 373–80.

2 Collins R, Peto R, Gray R, Parish S. Large-scale randomized evidence: trials and overviews. In: Weatherall DJ, Ledingham JGG, Warrell DA, eds. *Oxford Textbook of Medicine*, Vol. 1. Oxford: Oxford University Press, 1996: 21–32.

3 Teo KK, Yusuf S, Furberg CD. Effects of prophylactic antiarrhythmic drug therapy in acute myocardial infarction: an overview of results from randomized controlled trials. *JAMA* 1993; **270:** 1589–95.

4 The Cardiac Arrhythmia Suppression Trial II investigators. Effect of the antiarrhythmic agent moricizine on survival after myocardial infarction. *N Engl J Med* 1992; **327:** 227–33.

5 HIV Trialists' Collaborative Group. Zidovudine, didanosine, and zalcitabine in the treatment of HIV infection: meta-analyses of the randomised evidence. *Lancet* 1999; **353:** 2014–25.

6 Early Breast Cancer Trialists' Collaborative Group. Favourable and unfavourable effects on long-term survival of radiotherapy for early breast cancer: an overview of the randomised trials. *Lancet* 2000; **355:** 1757–70.

7 Early Breast Cancer Trialists' Collaborative Group. Effects of radiotherapy and of differences in the extent of surgery for early breast cancer on local recurrence and 15-year survival: an overview of the randomised trials. *Lancet* 2005; **366:** 2087–106.

8 Collins R, Gray R, Godwin J, Peto R. Avoidance of large biases and large random errors in the assessment of moderate treatment effects: the need for systematic overviews. *Stat Med* 1987; **6:** 245–50.

9 MacMahon S, Peto R, Cutler J, et al. Blood pressure, stroke, and coronary heart disease. Part 1, prolonged differences in blood pressure: prospective observational studies corrected for the regression dilution bias. *Lancet* 1990; **335:** 765–74.

10 Law MR, Wald NJ, Thompson SG. By how much and how quickly does reduction in serum cholesterol concentration lower risk of ischaemic heart disease? *BMJ* 1994; **308:** 367–73.

11 MacMahon S, Collins R. Reliable assessment of the effects of treatment on mortality and major morbidity, II: observational studies. *Lancet* 2001; **357:** 455–62.

12 Armitage P. The role of randomization in clinical trials. *Stat Med* 1982; **1:** 345–52.

13 Kunz R, Oxman AD. The unpredictability paradox: review of empirical comparisons of randomised and non-randomised clinical trials. *BMJ* 1998; **317:** 1185–90.

14 Keirse MJNC. Amniotomy or oxytocin for induction of labour: re-analysis of a randomized controlled trial. *Acta Obstet Gynecol Scand* 1988; **67:** 731–35.

15 Hansson L, Lindholm LH, Niskanen L, et al., for the Captopril Prevention Project (CAPPP) study group. Effect of angiotensin-converting-enzyme inhibition compared with conventional therapy on cardiovascular morbidity and mortality in hypertension: the Captopril Prevention Project (CAPPP) randomised trial. *Lancet* 1999; **353:** 611–16.

16 Peto R. Failure of randomisation by 'sealed' envelope. *Lancet* 1999; **354:** 73.

17 Benson K, Hartz AJ. A comparison of observational studies and randomized, controlled trials. *N Engl J Med* 2000; **342:** 1878–86.

18 Concato J, Shah N, Horwitz RI. Randomized, controlled trials, observational studies, and the hierarchy of research designs. *N Engl J Med* 2000; **342:** 1887–92.

19 Francis T Jr, Korns RF, Voight RB, et al. An evaluation of the 1954 poliomyelitis vaccine trials: summary report. *Am J Public Health* 1955; **45:** 1–50.

20 Pocock SJ, Elbourne DR. Randomized trials or observational tribulations? *N Engl J Med* 2000; **342:** 1907–09.

21 Chalmers TC, Matta RJ, Smith H Jr, Kunzler A-M. Evidence favoring the use of anticoagulants in the hospital phase of acute myocardial infarction. *N Engl J Med* 1977; **297:** 1091–96.

22 The Coronary Drug Project Research Group. Influence of adherence to treatment and response of cholesterol on mortality in the Coronary Drug Project. *N Engl J Med* 1980; **303:** 1038–41.

23 Cuzick J, Edwards R, Segnan N. Adjusting for non-compliance and contamination in randomized clinical trials. *Stat Med* 1997; **16:** 1017–29.

24 Antiplatelet Trialists' Collaboration. Collaborative overview of randomised trials of antiplatelet therapy. I: Prevention of death, myocardial infarction, and stroke by prolonged antiplatelet therapy in various categories of patients. *BMJ* 1994; **308:** 81–106.

25 ISIS-2 (Second International Study of Infarct Survival) Collaborative Group. Randomised trial of intravenous streptokinase, oral aspirin, both, or neither among 17 187 cases of suspected acute myocardial infarction: ISIS-2. *Lancet* 1988; **2:** 349–60.

26 Gruppo Italiano per lo Studio della Streptochinasi nell'Infarto Miocardico (GISSI). Effectiveness of intravenous thrombolytic treatment in acute myocardial infarction. *Lancet* 1986; **1:** 397–402.

27 Fibrinolytic Therapy Trialists' (FTT) Collaborative Group. Indications for fibrinolytic therapy in suspected acute myocardial infarction: collaborative overview of early mortality and major morbidity results from all randomised trials of more than 1000 patients. *Lancet* 1994; **343:** 311–22.

28 Food and Drug Administration. Final rule for professional labeling of aspirin, buffered aspirin, and aspirin in combination with antacid drugs (FR Doc 98-28519). *Federal Register* 1998; **63:** 56802–19.

29 Clarke M, Chalmers I. Discussion sections in reports of controlled trials published in general medical journals: islands in search of continents? *JAMA* 1998; **280:** 280–82.

30 Thompson SG. Why sources of heterogeneity in meta-analysis should be investigated. *BMJ* 1994; **309:** 1351–55.

31 Aspirin Myocardial Infarction Study Research Group. A randomized, controlled trial of aspirin in persons recovered from myocardial infarction. *JAMA* 1980; **243:** 661–69.

32 Cleland JGF, Bulpitt CJ, Falk RH, et al. Is aspirin safe for patients with heart failure? *Br Heart J* 1995; **74:** 215–19.

33 Flather MD, Yusuf S, Køber L, et al., for the ACE-inhibitor Myocardial Infarction Collaborative Group. Long-term ACE-inhibitor therapy in patients with heart failure or left-ventricular dysfunction: a systematic overview of data from individual patients. *Lancet* 2000; **355:** 1575–81.

34 Feinstein AR, Sosin DM, Wells CK. The Will Rogers phenomenon: stage migration and new diagnostic techniques as a source of misleading statistics for survival in cancer. *N Engl J Med* 1985; **312:** 1604–08.

35 West of Scotland Coronary Prevention Study Group. Influence of pravastatin and plasma lipids on clinical events in the West of Scotland Coronary Prevention Study (WOSCOPS). *Circulation* 1998; **97:** 1440–45.

36 Weber MA, Julius S, Kjeldsen SE, et al. Blood pressure dependent and independent effects of antihypertensive treatment on clinical events in the VALUE Trial. *Lancet* 2004; **363:** 2049–51.

37 Poulter NR, Wedel H, Dahlof B, et al., for the ASCOT Investigators. Role of blood pressure and other variables in the differential cardiovascular event rates noted in the Anglo-Scandinavian Cardiac Outcomes Trial-Blood Pressure Lowering Arm (ASCOT-BPLA). *Lancet* 2005; **366:** 907–13.

38 Yusuf S, Collins R, Peto R, et al. Intravenous and intracoronary fibrinolytic therapy in acute myocardial infarction: overview of results on mortality, reinfarction and side-effects from 33 randomized controlled trials. *Eur Heart J* 1985; **6:** 556–85.

39 Imperiale TF, Petrulis AS. A meta-analysis of low-dose aspirin for the prevention of pregnancy-induced hypertensive disease. *JAMA* 1991; **266:** 260–64.

40 CLASP (Collaborative Low-dose Aspirin Study in Pregnancy) Collaborative Group. CLASP: a randomised trial of low-dose aspirin for the prevention and treatment of pre-eclampsia among 9364 pregnant women. *Lancet* 1994; **343:** 619–29.

41 Knight M, Duley L, Henderson-Smart DJ, King JF. Antiplatelet agents for preventing and treating pre-eclampsia. In: *The Cochrane Library*, Issue 4. Oxford: Update Software, 2000.

42 Feldman AM, Bristow MR, Parmley WW, et al., for the Vesnarinone Study Group. Effects of vesnarinone on morbidity and mortality in patients with heart failure. *N Engl J Med* 1993; **329:** 149–55.

43 Cohn JN, Goldstein SO, Greenberg BH, et al., for the Vesnarinone Trial Investigators. A dose-dependent increase in mortality with vesnarinone among patients with severe heart failure. *N Engl J Med* 1998; **339:** 1810–16.

44 Edwards P, Arango M, Balica L, et al. CRASH trial collaborators. Final results of MRC CRASH, a randomised placebo-controlled trial of intravenous corticosteroid in adults with head injury – outcomes at 6 months. *Lancet* 2005; **365:** 1957–59.

45 Bucher HC, Guyatt GH, Cook RJ, et al. Effect of calcium supplementation on pregnancy-induced hypertension and pre-eclampsia: a meta-analysis of randomized controlled trials. *JAMA* 1996; **275:** 1113–17.

46 Levine RJ, Hauth JC, Curet LB, et al. Trial of calcium to prevent pre-eclampsia. *N Engl J Med* 1997; **337:** 69–76.

47 Chappelll LC, Seed PT, Briley AL, et al. Effects of antioxidants on the occurrence of pre-eclampsia in women at increased risk: a randomised trial. *Lancet* 1999; **354:** 810–16.

48 Poston L, Briley AL, Seed PT, et al. Vitamins in Pre-eclampsia (VIP) Trial Consortium. Vitamin C and vitamin E in pregnant women at risk for pre-eclampsia (VIP trial): randomised placebo-controlled trial. *Lancet* 2006; **367:** 1145–54.

49 Yusuf S, Collins R, MacMahon S, Peto R. Effects of intravenous nitrates on mortality in acute myocardial infarction: an overview of the randomised trials. *Lancet* 1988; **1:** 1088–92.

50 Gruppo Italiano per lo Studio della Sopravvivenza nell'Infarcto Miocardico. GISSI-3: effects of lisinopril and transdermal glyceryl trinitrate singly and together on 6-week mortality and ventricular function after acute myocardial infarction. *Lancet* 1994; **343:** 1115–21.

51 Teo KK, Yusuf S, Collins R, et al. Effects of intravenous magnesium in suspected acute myocardial infarction: overview of randomised trials. *BMJ* 1991; **303:** 1499–503.

52 ISIS-4 (Fourth International Study of Infarct Survival) Collaborative Group. ISIS-4: a randomised factorial trial assessing early oral captopril, oral mononitrate, and intravenous magnesium sulphate in 58 050 patients with suspected acute myocardial infarction. *Lancet* 1995; **345:** 669–85.

53 Kay R, Wong KS, Yu YL, et al. Low-molecular-weight heparin for the treatment of acute ischemic stroke. *N Engl J Med* 1995; **333:** 1588–93.

54 Gubitz G, Counsell C, Sandercock P, Signorini D. Anticoagulants for acute ischaemic stroke. *The Cochrane Library*, Issue 4. Oxford: Update Software, 1999.

55 Gelmers HJ. The effects of nimodipine on the clinical course of patients with acute ischemic stroke. *Acta Neurol Scand* 1984; **69:** 232–39.

56 Horn J, Limburg M. Calcium antagonists for acute ischemic stroke. In: *The Cochrane Library*, Issue 4. Oxford: Update Software, 2000.

57 Stephens NG, Parsons A, Schofield PM, et al. Randomised controlled trial of vitamin E in patients with coronary disease: Cambridge Heart Antioxidant Study (CHAOS). *Lancet* 1996; **347:** 781–86.

58 GISSI – Prevenzione Investigators (Gruppo Italiano per lo Studio della Sopravvivenza nell'Infarto Miocardico). Dietary supplementation with n-3 polyunsaturated fatty acids and vitamin E after myocardial infarction: results of the GISSI–Prevenzione trial. *Lancet* 1999; **354:** 447–55.

59 The Heart Outcomes Prevention Evaluation Study Investigators. Vitamin E supplementation and cardiovascular events in high-risk patients. *N Engl J Med* 2000; **342:** 154–60.

60 Heart Protection Study Collaborative Group. MRC/BHF Heart Protection Study of antioxidant vitamin supplementation in 20,536 high-risk individuals: a randomised placebo-controlled trial. *Lancet* 2002; **360:** 23–33.

61 Gurfinkel E, Bozovich G, Daroca A, et al., for the ROXIS Study Group. Randomised trial of roxithromycin in non-Q-wave coronary syndromes: ROXIS pilot study. *Lancet* 1997; **350:** 404–07.

62 O'Connor CM, Dunne MW, Pfeffer MA, et al. Investigators in the WIZARD Study. Azithromycin for the secondary prevention of coronary heart disease events: the WIZARD study: a randomized controlled trial. *JAMA* 2003; **290:** 1459–66.

63 Grayston JT, Kronmal RA, Jackson LA, et al. ACES Investigators. Azithromycin for the secondary prevention of coronary events. *N Engl J Med* 2005; **352:** 1637–45.

64 Cannon CP, Braunwald E, McCabe CH, et al. Pravastatin or Atorvastatin Evaluation and Infection Therapy–Thrombolysis in Myocardial Infarction 22 Investigators. Antibiotic treatment of *Chlamydia pneumoniae* after acute coronary syndrome. *N Engl J Med* 2005; **352:** 1646–54.
65 The EC/IC Bypass Study Group. Failure of extracranial–intracranial arterial bypass to reduce the risk of ischemic stroke: results of an international randomized trial. *N Engl J Med* 1985; **313:** 1191–200.
66 Goldring S, Zervas N, Langfitt T. The extracranial-intracranial bypass study: a report of the committee appointed by the American Association of Neurological Surgeons to examine the study. *N Engl J Med* 1987; **316:** 817–20.
67 Barnett HJM, Sackett D, Taylor DW, et al. Are the results of the extracranial–intracranial bypass trial generalizable? *N Engl J Med* 1987; **316:** 820–24.
68 Dickersin K. How important is publication bias? A synthesis of available data. *AIDS Edu Prev* 1997; **9:** 15–21.
69 Pocock SJ, Hughes MD. Estimation issues in clinical trials and overviews. *Stat Med* 1990; **9:** 657–71.
70 Yusuf S, Wittes J, Probstfield J, Tyroler HA. Analysis and interpretation of treatment effects in subgroups of patients in randomized clinical trials. *JAMA* 1991; **266:** 93–98.
71 Thiemann DR, Coresh J, Schulman SP, et al. Lack of benefit for intravenous thrombolysis in patients with myocardial infarction who are older than 75 years. *Circulation* 2000; **101:** 2239–46.
72 Berger AK, Radford MJ, Wang Y, Krumholz HM. Thrombolytic therapy in older patients. *J Am Coll Cardiol* 2000; **36:** 366–74.
73 White HD. Thrombolytic therapy in the elderly. *Lancet* 2000; **356:** 2028–30.
74 Baigent C, Keech A, Kearney PM, et al. Cholesterol Treatment Trialists' (CTT) Collaborators. Efficacy and safety of cholesterol-lowering treatment: prospective meta-analysis of data from 90,056 participants in 14 randomised trials of statins. *Lancet* 2005; **366:** 1267–78.
75 Tavazzi L, Tognoni G, Franzosi MG, et al. GISSI-HF Investigators. Rationale and design of the GISSI heart failure trial: a large trial to assess the effects of n-3 polyunsaturated fatty acids and rosuvastatin in symptomatic congestive heart failure. *Eur J Heart Fail* 2004; **6:** 635–41.
76 Kjekshus J, Dunselman P, Blideskog M, et al. CORONA Study Group. *Eur J Heart Fail* 2005; **7:** 1059–69.
77 Collins R, Peto R, MacMahon S, et al. Blood pressure, stroke, and coronary heart disease. Part 2, short-term reductions in blood pressure: overview of randomised drug trials in their epidemiological context. *Lancet* 1990; **335:** 827–38.
78 Rothwell PM, Warlow CP, on behalf of the European Carotid Surgery Trialists' Collaborative Group. Prediction of benefit from carotid endarterectomy in individual patients: a risk-modelling study. *Lancet* 1999; **353:** 2105–10.
79 Rothwell PM. Can overall results of clinical trials be applied to all patients? *Lancet* 1995; **345:** 1616–19.
80 Baigent C, Keech A, Kearney PM, et al., for the Cholesterol Treatment Trialists' (CTT) Collaborators. Efficacy and safety of cholesterol-lowering treatment: prospective meta-analysis of data from 90,056 participants in 14 randomised trials of statins. *Lancet* 2005; **366:** 1267–78.
81 Early Breast Cancer Trialists' Collaborative Group. Systemic treatment of early breast cancer by hormonal, cytotoxic, or immune therapy: 133 randomised trials involving 31 000 recurrences and 24 000 deaths among 75 000 women. *Lancet* 1992; **339:** 1–15, 71–85.
82 Davies C, McGale P, Peto R. Variation in use of adjuvant tamoxifen. *Lancet* 1998; **351:** 1487–88.
83 Early Breast Cancer Trialists' Collaborative Group. Tamoxifen for early breast cancer: an overview of the randomised trials. *Lancet* 1998; **351:** 1451–67.
84 Spiegelhalter DJ, Myles JP, Jones DR, Abrams KR. An introduction to Bayesian methods in health technology assessment. *BMJ* 1999; **319:** 508–12.
85 Layton AM, Ibbotson SH, Davies JA, Goodfield MJD. Randomised trial of oral aspirin for chronic venous leg ulcers. *Lancet* 1994; **344:** 164–65.
86 Forette F, Seux M-L, Staessen JA, et al., on behalf of the Syst-Eur Investigators. Prevention of dementia in randomised double-blind placebo-controlled Systolic Hypertension in Europe (Syst-Eur) trial. *Lancet* 1998; **352:** 1347–51.
87 Boaz M, Smetana S, Weinstein T, et al. Secondary prevention with antioxidants of cardiovascular disease in endstage renal disease (SPACE): randomised placebo-controlled trial. *Lancet* 2000; **356:** 1213–18.
88 Altman DG. Confidence intervals for the number needed to treat. *BMJ* 1998; **317:** 1309–12.
89 Mellin GW, Katzenstein M. The saga of thalidomide. *N Engl J Med* 1962; **267:** 1184–89.
90 Herbst AL, Ulfelder H, Poskanzer DC. Adenocarcinoma of the vagina: association of maternal stilbestrol therapy with tumor appearance in young women. *N Engl J Med* 1971; **284:** 878–81.
91 Khan MA, Herzog CA, St Peter JV, et al. The prevalence of cardiac valvular insufficiency assessed by transthoracic echocardiography in obese patients treated with appetite-suppressant drugs. *N Engl J Med* 1998; **339:** 713–18.

92 Rzany B, Correia O, Kelly JP, et al., for the Study Group of the International Case–Control Study on Severe Cutaneous Adverse Reactions. Risk of Stevens–Johnson syndrome and toxic epidermal necrolysis during first weeks of antiepileptic therapy: a case–control study. *Lancet* 1999; **353:** 2190–94.

93 Grady D, Rubin SM, Petitti DB, et al. Hormone therapy to prevent disease and prolong life in postmenopausal women. *Ann Intern Med* 1992; **117:** 1016–37.

94 Beral V, Banks E, Reeves G, Appleby P. Use of HRT and the subsequent risk of cancer. *J Epidemiol Biostat* 1999; **4:** 191–210.

95 Florey M, Florey H. General and local administration of penicillin. *Lancet* 1943; **1:** 387–97.

96 Harington M, Kincaid-Smith P, McMichael J. Results of treatment in malignant hypertension: a seven-year experience in 94 cases. *BMJ* 1959; **2:** 969–80.

97 Mahalanabis D, Choudhuri AB, Bagchi NG, et al. Oral fluid therapy of cholera among Bangladesh refugees. *Johns Hopkins Med J* 1973; **132:** 197–205.

98 Hennekens CH, Buring JE. Observational evidence. *Ann NY Acad Sci* 1993; **703:** 18–24.

99 Jick H, Zornberg GL, Jick SS, et al. Statins and the risk of dementia. *Lancet* 2000; **356:** 1627–31.

100 Chan KA, Andrade SE, Boles M, et al. Inhibitors of hydroxymethylglutaryl-coenzyme A reductase and risk of fracture among older women. *Lancet* 2000; **355:** 2185–88.

101 Lever AF, Hole DJ, Gillis CR, et al. Do inhibitors of angiotensin-I-converting enzyme protect against risk of cancer? *Lancet* 1998; **352:** 179–84.

102 Barrett-Connor E, Grady D. Hormone replacement therapy, heart disease, and other considerations. *Annu Rev Public Health* 1998; **19:** 55–72.

103 Onder G, Penninx BW, Balkrishnan R, et al. Relations between use of angiotensin-converting enzyme inhibitors and muscle strength and physical function in older women: an observational study. *Lancet* 2002; **359:** 926–30.

104 Hackham DG, Mamdani M, Li P, Redelmeier DA. Statins and sepsis in patients with cardiovascular disease: a population-based cohort analysis. *Lancet* 2006; **367:** 413–18.

105 Graham DJ, Campen D, Hui R, et al. Risk of acute myocardial infarction and sudden cardiac death in patients treated with cyclo-oxygenase 2 selective and non-selective non-steroidal anti-inflammatory drugs: nested case-control study. *Lancet* 2005; **365:** 475–81.

106 Sudbo J, Lee JJ, Lippman SM, et al. Non-steroidal anti-inflammatory drugs and the risk of oral cancer: a nested case-control study. *Lancet* 2005; **366:** 1359–66.

107 Soumerai SB, McLaughlin TJ, Spiegelman D, et al. Adverse outcomes of underuse of beta-blockers in elderly survivors of acute myocardial infarction. *JAMA* 1997; **277:** 15–21.

108 Yusuf S, Peto R, Lewis J, et al. Beta blockade during and after myocardial infarction: an overview of the randomized trials. *Prog Cardiovasc Dis* 1985; **27:** 335–71.

109 Doughty RN, Rodgers A, Sharpe N, MacMahon S. Effects of beta-blocker therapy on mortality in patients with heart failure: a systematic overview of randomized controlled trials. *Eur Heart J* 1997: **18:** 560–65.

110 CIBIS-II Investigators and Committees. The Cardiac Insufficiency Bisoprolol Study II (CIBIS II): a randomised trial. *Lancet* 1999; **353:** 9–13.

111 Hjalmarson A, Goldstein S, Fagerberg B, et al., for the MERIT-HF Study Group. Effects of controlled-release metoprolol on total mortality, hospitalizations, and well-being in patients with heart failure: the Metroprolol CR/XL Randomized Intervention Trial in Congestive Heart Failure (MERIT-HF). *JAMA* 2000; **283:** 1295–302.

112 Clarke R, Shipley M, Lewington S, et al. Underestimation of risk associations due to regression dilution in long-term follow-up of prospective studies. *Am J Epidemiol* 1999; **150:** 341–53.

113 Thurmer HL, Lund-Larsen PG, Tverdal A. Is blood pressure treatment as effective in a population setting as in controlled trials? Results from a prospective study. *J Hypertens* 1994; **12:** 481–90.

114 Collins R, MacMahon S. Blood pressure, antihypertensive drug treatment and the risks of stroke and of coronary heart disease. *Br Med Bull* 1994; **50:** 272–98.

115 Paganini-Hill A, Chao A, Ross RK, Henderson BE. Aspirin use and chronic diseases: a cohort study of the elderly. *BMJ* 1989; **299:** 1247–50.

116 Antiplatelet Trialists' Collaboration. Collaborative overview of randomised trials of antiplatelet therapy. I: Prevention of death, myocardial infarction, and stroke by prolonged antiplatelet therapy in various categories of patients. *BMJ* 1994; **308:** 81–106.

117 Barnett HJM, Taylor DW, Eliasziw M, et al., for the North American Symptomatic Carotid Endarterectomy Trial Collaborators. Benefit of carotid endarterectomy in patients with symptomatic moderate or severe stenosis. *N Engl J Med* 1998; **339:** 415–25.

118 Taylor DW, Barnett HJM, Haynes RW, et al., for the ASA and Carotid Endarterectomy (ACE) Trial Collaborators. Low-dose and high-dose acetylsalicylic acid for patients undergoing carotid endarterectomy: a randomised controlled trial. *Lancet* 1999; **353:** 2179–84.

119 Swan SH, Shaw GM, Schulman J. Reporting and selection bias in case-control studies of congenital malformations. *Epidemiology* 1992; **3:** 356–63.

120 Stewart A, Webb J, Hewitt D. A survey of childhood malignancies. *BMJ* 1958; **1:** 1495–508.

121 MacMahon B, Hutchinson GB. Prenatal x-ray and childhood cancer: a review. *Acta Unio Int Contra Cancrum* 1964; **20:** 1172–74.

122 Khoury MJ, James LM, Erickson JD. On the use of affected controls to address recall bias in case-controlled studies of birth defects. *Teratology* 1994; **49:** 273–81.

123 Collaborative Group on Hormonal Factors in Breast Cancer. Breast cancer and hormonal contraceptives: collaborative reanalysis of individual data on 53 297 women with breast cancer and 100 239 women without breast cancer from 54 epidemiological studies. *Lancet* 1996; **347:** 1713–27.

124 Bar-Oz B, Moretti ME, Mareels G, et al. Reporting bias in retrospective ascertainment of drug-induced embryopathy. *Lancet* 1999; **354:** 1700–01.

125 Psaty BM, Heckbert SR, Koepsell TD, et al. The risk of myocardial infarction associated with antihypertensive drug therapies. *JAMA* 1995; **274:** 620–25.

126 Blood Pressure Lowering Treatment Trialists' Collaboration. Effects of ACE inhibitors, calcium antagonists, and other blood-pressure-lowering drugs: results of prospectively designed overviews of randomised trials. *Lancet* 2003; **355:** 1955–64.

127 McClellan M, McNeil BJ, Newhouse JP. Does more intensive treatment of acute myocardial infarction in the elderly reduce mortality? Analysis using instrumental variables. *JAMA* 1994; **272:** 859–66.

128 Gargiullo PM, Kramarz P, DeStefano F, Chen RT. Principles of epidemiological research on drug effects. *Lancet* 1999; **353:** 501.

129 MacDonald TM, Evans JMM, Sullivan F, McMahon AD. Principles of epidemiological research on drug effects. *Lancet* 1999; **353:** 501–02.

130 Barbone F, McMahon AD, Davey PG, et al. Association of road-traffic accidents with benzodiazepine use. *Lancet* 1998; **352:** 1331–36.

131 Rubin DB. Estimating causal effects from large data sets using propensity scores. *Ann Intern Med* 1997; **127:** 757–63.

132 Barrett-Connor E. Hormone replacement therapy. *BMJ* 1998; **317:** 457–61.

133 Collaborative Group on Hormonal Factors in Breast Cancer. Breast cancer and hormone replacement therapy: collaborative reanalysis of data from 51 epidemiological studies of 52 705 women with breast cancer and 108 411 women without breast cancer. *Lancet* 1997; **350:** 1047–59.

134 Matthews KA, Kuller LH, Wing RR, et al. Prior to use of estrogen replacement therapy, are users healthier than nonusers? *Am J Epidemiol* 1996; **143:** 971–78.

135 Barrett-Connor E. Postmenopausal estrogen and prevention bias. *Ann Intern Med* 1991; **115:** 455–56.

136 Giovannucci E, Colditz GA, Stampfer MJ, Willett WC. Physical activity, obesity, and risk of colorectal adenoma in women (United States). *Cancer Causes Control* 1996; **7:** 253–63.

137 Hsia J, Langer R, Manson JE, et al., for the Women's Health Initiative Investigators. Conjugated equine estrogens and coronary heart disease. The Women's Health Initiative. *Arch Intern Med* 2006; **166:** 357–65.

138 Manson JE, Hsia J, Johnson KC, et al., for the Women's Health Initiative Investigators. Estrogen plus progestin and the risk of coronary heart disease. *N Engl J Med* 2003; **349:** 523–34.

139 Chlebowski RT, Hendrix SL, Langer RD, et al., for the WHI Investigators. Influence of estrogen plus progestin on breast cancer and mammography in healthy postmenopausal women. *JAMA* 2003; **289:** 3243–53.

140 Chlebowski RT, Wactawski-Wende J, Ritenbaugh C, et al., for the Women's Health Initiative Investigators. Estrogen plus progestin and colorectal cancer in postmenopausal women. *N Eng J Med* 2004; **350:** 991–1004.

141 The Women's Health Initiative Steering Committee. Effects of conjugated equine estrogen in postmenopausal women with hysterectomy. *JAMA* 2004; **291:** 1701–12.

142 Benson K, Hartz AJ. A comparison of observational studies and randomized, controlled trials. *N Engl J Med* 2000; **342:** 1878–86.

143 Concato J, Shah N, Horwitz RI. Randomized, controlled trials, observational studies, and the hierarchy of research designs. *N Engl J Med* 2000; **342:** 1887–92.

144 Pocock SJ, Elbourne DR. Randomized trials or observational tribulations? *N Engl J Med* 2000; **342:** 1907–09.

145 Moss AJ, Davis HT, Conrad DL, et al. Digitalis-associated cardiac mortality after myocardial infarction. *Circulation* 1981; **64:** 1150–56.

146 The Digitalis Investigation Group. The effect of digoxin on mortality and morbidity in patients with heart failure. *N Engl J Med* 1997; **336:** 525–33.

147 Lindsay SJ, Kearney MT, Prescott RJ, et al., for the UK Heart Investigation. Digoxin and mortality in chronic heart failure. *Lancet* 1999; **354:** 1003.

148 Spargias KS, Hall AS, Ball SG. Safety concerns about digoxin after acute myocardial infarction. *Lancet* 1999; **354:** 391–92.

149 Black N. Why we need observational studies to evaluate the effectiveness of health care. *BMJ* 1996; **312:** 1215–18.

150 McKee M, Britton A, Black N, et al. Interpreting the evidence: choosing between randomised and non-randomised studies. *BMJ* 1999; **319:** 312–15.

151 Report from the Boston Collaborative Drug Surveillance Program. Reserpine and breast cancer. *Lancet* 1974; **2:** 669–71.

152 Heinonen OP, Shapiro S, Tuominen L, Turunen MI. Reserpine use in relation to breast cancer. *Lancet* 1974; **2:** 675–77.

153 Horwitz RI, Feinstein AR. Exclusion bias and the false relationship of reserpine and breast cancer. *Arch Intern Med* 1985; **145:** 1873–75.

154 Pahor M, Guralnik JM, Ferrucci L, et al. Calcium-channel blockade and incidence of cancer in aged populations. *Lancet* 1996; **348:** 493–97.

155 Ad Hoc Subcommittee of the Liaison Committee of the World Health Organisation and the International Society of Hypertension. Effects of calcium antagonists on the risks of coronary heart disease, cancer and bleeding. *J Hypertens* 1997; **15:** 105–15.

156 Rodgers A, MacMahon S, Gamble G, et al., on behalf of the UKTIA Collaborative Group. Blood pressure and risk of stroke in patients with cerebrovascular disease. *BMJ* 1996; **313:** 147.

157 PROGRESS Collaborative Group. Randomised trial of a perindopril-based blood pressure lowering regimen among 6,105 individuals with previous stroke or transient ischaemic attack. *Lancet* 2001; **358:** 1033–41.

158 MacMahon S, Neal B, Rodgers A, Chalmers J. The PROGRESS trial three years later: time for more action, less distraction. BMJ 2004; **329:** 970–71.

159 Blood Pressure Lowering Treatment Trialists' Collaboration. Effects of different blood-pressure lowering regimens on major cardiovascular events: results of prospectively designed overviews of randomised trials. *Lancet* 2003; **362:** 1527–35.

160 Law MR, Wald NJ, Thompson SG. By how much and how quickly does reduction in serum cholesterol concentration lower risk of ischaemic heart disease? *BMJ* 1994; **308:** 367–73.

161 LaRosa JC, He JM, Vupputuri S. Effect of statins on risk of coronary disease: a meta-analysis of randomized controlled trials. *JAMA* 1999; **282:** 2340–46.

162 Pfeffer MA, Braunwald E, Moyé LA, et al., on behalf of the SAVE Investigators. Effect of captopril on mortality and morbidity in patients with left ventricular dysfunction after myocardial infarction: results of the survival and ventricular enlargement trial. *N Engl J Med* 1992; **327:** 669–77.

163 The SOLVD Investigators. Effect of enalapril on mortality and the development of heart failure in asymptomatic patients with reduced left ventricular ejection fractions. *N Engl J Med* 1992; **327:** 685–91.

164 The Heart Outcomes Prevention Evaluation Study Investigators. Effects of an angiotensin-converting-enzyme inhibitor, ramipril, on cardiovascular events in high-risk patients. *N Engl J Med* 2000; **342:** 145–53.

165 Peto R, Doll R, Buckley JD, Sporn MB. Can dietary beta-carotene materially reduce human cancer rates? *Nature* 1981; **290:** 201–08.

166 Buring J, Hennekens C. Retinoids and carotenoids. In: De Vita VT Jr, Hellman S, Rosenberg S, eds. *Cancer: Principles and Practice of Oncology*. Philadelphia, PA: JB Lippincott, 1993.

167 Hennekens CH, Buring JE, Manson JE, et al. Lack of effect of long-term supplementation with beta carotene on the incidence of malignant neoplasms and cardiovascular disease. *N Engl J Med* 1996; **334:** 1145–49.

168 Danesh J, Collins R, Appleby P, Peto R. Association of fibrinogen, C-reactive protein, albumin, or leukocyte count with coronary heart disease: meta-analyses of prospective studies. *JAMA* 1998; **279:** 1477–82.

169 Danesh J, Lewington S. Plasma homocysteine and coronary heart disease: systematic review of published epidemiological studies. *J Cardiol Risk* 1998; **5:** 229–32.

170 World Health Organization. *World Health Statistics Annual*. Geneva: WHO, 1996.

2

The lethal consequences of failing to make full use of all relevant evidence about the effects of medical treatments: the importance of systematic reviews

Iain Chalmers

Introduction

For nearly two centuries there have been arguments about the relevance of evidence derived from research involving groups of patients when treatment decisions are needed for individual patients.[1, 2] This book will help to promote much-needed clearer thinking about this issue. Only rarely is complete certainty justified about how a treatment will affect a particular patient. Half a century ago, not long after the birth of the randomised clinical trial, Austin Bradford Hill[3] drew attention to the inevitable guesswork involved in using the results of clinical trials to predict the effects of treatments in individuals:

> *Our answers from the clinical trial present ... a group reaction. They show that one group fared better than another, that given a certain treatment, patients, on the average, get better more frequently or rapidly, or both. We cannot necessarily, perhaps very rarely, pass from that to stating exactly what effect the treatment will have on a particular patient.* But there is, surely, no way and no method of deciding that. [My emphasis.][3]

How do I want this inevitable guesswork about the effects of treatment to be informed when I am a patient?[4] Very occasionally it will be possible to design research ('*n*-of-1' trials) to find out which of alternative treatments best suits me – absolutely specifically. More usually this kind of very specific information will not be available, even when my genotype becomes known.[5] Patients like me, and the clinicians to whom we look for personalised care, are clearly very interested in knowing which factors should be taken into account when assessing the applicability of average effects of treatments derived from studying groups of patients. Although it seems unlikely that 'just about every treatment does some good for someone', as some have suggested,[6, 7] I imagine I am not alone in wanting decisions about my treatment to be as individualised as possible. This is a tough challenge and later chapters in this book will deal with twin thorny problems: identifying which individuals are likely to benefit from or be harmed by treatments, and avoiding the false inferences that can result from biases and chance associations.[8–10]

The widely promulgated vision of general availability of individually tailored treatments seems still to be some way from being realised in practice. During the lifetime of this edition of this book at least, my clinician advisers and I will usually need to fall back on evidence derived from observing groups of patients who are more or less like me. Often this evidence will be informal, existing only inside the heads of my advisers, who will draw on their experience of treating other patients. I may want that kind of informal evidence to be taken into account in decisions about my treatment; but as there are many examples of such evidence having been dangerously misleading, I certainly want account to be taken of relevant research evidence.

Some people may suggest that I should not assume that evidence from research is relevant to me unless the people studied in the research can be shown to be very like me. My approach is different. I want to know whether there are reasons that could justify confidently dismissing – as irrelevant to me – estimates of effects derived from the best available research evidence on groups of people. These estimates might be dismissed either because I am confident that I am completely different from the people who participated in the research; or because the interventions available to me are not those that have been evaluated by researchers; or because the questions or the treatment outcomes which I rate as important have been ignored by researchers.[11]

When I say that I want 'relevant research evidence' to be taken into account in decisions about my treatment, what kind of evidence do I have in mind? Although very large randomised trials may often contribute the overwhelming weight of evidence on particular therapeutic questions, this is no reason to ignore evidence from smaller studies judged likely to be unbiased, particularly if they have been registered prospectively to reduce publication bias.[12] I want treatment decisions to be informed by synthesis of all the relevant evidence – synthesised rigorously in systematic reviews.

And I do mean *all* the relevant evidence. Biased underreporting of research can be lethal. For example, Cowley et al.,[13] to their great credit, reported in 1993 the results of a clinical trial of an antiarrhythmic drug in myocardial infarction actually done 13 years earlier.

> *Nine patients died in the lorcainide (drug) group and one in the placebo group ... When we carried out our study in 1980 we thought that the increased death rate that occurred in the lorcainide group was an effect of chance ... The development of lorcainide was abandoned for commercial reasons, and this study was therefore never published; it is now a good example of 'publication bias'. The results described here ... might have provided an early warning of trouble ahead.*[13]

The 'trouble ahead' to which they were referring was that, at the peak of their use, this class of drugs was causing tens of thousands of premature deaths every year in the USA alone.[14] Worldwide, the drugs seem likely to have caused hundreds of thousands of deaths.

Although most of the evidence of the dangers of biased underreporting of research has been sought and found among practice-orientated clinical research studies,[15] it appears that the results of an unpublished study might have provided a forewarning of the tragic consequences of using the drug TGN1412, which had life-threatening effects on six young, healthy volunteers in a study in London in early 2006.[16] Biased underreporting of preclinical research may also help to explain the high and increasing failure of proposals for new drugs to survive assessment in early clinical studies.[17]

As far as possible, therefore, whether in early or late studies of treatments, systematic reviews should take account of *all* the relevant data – published and unpublished. Systematic reviews based on these data can show that when the results of studies addressing the same or similar questions appear to differ, the apparent differences (even in the results of large studies) are compatible with the effects of chance.[18] And when chance is an unlikely explanation for differing results of apparently similar trials, systematic reviews can be used to explore and possibly explain the differences in ways that may improve understanding of how to individualise treatment. Systematic reviews can also be used to test hypotheses generated by unexpected results in individual trials. For example, after a trial had found an unpredicted, statistically significantly higher rate of breast cancer in women who had received a lipid-lowering drug,[19] a systematic review of all similar studies provided reassurance that the observation was very likely to have reflected chance.[20]

Of course, the term 'systematic review' begs the question – what system? As with reports of any scientific investigation, the expectation of readers should be that reports of systematic reviews will contain descriptions of the materials and methods used by researchers to address clearly stated questions, in ways that reduce distortions from biases and the play of chance. The term 'systematic review' means for me 'the application of strategies that *limit bias* [my emphasis] in the assembly, critical appraisal, and synthesis of all relevant studies on a specific topic'.[21] Meta-analysis – 'statistical synthesis of the data from separate but similar studies leading to a quantitative summary of the pooled results'[21] – may or may not be a component of systematic reviews, but it does nothing to reduce bias. If appropriate and possible, however, it can often reduce the likelihood of our being misled by the effects of the play of chance, as Karl Pearson demonstrated more than a century ago.[22]

For questions about the effects of healthcare interventions, a key issue concerns the kind of primary studies that will be eligible for inclusion in systematic reviews. Some interventions have dramatic effects that can be confidently identified without carefully controlled research.[23] Unbiased, confident detection of the more modest effects of most interventions, however, requires sufficiently large studies that have used randomisation and other measures to minimise biases. That is why this book emphasises the importance of randomised trials. There are many examples of the dangers of basing treatment decisions on non-randomised studies. An example relevant to a later section in this chapter is a non-randomised study reported by Horwitz and Feinstein:[24] the results of their analysis encouraged the use of a class of drugs that turned out to be lethal.[14]

Because people have not taken sufficiently seriously the need to make full use of *all* the relevant research evidence, readers of research reports have been misled by biases and the play of chance, patients have suffered and died unnecessarily, and resources for healthcare and health research have been wasted. It was against this background that

2 The consequences of failing to fully use all relevant evidence

Peter Rothwell asked me to stress in this chapter 'the absolute importance of research synthesis in determining the overall effects of treatment, and the fact that this has to be the starting point for any further consideration of who might benefit most.' (P. Rothwell, personal communication, 2 September 2005).

The scandalous failure of biomedical science to cumulate evidence scientifically

Four decades ago, one of the pioneers of randomised trials, Austin Bradford Hill, suggested that readers of published reports of research want their authors to provide the answers to four basic questions: 'Why did you start; what did you do; what did you find; and what does it mean anyway?'[25] As a result of the adoption of reporting guidelines such as those recommended by the CONSORT Group,[26] it has become more likely that readers of research reports will have satisfactory answers to Hill's second and third questions – What did you do? and What did you find? – but satisfactory answers to Hill's first and fourth questions are much rarer.

To answer Bradford Hill's first question – Why did you start? – readers need to be reassured that new research has been done because, at the time it was initiated, important questions could not be answered satisfactorily with existing evidence. Systematic reviews of existing evidence have sometimes raised serious ethical questions, for example, about the continued use of placebos or no treatment controls.[27, 29] Although these problems have been exposed repeatedly over the past quarter century, a recent survey showed that researchers still do not, in general, review existing evidence systematically when designing controlled trials.[30] Indeed, some of them state bluntly that they see no need to do this (A. Sutton, personal communication, 2 December 2005). Even among those who take a formal Bayesian approach to the design of controlled trials, the fairly basic step of using a systematic review of existing evidence to estimate the likely size of a treatment difference seems often to be overlooked.[31] Although applicants to some research funding bodies are required[32] or being urged[33] to show how their proposals build on systematic reviews of existing evidence, the unjustified duplication of research illustrated in the examples given later in this chapter make clear that many research funders are not taking sufficiently seriously their responsibilities to husband limited resources for research efficiently and ethically.

Research funding organisations, research ethics committees, journals and drug licensing authorities have all been challenged to accept the responsibilities implied by their authority to reduce this form of research misconduct.[34, 35] The situation would improve if there was less institutionalised reverence for the current systems of peer review operated by research funders and editors of journals. The failure of authors to mention relevant previous work is a widespread form of research malpractice.[36] Fifteen years ago, Chalmers et al.[37] suggested that, when submitting reports for review, investigators should be required by journals to provide evidence that they have made a thorough search for relevant previous work. Such a requirement might both improve the relevance and quality of research conducted and help to reduce the frequency of undeclared duplicate publication, as well as improve detection of plagiarism.[38] Yet very few funders and journal editors appear to have taken seriously that suggestion, or

Jefferson and co-workers'[39, 40] related proposal that, until proved otherwise, a research proposal or a submitted manuscript should be viewed as one member of a population of related studies, and judged in the context of a systematic review of the other member studies in that population.

Research ethics committees have done little to protect patients from the adverse effects of this scientific sloppiness. Ten years have passed since research ethics committees were challenged publicly to recognise that they were behaving unethically if they did not take steps to satisfy themselves that they were approving research that had been designed in the light of systematic reviews of existing evidence;[34] yet there is very little evidence that they have taken this challenge seriously.[41, 42] The failure of research ethics committees to hold research funders and researchers to account in this respect can sometimes result in dramatic tragedies. For example, Ellen Roche, a young woman volunteer in a physiological experiment at Johns Hopkins Medical School, died because the design of the experiment in which she had been asked to participate had not been informed by a systematic review of relevant pre-existing evidence about the hazards of inhaled hexamethonium.[43] The researchers had depended on Medline in their search for relevant evidence about the effects of inhaling the drug, so they were only aware of material published after 1965.[44] Pre-1966 evidence about the risks associated with inhaled hexamethonium was available in *The Cochrane Library* and other sources.[45] Researchers should be more ready to call on the skills of information scientists to help them avoid embarking on ill-conceived or frankly unnecessary research.[46]

What about Bradford Hill's fourth question – 'What does it mean, anyway?' Getting a reliable answer to this question is of great importance to consumers of research evidence because it is the 'bottom line', and so may influence choices, practices or policies. Lord Rayleigh, professor of physics at Cambridge University, had something to say about this in his presidential address to the 54th Meeting of the British Association for the Advancement of Science in Montreal in 1884:

> *If, as is sometimes supposed, science consisted in nothing but the laborious accumulation of facts, it would soon come to a standstill, crushed, as it were, under its own weight ... The work which deserves, but I am afraid does not always receive, the most credit is that in which discovery and explanation go hand in hand, in which not only are new facts presented, but their relation to old ones is pointed out.*[47]

More than a century later, researchers and journal editors in most fields of scientific investigation have not taken his admonition seriously. Authors have too rarely assessed systematically the relation between 'new facts' and 'old facts' in the discussion sections of their reports of new research.[48] Even reports of randomised trials published in the most prestigious general medical journals leave Bradford Hill's fourth question inadequately addressed (table 2.1).

All new research – whether basic or applied – should be designed in the light of scientifically defensible syntheses of existing research evidence, and reported setting

Classification	May 1997 (*n* = 26)	May 2001 (*n* = 33)	May 2005 (*n* = 18)
First trial addressing the question	1	3	3
Contained an updated systematic review integrating the new results	2	0	0
Discussed a previous review but did not attempt to integrate the new results	4	3	5
No apparent systematic attempt to set the results in the context of other trials	19	27	10

**The Lancet, New England Journal of Medicine, BMJ, JAMA* and *Annals of Internal Medicine*. Data from Clarke and co-workers.[49–51]

Table 2.1: **Classification of discussion sections in reports of randomised controlled trials published in May 1997, May 2001 and May 2005 in five general medical journals***

the new evidence 'in the light of the totality of the available evidence'.[26] This makes clear to readers what contribution – if any – new studies have made to knowledge.

As an illustration of the failure of researchers to take account of relevant evidence when designing and reporting new research, consider an analysis of reports of trials assessing the effect of aprotinin on the use of perioperative blood transfusion.[52] The first trial was reported in *The Lancet* in 1987, and showed a dramatically lower use of blood transfusions among patients who had received aprotinin than among control patients.[53] This difference was confirmed in 14 trials done over the subsequent 5 years. Yet, over the subsequent decade, a further 49 trials were reported. Figure 2.1 shows an analysis of the extent to which the authors of the reports of the 64 trials published by 2002 had cited relevant earlier trials. The shocking message in the figure is that, between 1987 and 2002, the proportion of relevant previous reports cited in successive reports of trials of aprotinin fell from a high of 33% to only 10% among the most recent reports. Furthermore, only seven of 44 subsequent reports referenced the report of the largest trial (which was 28 times larger than the median trial size); and most of the reports failed to reference either of the systematic reviews of relevant trials published in 1994 and 1997, respectively.

The human consequences of biomedicine's failure to cumulate evidence systematically

A pioneering study reported by Antman et al. in the *Journal of the American Medical Association* in 1992[28] used the technique of cumulative meta-analysis of randomised trials to show how much more would have been confidently known about the effects of treatments for myocardial infarction had successive trials set new results in the context of up-to-date systematic reviews of other relevant evidence. Figure 1 in their paper (reproduced here in figure 2.2) shows this, using data on the effects of beta-blockade for secondary prevention of myocardial infarction.

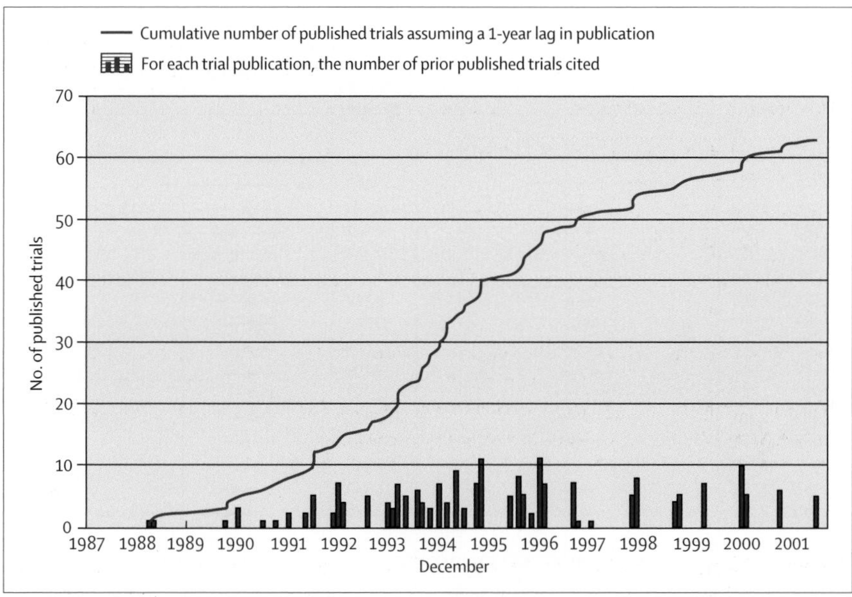

***Figure* 2.1: Citations of relevant prior publications in 64 reports of randomised trials of aprotinin, 1988–2002. (Reproduced from Fergusson et al.[52] by permission of the Society for Clinical Trials.)**

Figure 2.2(A) shows a now-familiar 'forest plot' presenting the results of 17 controlled trials comparing rates of death among patients receiving a beta-blocker drug with death rates among patients allocated to control. Along with the date of publication and number of participants in each trial, the results are represented by horizontal lines (confidence intervals) – the shorter the line, the more certain the result, reflecting the greater numbers of outcome events experienced by patients participating in that trial. The vertical line indicates the position around which the horizontal lines would cluster if the two treatments compared in the trials had similar effects. If a horizontal line touches or crosses the vertical line, it means that that particular trial found no statistically significant difference between the outcome of the drug group and that of the control group. Only two of these 17 trials individually yielded statistically significant estimates, which suggested that beta-blockers after myocardial infarction reduce mortality. However, it is not difficult to see that the horizontal lines tend to lie to the left of the vertical line. And indeed, when data derived from all 20 138 patients who participated in these studies is taken into account using meta-analysis, clear evidence emerges (shown by the bottom line) that these drugs have important beneficial effects.

Figure 2.2(B), which has a different horizontal scale to make it easier to see the confidence intervals, presents an analysis based on the same 20 138 patients in the same 17 trials, but arrayed in a different way – as a cumulative meta-analysis. This plot shows how estimates of the effects of beta-blockers would have looked had they been updated in the discussion sections of successive reports of each new trial. It shows that, had each of the successive reports published between 1972 and 1981 done this, chance would have

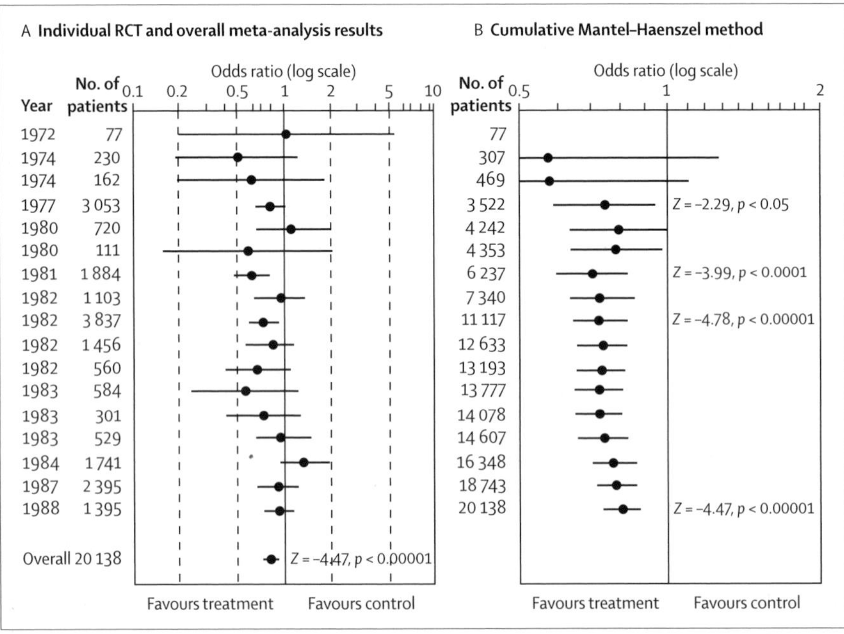

Figure 2.2: (A) Standard and (B) cumulative meta-analyses of the results of 17 randomised control trials of the effects of oral beta-blockers for secondary prevention of mortality in patients surviving a myocardial infarction. (Reproduced from Antman et al.,[28] with permission. Copyright American Medical Association © 1992. All rights reserved.)

been ruled out very confidently by 1981, after only six trials involving a total of 6237 patients had been reported. Although it may have been reasonable to do a few more placebo-controlled trials of these drugs, it is scientifically and ethically highly questionable whether nearly 14 000 patients needed to participate in further such studies.

Beta-blockade after myocardial infarction was just one of a number of treatments for myocardial infarction which Antman et al. evaluated in this way. For example, although strong evidence about the beneficial effects of thrombolytic therapy in myocardial infarction could, in principle, have been available by the mid-1970s, and a systematic review of this evidence was published in the *New England Journal of Medicine* in 1982,[54] the beneficial effects of thrombolysis were not mentioned at all in most textbooks until the late 1980s, and even when thrombolysis was mentioned, it was sometimes dismissed as unproven.[55]

The analyses done by Antman et al.[28] showed how science's failure to cumulate evidence scientifically had led to lethally incorrect advice in textbooks between 1960 and 1990: not only had advice on some life-saving therapies been delayed for more than a decade, but other treatments had been recommended long after controlled research had shown them to be harmful. An example of delayed recognition of lethal effects concerns prophylactic use of antiarrhythmic drugs in myocardial infarction. Hundreds of thousands of premature deaths would have been prevented if the hazards had been recognised earlier. Although there was evidence from the 1970s showing that these drugs did indeed reduce arrhythmias,[56] doubts about their effectiveness in reducing death were first raised in a systematic review of 14 randomised trials published in the early 1980s.[57] By the late 1980s two further systematic reviews had confirmed not only that there was no evidence that these drugs had beneficial effects on mortality, but that they were probably lethal.[58, 59] By the time that their lethal potential had become generally accepted in the early 1990s, more than 50 randomised controlled trials involving 23 229 patients had been reported.[60] If each new report of the many randomised trials of a class 1 antiarrhythmic drug had set new results in the context of a systematic review of the results of all previous trials – in other words, if scientists had cumulated evidence scientifically – the lethal potential of these drugs could have been widely recognised a decade earlier. As already noted, it has been estimated that, at the peak of their use in the late 1980s, these drugs were causing tens of thousands of deaths every year in the USA[14] – comparable annual numbers of deaths to the *total* number of Americans who died in the Vietnam war.

There are now many examples of the consequences for patients of failure to cumulate evidence scientifically. It is obviously particularly important to identify treatments with harmful effects more efficiently, for example, postoperative radiotherapy in non-small-cell lung cancer,[61] and treatments with toxic effects which confer no advantage compared with less toxic alternatives, as systematic reviews have demonstrated in respect of treatments for ovarian cancer.[62]

A further illustration of the way in which beneficial effects of treatments will be missed unless evidence is cumulated scientifically concerns the long delay in recognising one of the most effective and cost-effective interventions for preventing neonatal morbidity and mortality.[63–68] In 1969, Liggins[69] reported his observation that ewes in whom he had induced labour prematurely with steroids had given birth to lambs who, unexpectedly, had air in their lungs. Liggins and Howie promptly began a randomised, placebo-controlled trial to assess the effect of giving a short course of corticosteroids to pregnant women who were expected to deliver prematurely. Within 3 years of the report on neonatal lambs they had reported a statistically significant lower infant morbidity and mortality in infants born to mothers who had received steroids compared with those who had received placebo.[70]

Many additional, smaller trials were done, and systematic reviews of these done in the 1980s[63, 64] made clear the important beneficial effects of prenatal corticosteroids (the results of the first seven trials form the basis of the logo of The Cochrane Collaboration; figure 2.3). More than 20 years after the initial trial had been published, in the light of continuing uncertainty among practitioners about the value of the treatment, the National Institutes of Health convened a consensus conference to assess the evidence. A cumulative meta-analysis prepared for the conference showed that, had scientists cumulated evidence systematically in reports of successive trials, there would have been little room for doubt about the importance of the treatment for at least the previous 15 years.[71] An account of the missed opportunities to reduce neonatal morbid-

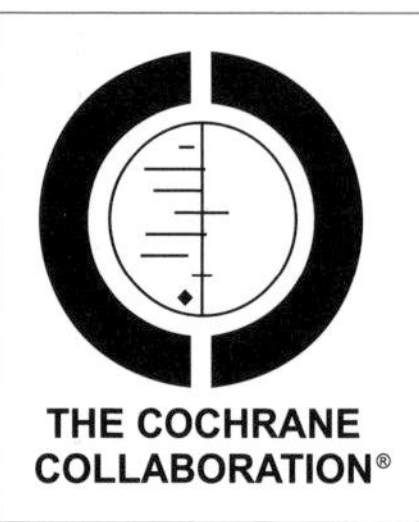

Figure 2.3: The Cochrane Collaboration logo. (Reproduced with permission of The Cochrane Collaboration.)

ity and mortality (and the costs of neonatal intensive care) is available in the proceedings of a Wellcome Trust Witness Seminar.[72]

Some medical interventions with plausible effects have been promulgated very widely without evidence from randomised trials that they are likely to do more good than harm. In these circumstances, if systematic reviews have made explicit the absence of relevant evidence from randomised trials, it is clearly important to promote the needed trials, as was done eventually to assess the long-term effects of hormone replacement therapy, for example. In some circumstances, however, randomised trials of sufficient size may be particularly difficult to organise, and it may be necessary to rely on systematic reviews of evidence derived from the studies of the best available observational data.

One such example relates to advice to put infants to sleep on their fronts (prone) in the belief that this would reduce the risk of death from choking. Based on untested logic, this advice was promulgated between the mid-1950s and the late-1980s,[73] notably by one of the most influential paediatricians during this era, Dr Benjamin Spock, whose book *Baby and Child Care* had become a multimillion-copy best seller. From the 1958 edition of the book he recommended front sleeping because, he suggested, babies sleeping on their backs are more likely to choke if they vomit.

Partly because of the dramatic impact of the 'Back to Sleep' campaigns launched in the late 1980s and early 1990s, we now know that influential earlier promulgation of front sleeping advice by Spock and others led to tens of thousands of avoidable cot deaths.[73] It is an example of the dangers of introducing new practices on the basis of theory unsupported by evidence. In addition, however, it is a further example of the consequences of failure of researchers to develop a cumulative science. As Gilbert et al. have shown,[73] advice promulgated for nearly half a century to put infants to sleep on the front was contrary to evidence available from 1970 that this was likely to be harmful. They estimate that systematic review of the evidence as it accumulated (figure 2.4) would have led to earlier recognition of the risks of sleeping on the front and might have prevented over 10 000 infant deaths in the UK and at least 50 000 in Europe, the USA and Australasia.

Although the above examples of failure to cumulate evidence systematically using methods to reduce biases and the play of chance are all from clinical and epidemiological research, it would be wrong to leave the impression that it is only within these spheres that there should be cause for concern about the failure of scientists to cumu-

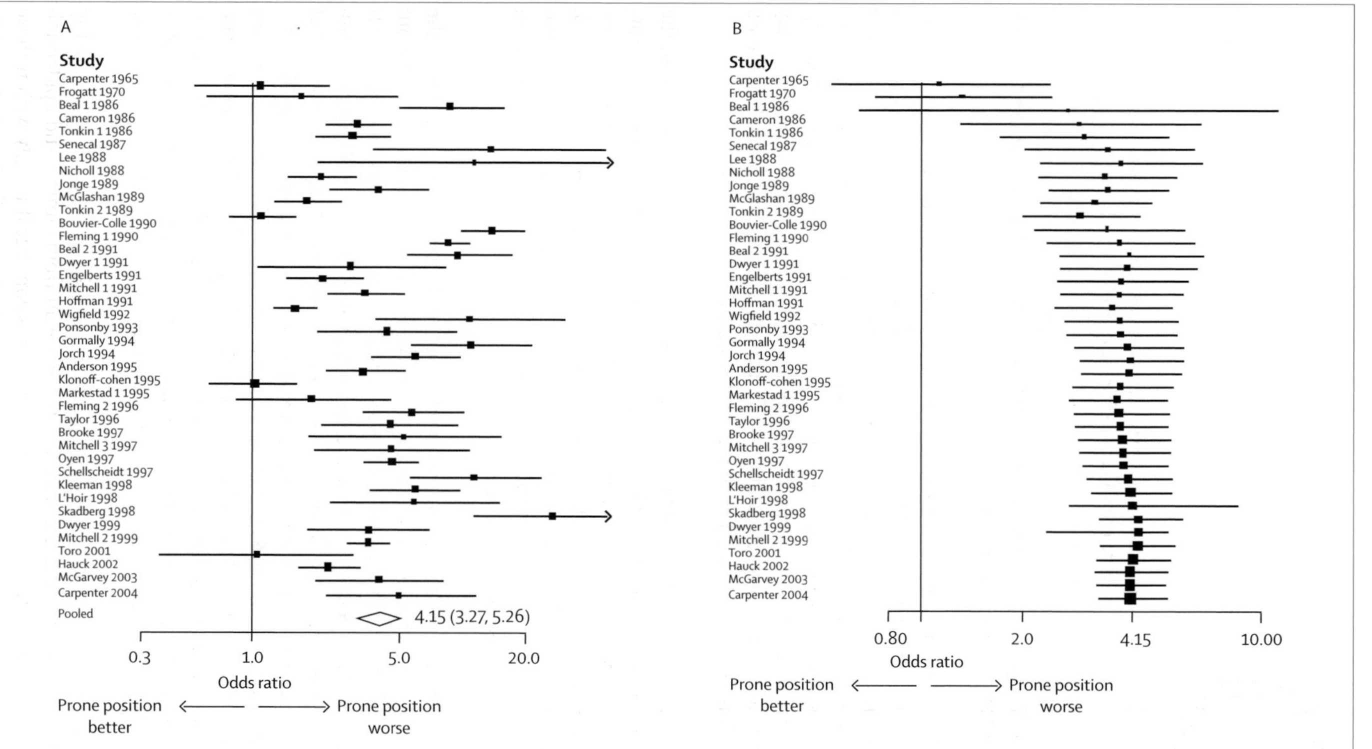

Figure 2.4: **(A) Odds ratios and pooled odds ratio and (B) cumulative odds ratios for front versus non-front sleeping position in comparisons of cases of sudden infant death syndrome (SIDS) and controls. (Reproduced from Gilbert et al.,[73] with permission of Oxford University Press and the International Epidemiological Association.)**

late scientifically. On the contrary, this issue is only now beginning to be addressed in preclinical research.

Failure to cumulate evidence systematically from experiments using animal models of human disease, for example, is not only bad science, it too can have adverse consequences for patients. Because it had been shown that calcium influx into areas of brain affected by acute ischaemic stroke led to cell death, it was thought that drugs that blocked calcium might protect the brain from damage. Based on selected reports of the early animal evidence, randomised clinical trials were begun. However, a systematic review of the evidence generated from randomised trials involving nearly 8000 patients found no evidence of any beneficial effects of nimodipine.[74] This finding prompted the authors to investigate the evidence from animal experiments. They concluded:

> *The results of this review did not show convincing evidence to substantiate the decision to perform trials with nimodipine in large numbers of patients. There were no differences between the results of the animal experiments and clinical studies. Surprisingly, we found that animal experiments and clinical studies ran simultaneously.*[75]

Had researchers using animal models of acute ischaemic stroke cumulated emerging evidence about the effects of nimodipine scientifically, it seems unlikely that it would have been judged worth inviting thousands of patients to participate in resource-intensive clinical trials of the drug. It is even more bizarre that animal experiments of nimodipine continued to be done for a considerable time after clinical trials had been initiated.[75]

Worrying examples of this kind have prompted challenges to animal researchers to be more systematic in developing the evidence base for their work.[76, 77] Systematic reviews of animal studies of six treatments that had been shown in systematic reviews of clinical trials to be either beneficial or to be harmful revealed a mixed picture of concordance and contradiction.[78] Formal assessment of the quality of animal research is beginning to yield some unsettling evidence.[79, 80] In 2002, for example, Bebarta et al.[81] showed that animal studies that had not used randomisation and blinding were more likely to have reported a difference between study groups than were studies that had used these methods to control biases – a comparable finding to that shown several years earlier in similar research analysing trials involving patients.[82] Assessment of the scientific quality of reviews of animal research also reveals serious deficiencies:[83] a large majority (i) did not specify a testable hypothesis, (ii) applied language restrictions, and (iii) failed to assess the possibility of publication bias or explore other reasons for heterogeneity. In only half of the reviews was the validity of component studies assessed.

A report on the ethics of research involving animals published by the Nuffield Council on Bioethics[84] in 2005 leaves little room for doubt that a serious problem exists, and that it must be addressed. The report notes the relative scarcity of systematic reviews and meta-analyses to evaluate more fully the predictability and transferability of animal models, and recommends that:

> *Since the scientific evaluation of animal research is fundamental to the cost–benefit assessment of any research, we recommend that the Home Office, in collaboration with major funders of such research such as the Wellcome Trust, the MRC, the BBSRC, animal protection groups and industry associations such as the ABPI, should consider ways of funding and carrying out these reviews.*[84]

At the time of writing, only the NHS Research and Development Programme, which does not fund research involving animals but has an unparalleled track record of supporting systematic reviews, has taken steps in response to this recommendation.[78]

Meeting the needs of clinicians and patients more effectively

When will readers of reports of clinical research be able to expect to find answers to the fourth of the questions posed by Bradford Hill in 1965 – 'What does it mean anyway?'[25] It is not that there are no examples showing how new results can be set systematically in the context of other evidence. Some of these examples go back centuries. Indeed, in many respects James Lind did a better job of this in his book on scurvy published in 1753 than many researchers and journals do today.[85] Although they remain rare, however, there are examples of discussion sections of clinical trials containing systematic reviews in more recent times (see, e.g., Saunders et al.[86]). In days when space was at a premium in printed journals, editors complained that this would use too many of the journals' pages. For example, in 1986, an editorial in *The Lancet* referred to the meta-analysis presented in the discussion section of the 10-page report of the ISIS-1 trial as a 'lengthy tailpiece'. While acknowledging that 'there is a good case for such analyses', the editorial went on to make clear that 'if anyone suggests that they should become a regular feature of clinical trial reports *The Lancet* will lead the opposition'.[87]

As was pointed out in response at the time, however, these problems are not insuperable in an age of electronic publishing.[88, 89] The expectation that a report of a new randomised trial will begin by reference to the systematic review(s) that prompted the investigators to embark on the study, and end by setting the new results in the context of an up-to-date systematic review of trials relevant at the time of publication, does not imply that the introductory and discussion sections of every report of a randomised trial should contain a full account of the material, methods and findings of the reviews. The technology already exists to link to relevant, up-to-date systematic reviews published elsewhere.[90–93]

As an example of the kind of process and report of research needed, consider recent research on the effects of systemic steroids given to people with acute traumatic brain injury. A systematic review of existing evidence – published and unpublished – was done in the late 1990s as part of a programme of reviews assessing evidence of the effects of interventions in injured patients. As shown in figure 2.5(A), the review revealed uncertainty about whether this treatment did more good than harm,[94] and this uncertainty was reflected in variations in the extent to which systematic steroids were used in clinical practice. Because this uncertainty related to a problem of global signifi-

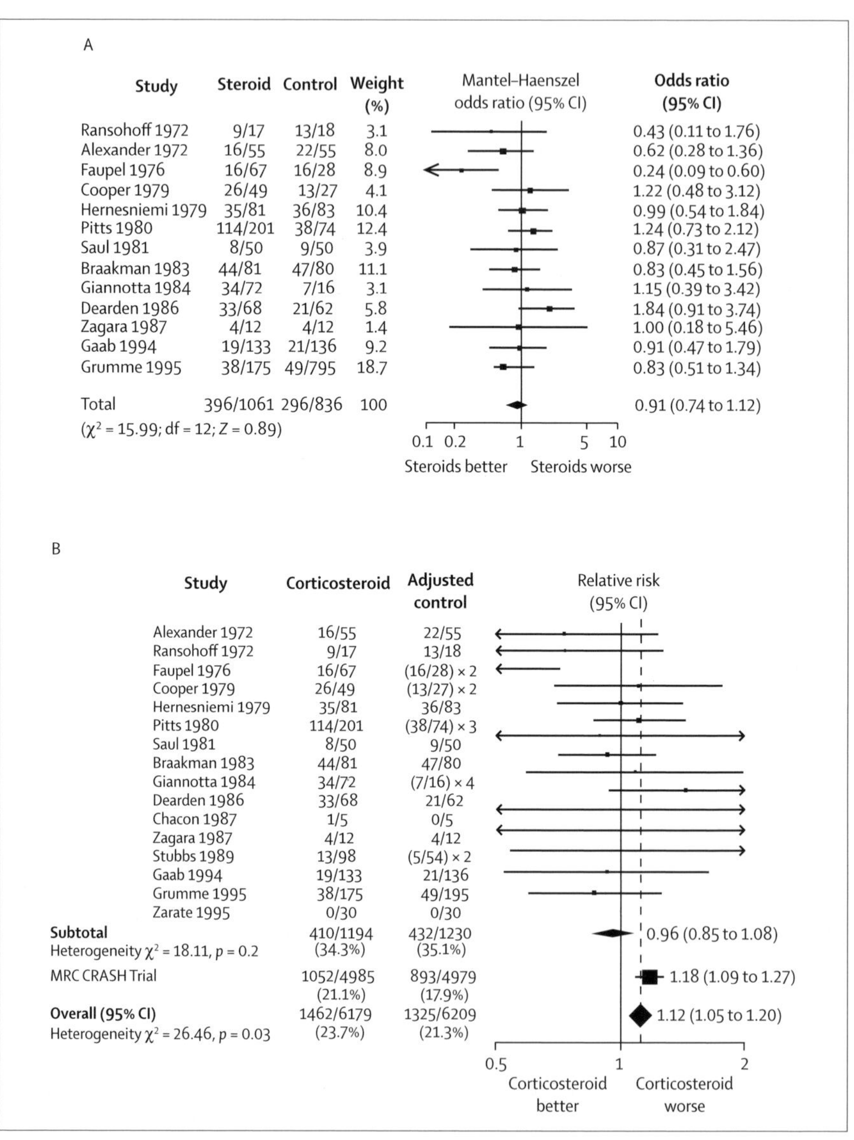

***Figure 2.5*: Systematic reviews and meta-analyses of the effect of systemic corticosteroids in acute traumatic brain injury in 1997, 2004 and 2005. ((A) Reproduced from Alderson and Roberts,[94] with permission of the *British Medical Journal*. (B) Reprinted from CRASH Trial Collaborators,[95] copyright 2001, with permission from Elsevier. (C) Reproduced from Alderson and Roberts,[96] with permission of The Cochrane Collaboration.)**

cance, a proposal for a large, multinational, randomised trial to address the uncertainty was submitted to the British Medical Research Council. The proposal met the Council's

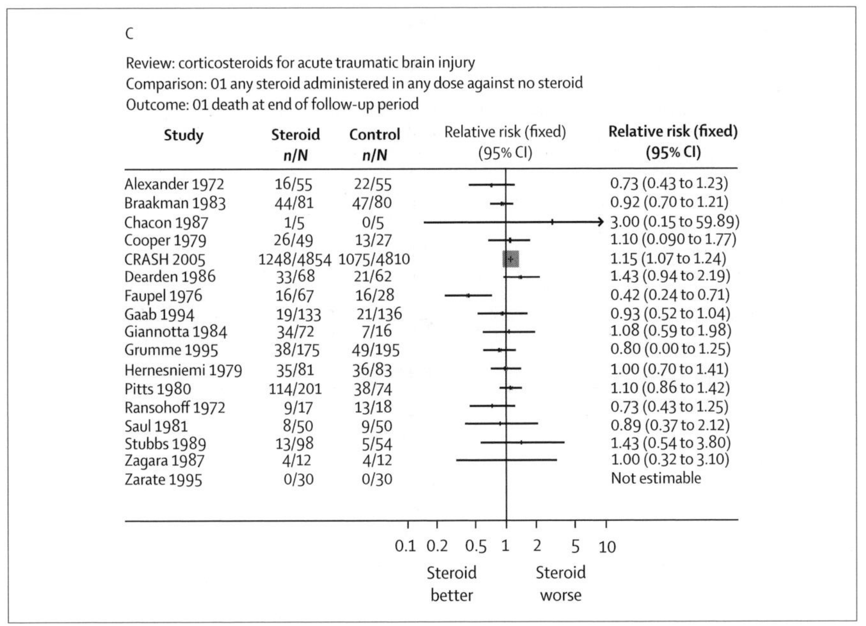

Figure 2.5: Continued.

requirement[32] that the applicants should show, by reference to systematic reviews, why the trial was needed. Funding was agreed, and the results of the trial were subsequently reported in *The Lancet.*[95] This commissioning process and the report of the trial is exemplary because: (i) it refers to current uncertainty about the effects of a treatment, as manifested in the systematic review of all the existing evidence (published and unpublished), and in variations in clinical practice; (ii) the systematic review was a pre-requisite required by the funding agency approached to support further research to address the uncertainty; (iii) the introduction of the trial report provides this background information, and notes that the trial protocol had been published; (iv) the discussion section of the report sets the new evidence in the context of an updated systematic review of all the evidence (figure 2.5(B)), thus providing readers with all the evidence needed for action to prevent thousands of iatrogenic deaths; and (v) the electronically published version of the relevant review in the Cochrane Library was updated promptly to take account of the new evidence[96] (figure 2.5(C)).

After giving examples of the adverse human consequences of the failure of biomedical scientists to cumulate scientifically in this way, editors at *The Lancet* wrote as follows:

> *In recognition that journal editors have a key part to play in ensuring that published research is presented in a way that clearly illustrates why it was necessary and what impact a particular trial has on the existing state of knowledge,* The Lancet *has decided to update its policies in this area. From August, 2005, we will require*

> *authors of clinical trials submitted to* The Lancet *to include a clear summary of previous research findings, and to explain how their trial's findings affect this summary. The relation between existing and new evidence should be illustrated by direct reference to an existing systematic review and meta-analysis. When a systematic review or meta-analysis does not exist, authors are encouraged to do their own. If this is not possible, authors should describe in a structured way the qualitative association between their research and previous findings.*[97]

The Lancet report of the ESPRIT trial is a welcome example of this policy being implemented in practice. The introduction in the report explained that the rationale for the trial had been uncertainty, made clear in systematic reviews of existing data, about the secondary preventive value of combined dipyridamole and aspirin in cerebral ischaemia of arterial origin. The discussion section of the new trial incorporated the new results in an updated systematic review, enabling the authors to conclude with the clinically important statement that: 'The ESPRIT results, combined with the results of previous trials, provide sufficient evidence to prefer the combination regimen of aspirin plus dipyridamole over aspirin alone'.[98]

These are important examples of what is needed, but if the fullest possible use is to be made of research evidence to inform treatment decisions in individual patients, more analyses based on individual patient data are needed, such as those pioneered by the Antiplatelet Trialists' Collaboration,[18] the Early Breast Cancer Trialists' Collaborative Group[99] and the Advanced Ovarian Cancer Trialists' Group.[100] These collaborative re-analyses provide the additional flexibility needed to explore and confirm some of the real modifiers of treatment effects that can help clinicians and patients to individualise treatment decisions.

Glass, who coined the word meta-analysis in 1976,[101] observed 25 years later that 'meta-analysis was created out of the need to extract useful information from the cryptic records of inferential data analyses in the abbreviated reports of research in journals and other printed sources'.[102] He had not imagined that it would still be necessary, a quarter of a century later, to rely on such sources (G. V. Glass, personal communication, 21 November 2001). If understanding how to use the results of randomised trials to inform decisions in personalised medicine really was the priority it should be, research synthesis should, by now, have become based on publicly accessible archives of raw data.[91] Indeed, responding to growing evidence that the current model of publishing clinical trials is hopelessly perverted, Smith and Roberts[103] have suggested it should be abandoned in favour of a radical new approach based on cumulating data in publicly accessible databases. As they and others[104] have made clear, however, these changes will require less selfish and secretive attitudes within the biomedical research community.

Conclusion

As Lord Balfour's remarks in 1884 make clear, the concept of research synthesis is not new. In addition to medicine, there have been systematic reviews in such diverse topics as advertising, agriculture, archaeology, astronomy, biology, chemistry, criminology, ecology, education, entomology, law, manufacturing, parapsychology, psychology, public policy, zoology and even eyewitness accounts of the Indian rope trick.[105] Reports of systematic reviews are cited more frequently than reports of other types of clinical research, including randomised trials, and this trend has been becoming stronger.[106] Furthermore, systematic reviews are likely to be a highly cost-effective form of research;[107] in particular, where there are several underpowered trials a systematic review can provide the needed power at a fraction of the cost of a 'mega-trial'.

Yet recognition that science is cumulative and that scientists need to cumulate scientifically using systematic reviews is still not accepted by many of the influential people who occupy the towering heights of biomedical academia.[108, 109] Some have felt the need to lampoon the very notion of systematic reviews – 'meta-analysis, shmeta-analysis',[110] 'statistical alchemy for the 21st century'.[111] Indeed, one senior academic has written: 'The idea of a systematic review is a nonsense, and the sooner those advocates of it are tried at the International Court of Human Rights at the Hague (or worse still, sent for counselling), the better'.[112]

These dismissive attitudes can have dangerous consequences. A systematic review and meta-analysis which had found no support for the widely promoted claim that post-menopausal hormone therapy prevents cardiovascular events[113] prompted the dean of a medical school to comment in a *BMJ* editorial: 'The correspondence columns this week will also reinforce readers' wariness of meta-analysis ... For one I shall continue to tell my patients that hormone replacement therapy is likely to help prevent coronary disease'.[114] Attitudes such as this can have important adverse consequences for patients, as illustrated with the evidence presented in this chapter, and because they can lead to such outcomes, those who wield power within the biomedical research community should either publicly defend their failure to take effective action, or act more forcefully to change the unacceptable state of affairs described in this chapter and elsewhere.[109, 115]

Editors at *The Lancet* commented on the situation as follows:

> *Unnecessary and badly presented clinical research injures volunteers and patients as surely as any other form of bad medicine, as well as wasting resources and abusing the trust placed in investigators by their trial participants. Those who say that systematic reviews and meta-analyses are not 'proper research' are wrong; it is clinical trials done in the absence of such reviews and meta-analyses that are improper, scientifically and ethically. Investigators and organisations who undertake and coordinate reviews and meta-analyses now need the funding and recognition they deserve if public trust in biomedical research is to be maintained and resources used in an effective way.*[97]

The changes needed undoubtedly pose a challenge to researchers who are successful under the existing system. It requires them to undertake systematic reviews before applying for funds to do additional primary research, and to update those reviews when they come to publish the results of new studies, and to collaborate with others doing related studies. This will be a new discipline for many of them, so it is easy to understand why they would oppose the changes needed.[116] It seems probable, however, that those who tacitly defend the status quo will increasingly have to defend their positions to the public. Articles in the lay press[117, 118] and popular books written for a lay readership[119] are beginning to draw attention to the issues discussed in this chapter. If research funders, academia, researchers, research ethics committees and scientific journals do not start to deal with the problems outlined in this chapter, the public seems likely to ask increasingly why they are acquiescing in what is clearly an indefensible state of affairs.

Systematic reviews are not a panacea: their results are a necessary but insufficient basis for informing policies in healthcare and treatment decisions in individual patients.[120] Furthermore, an increasing body of empirical research is beginning to explore the reasons why separate systematic reviews purportedly addressing the same question come to differing conclusions. Sometimes, for example, this may because the questions addressed are different; sometimes because the searches for potentially eligible studies differ in thoroughness; sometimes because of variations in inclusion criteria, or access to unpublished information; and sometimes because of differing spins put on essentially the same body of empirical evidence. The science of research synthesis is still young, and that is one of the reasons why current methodological discussions and research, and the insights that are emerging, make it a fulfilling field to work in and to develop.

That said, clinicians and patients need to be able to draw on syntheses of research evidence conducted to the highest standards possible, and the analyses in these systematic reviews should be able to draw on *all* the relevant research evidence. To increase the likelihood of making progress towards individualising treatment decisions, research syntheses must increasingly be based on collaborative analyses using individual patient data, as illustrated nicely in a recent reanalysis of controlled trials of treatment for otitis media,[121] improving on an influential earlier systematic review.

The scientific and ethical consequences of failure to take sufficiently seriously research synthesis, biased underreporting of clinical research, and access to the most useful data are that patients (and the public more generally) suffer directly and indirectly; policymakers, practitioners and patients have inadequate information to guide their choices among alternatives for individual patients; and limited resources for healthcare and new research are used inefficiently.

Acknowledgments

I am grateful to Doug Altman, Amanda Burls, Luis-Gabriel Cuervo, Frank Davidoff, Matthias Egger, Paul Glasziou, Andrew Herxheimer, Chris Hyde, Tom Jefferson, David Mant, Tom Marshall, Drummond Rennie, Peter Rothwell, David Sackett, Josie Sandercock, David Schriger, Loes van Bokhoven, Floris van de Laar and Simon Wessely for helpful discussion of the ideas and material presented in this chapter.

References

1 Poisson, Dulong, Larrey et Double. Recherches de statistique sur l'affection calculeuse, par M. le docteur Civiale. *Comptes rendus hebdomadaires des séances de l'Académie de Sciences.* Paris: Bachelier, 1835, 167–177. [Statistical research on conditions caused by calculi by Doctor Civiale. Translated and reprinted in *Int J Epidemiol* 2001; **30:** 1246–49.]

2 Mant D. Can randomised trials inform clinical decisions about individual patients? *Lancet* 1999; **353:** 743–46.

3 Bradford Hill A. The clinical trial. *N Engl J Med* 1952; **247:** 113–19.
4 Chalmers I. What do I want from health research and researchers when I am a patient? *BMJ* 1995; **310:** 1315–1318.
5 Baker SG, Kaprio J. Common susceptibility genes for cancer: search for the end of the rainbow. *BMJ* 2006; **332:** 1150–52.
6 New B. Defining a package of healthcare services the NHS is responsible for. The case for. *BMJ* 1997; **314:** 503–05.
7 Klein R. Defining a package of healthcare services the NHS is responsible for. The case against. *BMJ* 1997; **314:** 505–09.
8 Oxman AD, Guyatt GF. A consumer's guide to subgroup analyses. *Ann Intern Med* 1992; **116:** 78–84.
9 Glasziou P, Irwig L. An evidence-based approach to individualising patient treatment. *BMJ* 1995; **311:** 1356–59.
10 Bracken M. Genomic epidemiology of complex disease: the need for an evidence-based electronic approach to research synthesis. *Am J Epidemiol* 2005; **162:** 1–5.
11 Chalmers I. A patient's attitude to the use of research evidence to guide individual choices and decisions in health care. *Clin Risk* 2000; **6:** 227–30.
12 Schulz KF, Grimes DA. Sample size calculations in randomised trials: mandatory and mystical. *Lancet* 2005; **365:** 1348–53.
13 Cowley AJ, Skene A, Stainer K, Hampton JR. The effect of lorcainide on arrhythmias and survival in patients with acute myocardial infarction: an example of publication bias. *Int J Cardiol* 1993; **40:** 161–66.
14 Moore T. *Deadly Medicine*. New York: Simon and Schuster, 1995.
15 Chalmers I. From optimism to disillusion about commitment to transparency in the medico-industrial complex. *J R Soc Med* 2006; **99:** 337–41.
16 Jack A. Call to release human drug trial. *Financial Times,* 8 August 2006.
17 Global R&D performance metrics programme: industry success rates report. *CMR International,* May 2005, p 7.
18 Antiplatelet Trialists' Collaboration. Secondary prevention of vascular disease by prolonged anti-platelet treatment. *BMJ* 1988; **296:** 320–31.
19 Sacks FM, Pfeffer MA, Moye LA, et al. The effect of pravastatin on coronary events after myocardial infarction in patients with average cholesterol levels. Cholesterol and Recurrent Events Trial investigators. *N Engl J Med* 1996; **335:** 1001–09.
20 Bonovas S, Filioussi K, Tsavaris N, Sitaras NM. Use of statins and breast cancer: a meta-analysis of seven randomized clinical trials and nine observational studies. *J Clin Oncol* 2005; **23:** 8606–12.
21 Last JM. *A Dictionary of Epidemiology*. Oxford: Oxford University Press, 2001.
22 Pearson K. Report of certain enteric fever inoculation statistics. *BMJ* 1904; **3:** 1245–46.
23 Glasziou P, Chalmers I, Rawlins M, McCulloch P. When are randomized trials unnecessary? *BMJ* 2007; **334:** 349–51.
24 Horwitz RI, Feinstein AR. Improved observational method for study therapeutic efficacy: suggestive evidence that lidocaine prophylaxis prevents death in myocardial infarction. *JAMA* 1981; **246:** 2455–59.
25 Hill AB. Cited in: The reasons for writing. *BMJ* 1965; **2:** 870–72.
26 Begg C, Cho M, Eastwood S, et al. Improving the quality of reporting of randomized controlled trials. The CONSORT statement. *JAMA* 1996; **276:** 637–39.
27 Baum ML, Anish DS, Chalmers TC, et al. A survey of clinical trials of antibiotic prophylaxis in colon surgery: evidence against further use of no-treatment controls. *N Engl J Med* 1981; **305:** 795–99.
28 Antman EM, Lau J, Kupelnick B, et al. A comparison of results of meta-analyses of randomized control trials and recommendations of clinical experts. *JAMA* 1992; **268:** 240–48.
29 Aspinall RL, Goodman NW. Denial of effective treatment and poor quality of clinical information in placebo controlled trials of ondansetron for postoperative nausea and vomiting: a review of published trials. *BMJ* 1995; **311:** 844–46.
30 Cooper NJ, Jones DR, Sutton AJ. The use of systematic reviews when designing studies. Clin Trials 2005; **2:** 260–64.
31 Chalmers I, Matthews R. What are the implications of optimism bias in clinical research? *Lancet* 2006; **367:** 449–50.
32 O'Toole L. Using systematically synthesized evidence to inform the funding of new clinical trials – the UK Medical Research Council approach. Paper presented at the 6th International Cochrane Colloquium, Baltimore, MD, 22–26 October 1998.
33 Kramer BS, Wilentz J, Alexander D, et al. Getting it right: being smarter about clinical trials. *PLoS Med* 2006; **3:** e144.

34 Savulescu J, Chalmers I, Blunt J. Are research ethics committees behaving unethically? Some suggestions for improving performance and accountability. *BMJ* 1996; **313:** 1390–93.
35 Rothman KJ, Michels KB. The continuing unethical use of placebo controls. *N Engl J Med* 1994; **331:** 384–89.
36 Smith AJ, Goodman NW. The hypertensive response to intubation. Do researchers acknowledge previous work? *Can J Anaesth* 1997; **44:** 9–13.
37 Chalmers TC, Frank CS, Reitman D. Minimizing the three stages of publication bias. *JAMA* 1990; **263:** 1392–95.
38 Chalmers I. Role of systematic reviews in detecting plagiarism: case of Asim Kurjak. *BMJ* 2006; **333:** 594–96.
39 Jefferson T, Deeks J. The use of systematic reviews for editorial peer reviewing: a population approach. In: Godlee F, Jefferson T, eds. *Peer Review in Health Sciences.* London: BMJ Books, 1999: 224–34.
40 Jefferson T, Shashok K. Journals: how to decide what's worth publishing. Nature 2003; **421:** 209–10.
41 Chalmers I. Lessons for research ethics committees. *Lancet* 2002; **359:** 174.
42 Mann H, Djulbegovic B. Why comparisons must address genuine uncertainties. James Lind Library, 2005. Available at: http://www.jameslindlibrary.org/trial_records/21st_Century/djulbegovic/djulbegovic_commentary.html (accessed February 2007).
43 Savulescu J, Spriggs M. The hexamethonium asthma study and the death of a normal volunteer in research. *J Med Ethics* 2002; **28:** 3–4.
44 McLellan F. 1966 and all that – when is a literature search done? *Lancet* 2001; **358:** 646.
45 Clark O, Clark L, Djulbegovic B. Is clinical research still too haphazard? *Lancet* 2001; **358:** 1648.
46 Florance V, Davidoff F. The informationist: a new health profession? *Ann Intern Med* 2000; **132:** 996–98.
47 Rayleigh, The Right Hon Lord. Presidential address at the 54th Meeting of the British Association for the Advancement of Science, Montreal, August/September 1884. London: John Murray, 1885: 3–23.
48 Chalmers I, Hedges LV, Cooper H. A brief history of research synthesis. *Evaluation Health Professions* 2002; **25:** 12–37.
49 Clarke M, Chalmers I. Discussion sections in reports of controlled trials published in general medical journals: islands in search of continents? *JAMA* 1998; **280:** 280–82.
50 Clarke M, Alderson P, Chalmers I. Discussion sections in reports of controlled trials published in general medical journals. *JAMA* 2002; **287:** 2799–801.
51 Clarke M, Hopewell S, Chalmers I. Reports of clinical trials should begin and end with up-to-date systematic reviews of other relevant evidence: a status report. *J R Soc Med* 2007; **100:** 187–90.
52 Fergusson D, Glass KC, Hutton B, Shapiro S. Randomized controlled trials of aprotinin in cardiac surgery: using clinical equipoise to stop the bleeding. *Clin Trials* 2005; **2:** 218–32.
53 Royston D, Bidstrup BP, Taylor KM, Sapsford RN. Effect of aprotinin on the need for blood transfusion after repeat open-heart surgery. *Lancet* 1987; **2:** 1289–91.
54 Stampfer MJ, Goldhaber SZ, Yusuf S, et al. Effect of intravenous streptokinase on acute myocardial infarction: pooled results from randomized trials. *N Engl J Med* 1982; **307:** 1180–82.
55 Pentecost A. Myocardial infarction. In: Weatherall DJ, Ledingham JGG, Warrell DA, eds. *Oxford Textbook of Medicine,* 2nd edn. Oxford: Oxford University Press, 1987: 13.173.
56 Sheridan DJ, Crawford L, Rawlins MD, Julian DG. Antiarrhythmic action of lignocaine in early myocardial infarction. Plasma levels after combined intramuscular and intravenous administration. *Lancet* 1977; **1:** 824–25.
57 Furberg CD. Effect of anti-arrhythmic drugs on mortality after myocardial infarction. *Am J Cardiol* 1983; **52:** 32C–36C.
58 Hine LK, Laird N, Hewitt P, Chalmers TC. Meta-analytic evidence against prophylactic use of lidocaine in acute myocardial infarction. *Arch Intern Med* 1989; **149:** 2694–98.
59 MacMahon S, Collins R, Peto R, et al. Effects of prophylactic lidocaine in suspected acute myocardial infarction. An overview of results from the randomized, controlled trials. *JAMA* 1988; **260:** 1910–16.
60 Teo KK, Yusuf S, Furberg CD. Effects of prophylactic anti-arrhythmic drug therapy in acute myocardial infarction. *JAMA* 1993; **270:** 1589–95.
61 PORT Meta-analysis Trialists Group. Post-operative radiotherapy in non-small cell lung cancer: systematic review and meta-analysis of individual patient data from nine-randomised controlled trials. *Lancet* 1998; **352:** 257–63.
62 Sandercock J, Parmar MKB, Torri V, Qian W. Chemotherapy for advanced ovarian cancer: paclitaxel, cisplatin and the evidence. *Br J Cancer* 2002; **87:** 815–24.
63 Crowley PA. Corticosteroids in pregnancy: the benefits outweigh the costs. *J Obstet Gynaecol* 1981; **1:** 147–50.
64 Crowley PA. Promoting pulmonary maturity. In: Chalmers I, Enkin M, Keirse MJNC, eds. *Effective Care in Pregnancy and Childbirth.* Oxford: Oxford University Press, 1989: 746–64.

65 Crowley P, Chalmers I, Keirse MJNC. The effects of corticosteroid administration before preterm delivery: an overview of the evidence from controlled trials. *Br J Obstet Gynaecol* 1990; **97:** 11–25.

66 Mugford M, Piercy J, Chalmers I. Cost implications of different approaches to the prevention of respiratory distress syndrome. *Arch Dis Child* 1991; **66:** 757–64.

67 Crowley PA. Antenatal corticosteroid therapy: a meta-analysis of the randomized trials, 1972–1994. *Am J Obstet Gynaecol* 1995; **173:** 322–35.

68 Hanney S, Mugford M, Grant J, Buxton M. Assessing the benefits of health research: lessons from research into the use of antenatal corticosteroids for the prevention of neonatal respiratory distress syndrome. *Soc Sci Med* 2005; **60:** 937–47.

69 Liggins GC. Premature delivery of lambs infused with glucocorticoids. *J Endocrinol* 1969; **45:** 515–23.

70 Liggins GC, Howie RN. A controlled trial of antepartum glucorticoid treatment for the prevention of the respiratory distress syndrome in premature infants. *Pediatrics* 1972; **50:** 515–25.

71 Sinclair JC. Meta-analysis of randomized trials antenatal corticosteroid therapy for the prevention of respiratory distress syndrome: discussion. *Am J Obstet Gynaecol* 1995; **173:** 335–44.

72 Reynolds L, Tansey EM. *Prenatal Corticosteroids for Reducing Morbidity and Mortality after Preterm Birth.* London: Wellcome Trust, 2005.

73 Gilbert R, Salanti G, Harden M, See S. Infant sleeping position and the sudden infant death syndrome: systematic review of observational studies and historical review of clinicians' recommendations from 1940–2000. *Int J Epidemiol* 2005; **34:** 74–87.

74 Horn J, Limburg M. Calcium antagonists for acute ischemic stroke (Cochrane Review). In: *The Cochrane Library*, Issue 3. Oxford: Update Software, 2001.

75 Horn J, de Haan RJ, Vermeulen M, et al. Nimodipine in animal model experiments of focal cerebral ischaemia: a systematic review. *Stroke* 2001; **32:** 2433–38.

76 Sandercock P, Roberts I. Systematic reviews of animal experiments. *Lancet* 2002; **2:** 586.

77 Pound P, Ebrahim S, Sandercock P, et al. Where is the evidence that animal research benefits humans? *BMJ* 2004; **328:** 514–17.

78 Perel P, Roberts I, Sena E, et al. Comparison of treatment effects between animal experiments and clinical trials: systematic review. *BMJ* 2007; **334:** 197–200.

79 Khan KS, Mignini L. Surveying the literature from animal experiments: avoidance of bias is objective of systematic review, not meta-analysis. *BMJ* 2005; **331:** 110–11.

80 Macleod MR, Ebrahim S, Roberts I. Surveying the literature from animal experiments: systematic reviews and meta-analysis are important contributions. *BMJ* 2005; **331:** 110.

81 Bebarta V, Luyten D, Heard K. Emergency medicine animal research: does use of randomization and blinding affect the results? *Academic Emerg Med* 2003; **10:** 684–87.

82 Schulz KF, Chalmers I, Hayes RJ, Altman DG. Empirical evidence of bias: dimensions of methodological quality associated with estimates of treatment effects in controlled trials. *JAMA* 1995; **273:** 408–12.

83 Mignini LE, Khan KS. Methodological quality of systematic reviews of animal studies: a survey of reviews of basic research. *BMC Med Res Methodol* 2006; **6:** 10 [DOI: 10.11186/1471–2288/6/10].

84 Nuffield Council on Bioethics. *The Ethics of Research Involving Animals.* London: Nuffield Foundation, 2005.

85 Milne I, Chalmers I. Documenting the evidence: the case of scurvy. Bull WHO 2004; **82:** 791–92.

86 Saunders MC, Dick JS, Brown IMcL, et al. The effects of hospital admission for bed rest on the duration of twin pregnancy: a randomised trial. *Lancet* 1985; **2:** 793–95.

87 Editorial. Intravenous beta-blockade during acute myocardial infarction. *Lancet* 1986; **2:** 79–80.

88 Chalmers I. Electronic publications for updating controlled trial reviews. *Lancet* 1986; **2:** 287.

89 Chalmers I. Improving the quality and dissemination of reviews of clinical research. In: Lock S, ed. The Future of Medical Journals: In *Commemoration of 150 Years of the British Medical Journal.* London: BMJ Books, 1991: 127–46.

90 Huth EJ. Quality in the electronic age. *Eur Sci Editing* 1997; **23:** 41–42.

91 Chalmers I, Altman DG. How can medical journals help prevent poor medical research? Some opportunities presented by electronic publishing. *Lancet* 1999; **353:** 490–93.

92 Chalmers I. Using systematic reviews and registers of ongoing trials for scientific and ethical trial design, monitoring, and reporting. In: Egger M, Davey Smith G, Altman D, eds. *Systematic Reviews in Health Care: Meta-Analysis in Context*, 2nd edn of Systematic Reviews. London: BMJ Books, 2001: 429–43.

93 Clarke M. Doing new research? Don't forget the old. Nobody should do a trial without reviewing what is known. *PLoS Med* 2004; **1:** 100–02.

94 Alderson P, Roberts I. Corticosteroids in acute traumatic brain injury: systematic review of randomised controlled trials. *BMJ* 1997; **314:** 1855–59.

95 CRASH Trial Collaborators. Effect of intravenous corticosteroids on death within 14 days in 10 008 adults with clinically significant head injury (MRC CRASH Trial): a randomised placebo-controlled trial. *Lancet* 2004; **364:** 1321–28.

96 Alderson P, Roberts I. Corticosteroids in acute traumatic brain injury. *Cochrane Database of Systematic Reviews*, 2005, Issue 1. Art. No.: CD000196 [DOI: 10.1002/14651858.CD000196.pub2].

97 Young C, Horton R. Putting clinical trials into context. *Lancet* 2005; **366:** 107–08.

98 ESPRIT Study Group. Aspirin plus dipyridamole versus aspirin alone after cerebral ischaemia of arterial origin (ESPRIT): randomised controlled trial. *Lancet* 2006; **367:** 1665–73.

99 Early Breast Cancer Trialists' Collaborative Group. Effects of adjuvant tamoxifen and of cytotoxic therapy on mortality in early breast cancer: and overview of 62 randomized trials among 28,896 women. *N Engl J Med* 1988; **319:** 1681–92.

100 Advanced Ovarian Cancer Trialists' Group. Chemotherapy in advanced ovarian cancer: an overview of randomised clinical trials. *BMJ* 1991; **303:** 884–93.

101 Glass GV. Primary, secondary and meta-analysis of research. *Educational Researcher* 1976; **10:** 3–8.

102 Glass GV. Meta-analysis at 25 January 2000. Available at: http://glass.ed.asu.edu/gene/papers/meta25.html (accessed February 2007).

103 Smith R, Roberts I. Patient safety requires a new way to publish clinical trials. *PLoS Clin Trials* 2006, May, e6.

104 Vickers AJ. Whose data set is it anyway? Sharing raw data from randomized trials. *Trials* 2006; **7:** 15 [DOI: 10.1186/1745-6215-7-15].

105 Petticrew M. Systematic reviews from astronomy to zoology: myths and misconceptions. *BMJ* 2001; **322:** 98–101.

106 Patsopoulos NA, Analatos AA, Ioannidis JP. Relative citation impact of various study designs in the health sciences. *JAMA* 2005; **293:** 2362–66.

107 Glasziou P, Djulbegovic B, Burls A. Are systematic reviews more cost-effective than randomized trials? *Lancet* 2006; **367:** 2057–58.

108 Alderson P, Gliddon L, Chalmers I. Academic recognition of critical appraisal and systematic reviews in British postgraduate medical education. *Med Educ* 2003; **37:** 386–87.

109 Chalmers I. Academia's failure to support systematic reviews. *Lancet* 2005; **365:** 469.

110 Shapiro S. Meta-analysis/shmeta-analysis. *Am J Epidemiol* 1994; **140:** 771–78.

111 Feinstein AR. Meta-analysis: statistical alchemy for the 21st century. *J Clin Epidemiol* 1995; **48:** 71–79.

112 Rees J. Two cultures? *J Am Acad Dermatol* 2002; **46:** 313–14.

113 Hemminki E, McPherson K. Impact of postmenopausal hormone therapy on cardiovascular events and cancer: pooled data from clinical trials. *BMJ* 1997; **315:** 149–53.

114 Naylor CD. Meta-analysis and the meta-epidemiology of clinical research. *BMJ* 1997; **315:** 617–19.

115 Chalmers I. The scandalous failure of science to cumulate evidence scientifically. *Clin Trials* 2005; **2:** 229–31.

116 Marshall T. Scientific knowledge in medicine: a new clinical epistemology? *J Evaluation Clin Pract* 1997; **3:** 133–38.

117 Brown D. Superfluous medical studies called into question. *The Washington Post*, 2 January 2006: A06.

118 Matthews R. No way to treat a patient: tens of thousands of people have been subjected to unnecessary drug trials. *New Scientist*, 9 July 2006: 19.

119 Evans I, Thornton H, Chalmers I. *Testing Treatments: Better Research for Better Healthcare.* London: British Library, 2006.

120 Chalmers I. The Cochrane Collaboration: preparing, maintaining and disseminating systematic reviews of the effects of health care. In: Warren KS, Mosteller F, eds. Doing more good than harm: the evaluation of health care interventions. *Ann NY Acad Sci* 1993; **703:** 156–63.

121 Rovers M, Glasziou P, Appelman C, et al. Antibiotics for acute otitis media: a meta-analysis with individual patient data. *Lancet* 2006; **368:** 1429–35.

Section 2

Is the trial relevant to this patient?

3

Assessment of the external validity of randomised controlled trials

Peter M. Rothwell

Introduction

> *Between measurements based on RCTs and benefit ... in the community there is a gulf which has been much under-estimated.* (A. L. Cochrane, 1971[1])
>
> *At its best a trial shows what can be accomplished with a medicine under careful observation and certain restricted conditions. The same results will not invariably or necessarily be observed when the medicine passes into general use.* (A. Bradford Hill, 1984[2])

As discussed in Chapters 1 and 2, randomised controlled trials (RCTs) and systematic reviews are the most reliable methods of determining the effects of treatment and many serious errors have resulted from relying on other types of evidence. They must be internally valid (i.e. design and conduct must eliminate the possibility of bias),[3,4] but to be clinically useful the result must also be relevant to a definable group of patients in a particular clinical setting; this is generally termed *external validity*, *applicability* or *generalisability*. The beneficial effects of some interventions, such as blood pressure lowering in chronic uncontrolled hypertension, have been shown to be generalisable to the vast majority of patients and settings, but the effects of other interventions can be very dependent on factors such as the characteristics of the patient, the method of application of the intervention and the setting of treatment. How these factors are taken into account in the design and performance of an RCT and in the reporting of the results can have a major impact on external validity.

Lack of consideration of external validity is the most frequent criticism by clinicians of RCTs, systematic reviews and guidelines,[5–13] and is one explanation for the widespread underuse in routine practice of treatments that have been shown to be beneficial in trials and are recommended in guidelines.[14–26] Neither Cochrane nor Bradford Hill were practising clinicians, but they understood the limitations of the methodology that they had pioneered. Yet, although what little systematic evidence we now have confirms that RCTs do often lack external validity,[27–41] the issue is neglected by current researchers, medical journals, funding agencies, ethics committees, the pharmaceutical industry and governmental regulators alike (panel 3.1).[42–50] Admittedly, assessment of external validity is complex and requires clinical rather than statistical expertise, but it is vital if treatments are to be used correctly in as many patients as possible in routine clinical practice. We cannot expect the results of RCTs and systematic reviews to be relevant to all patients and all settings (that is not what is meant by external validity), but they

Panel 3.1: Evidence of the neglect of consideration of external validity of RCTs and systematic reviews

- Research into internal validity of RCTs and systematic reviews far outweighs research into how results should best be used in practice[42, 43]
- Rules governing the performance of trials, such as good clinical practice,[44] do not cover issues of external validity
- Drug licensing bodies, such as the US Food and Drug Administration, do not require evidence that a drug has a *clinically useful* treatment effect, or a trial population that is representative of routine clinical practice[45]
- Guidance on the design and performance of RCTs from funding agencies, such as that from the UK Medical Research Council,[46, 47] makes virtually no mention of issues related to external validity
- Guidance from ethics committees, such as that from the UK Department of Health,[48] indicates that clinical research should be internally valid, and raises some issues that relate to external validity, but makes no explicit recommendations about the need for results to be generalisable to future patients
- Guidelines on the reporting of RCTs and systematic reviews focus mainly on internal validity and give very little space to external validity[49, 50]
- None of the many scores for judging the 'quality' of RCTs addresses external validity adequately[31]
- There are no accepted guidelines on how external validity of RCTs should be assessed

should at least be designed and reported in a way that allows clinicians to judge to whom they can reasonably be applied.

This chapter considers how external validity should be assessed. Panel 3.2 lists some of the important potential determinants of external validity, each of which is reviewed briefly below. Many of the considerations will only be relevant in certain types of trial, for certain interventions or in certain clinical settings, but they can each sometimes undermine external validity. Moreover, the list is not exhaustive and requires more detailed annotation and explanation than is possible in a single chapter. Illustrative examples are drawn mainly from treatments for cerebrovascular or cardiovascular disease but the general principles are relevant to all areas of medicine and surgery.

Inevitable limits on external validity

RCTs and systematic reviews are the most reliable methods of determining moderate treatment effects, but external validity is inevitably less than perfect, at least in theory, because these studies do not actually aim to measure the benefit that will be derived from treatment in clinical practice. The response to and/or compliance with a treatment can be influenced strongly by the doctor–patient relationship,[51–53] placebo effects[54, 55] and patient preference.[56–58] Yet, trialists rightly try where possible to exclude any influence of these factors by blinded treatment allocation, placebo control, and exclusion of patients or clinicians who have strong treatment preferences. These procedures increase

Panel 3.2: **Some of the main issues that potentially affect external validity and which should be addressed in reports of the results of RCTs or systematic reviews and be considered by clinicians**

Setting of the trial
- Healthcare system
- Country
- Recruitment from primary, secondary or tertiary care
- Selection of participating centres
- Selection of participating clinicians

Selection of patients
- Methods of pre-randomisation diagnosis and investigation
- Eligibility criteria
- Exclusion criteria
- Placebo run-in period
- Treatment run-in period
- 'Enrichment' strategies
- Ratio of randomised patients to eligible non-randomised patients in participating centres
- Proportion of patients who declined randomisation

Characteristics of randomised patients
- Baseline clinical characteristics
- Racial group
- Uniformity of underlying pathology
- Stage in the natural history of their disease
- Severity of disease
- Comorbidity
- Absolute risks of a poor outcome in the control group

Differences between the trial protocol and routine practice
- Trial intervention
- Timing of treatment
- Appropriateness/relevance of control intervention
- Adequacy of non-trial treatment – both intended and actual
- Prohibition of certain non-trial treatments
- Therapeutic or diagnostic advances since trial was performed

Outcome measures and follow-up
- Clinical relevance of surrogate outcomes
- Clinical relevance, validity and reproducibility of complex scales
- Effect of intervention on most relevant components of composite outcomes
- Who measured outcome
- Use of patient-centred outcomes
- Frequency of follow-up
- Adequacy of the length of follow-up

Adverse effects of treatment
- Completeness of reporting of relevant adverse effects
- Rates of discontinuation of treatment
- Selection of trial centres and/or clinicians on the basis of skill or experience
- Exclusion of patients at risk of complications
- Exclusion of patients who experienced adverse effects during a run-in period
- Intensity of trial safety procedures

the internal validity of an RCT, but will often lead to underestimation of the benefits of treatment in clinical practice, particularly for patient-centred outcomes.

Patient preference can cause particular problems for external validity. For example, some women with early breast cancer have a strong preference for lumpectomy, whereas others are far happier that perhaps 'all the cancer has been removed' by a mastectomy. However, only women who did not have a strong preference for one treatment or the other could be recruited into the relevant RCTs, and as few as 10% agreed to have their treatment chosen at random.[59] If RCTs show a major advantage for one treatment, then external validity is not a problem. Difficulties arise when one treatment is only moderately more effective but the patient has a strong 'gut' preference for the less effective option. Would the results of the breast surgery RCTs, particularly in relation to psychological well-being, have been the same if such patients had been randomised?

These inevitable limitations by no means invalidate the results of RCTs and systematic reviews, and they are mentioned here partly for the sake of completeness, but the importance of patient preference, placebo effects and the doctor–patient relationship outside trials should not be underestimated – a fact that is perhaps best illustrated by the popularity of 'alternative' therapies, such as homeopathy, in which such factors are the only active ingredients. The remainder of this chapter will concentrate on those factors in the design and reporting of RCTs and systematic reviews that limit external validity but which are not unavoidable.

The setting of the trial

There is often concern about the generalisability of trials performed in secondary or tertiary care to practice in primary care,[26–29] but there are several other ways in which the setting of an RCT can affect external validity.

The healthcare system

Differences between healthcare systems can affect external validity. For example, in the European Carotid Surgery Trial (ECST),[60] an RCT of endarterectomy for recently symptomatic carotid stenosis, there were national differences in the time before which patients were investigated, with a median delay from last symptoms to randomisation of more than 2 months in the UK, for example, compared with 3 weeks in Belgium and Holland. Figure 3.1 shows that separate trials in these different healthcare systems would have produced very different results – due to the shortness of the time window for prevention of stroke.[61] These differences were not mentioned in any of the ECST publications or in any subsequent guidelines. Similar differences in performance between healthcare systems will exist for other conditions, and there is, of course, the broader issue of how the findings of trials done in the developed world apply in the developing world.

The country

Even if the healthcare systems are similar, other national differences can still affect generalisability. Continuing with the example of cerebrovascular disease, there are many differences between countries in methods of diagnosis and management,[62] as

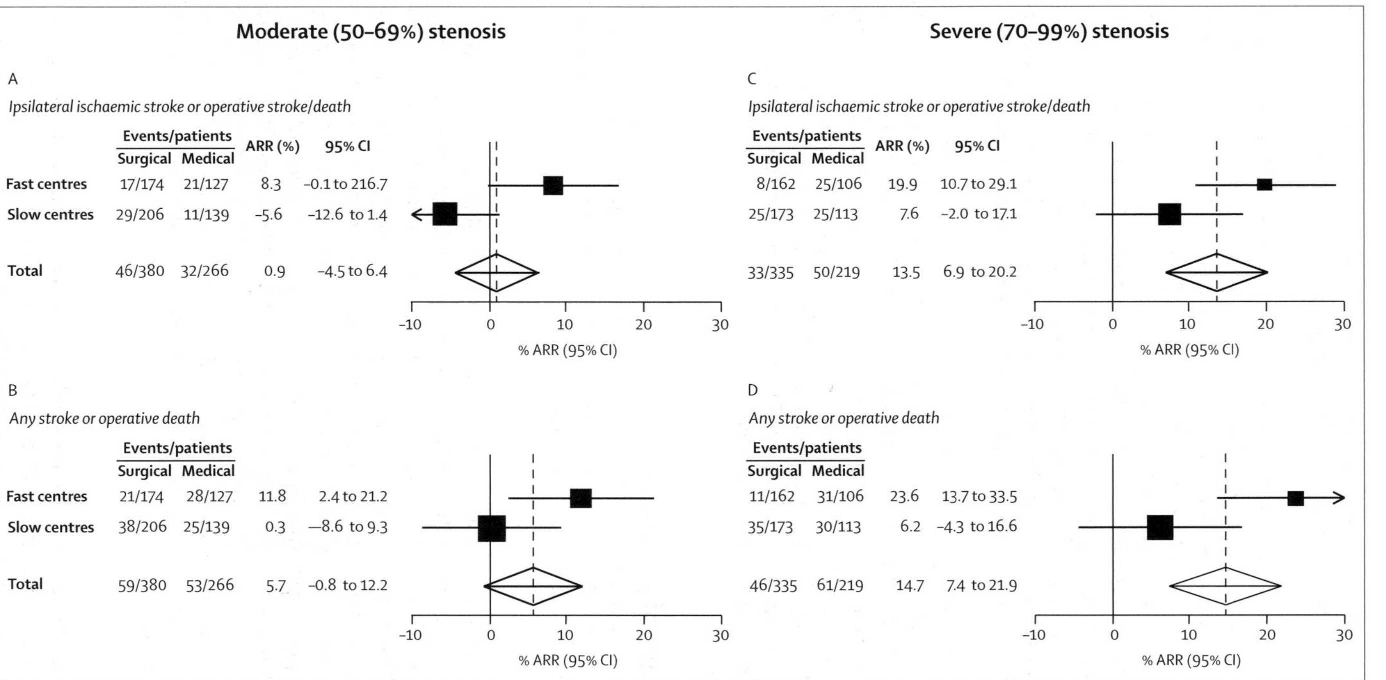

Figure 3.1: **The absolute risk reductions (ARR) in the 5-year risks of ipsilateral ischaemic stroke (A, C) and any stroke or death (B, D) with surgery in European Carotid Surgery Trial[60] centres in which the median delay from last symptomatic event to randomisation was ≤ 50 days (fast centres) compared with centres with a longer delay (slow centres). Data are shown separately for patients with moderate (50–69%) and severe (70–99%) carotid stenosis. (Reprinted from Rothwell,[146] copyright 2005, with permission from Elsevier.)**

well as important racial differences in pathology and natural history,[63] all of which could affect the external validity of trial results. In particular, there are often striking national differences in the use of ancillary 'non-trial' treatments. In one international RCT of aspirin and heparin in nearly 20 000 patients with acute ischaemic stroke, it was noted that glycerol was used in 50% of the 1473 patients in Italy versus 3% elsewhere, steroids in 32% of the 225 patients in Turkey versus 4% elsewhere, and haemodilution in 44% of the 597 patients in Austria and the Czech Republic versus 3% elsewhere.[64] Even more extreme differences between countries were recorded in the use of two important non-trial surgical techniques in the ECST (figure 3.2).[65] For both techniques there is independent evidence that their use does affect operative risk. Other differences between countries in the methods of diagnosis and management of disease, which can be substantial, or important racial differences in pathology and natural history of disease, also affect the external validity of RCTs. A good example is the heterogeneity of results of trials of BCG in the prevention of tuberculosis, with a progressive loss of

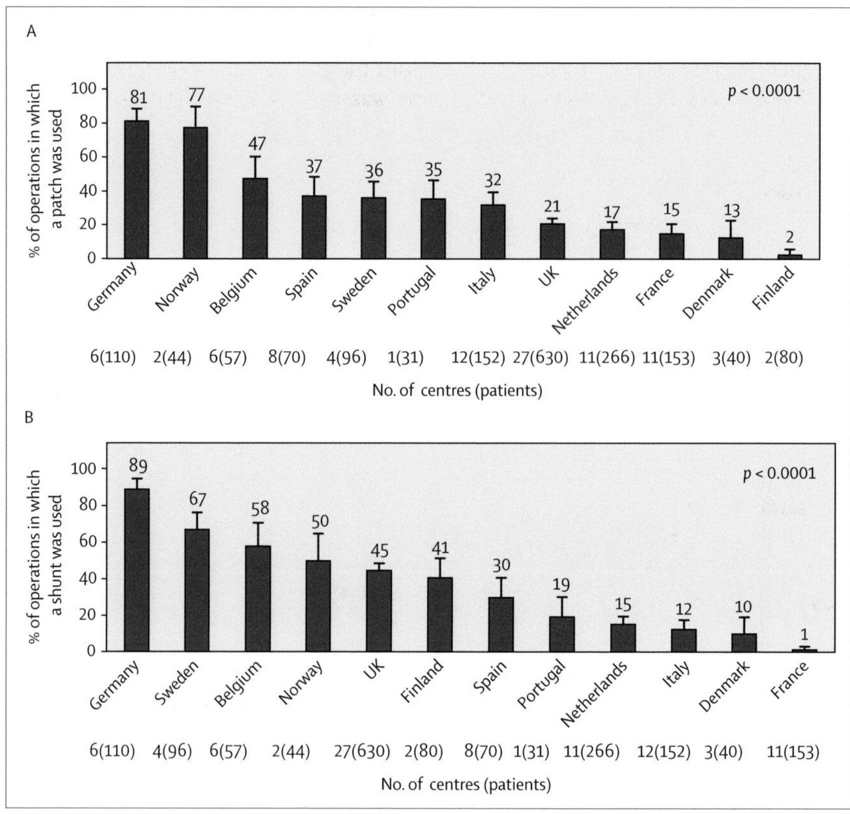

***Figure* 3.2: Variation in rate of use of two ancillary surgical techniques used during carotid endarterectomy ((A) patch angioplasty; (B) intraoperative shunt) by country in the ECST.[60] (Reprinted from Rothwell,[146] copyright 2005, with permission from Elsevier.)**

efficacy ($p < 0.0001$) with decreasing latitude.[66] The substantial racial differences in genetic determinants of drug response are discussed in Chapter 10. Overall, however, RCTs done in one country probably are for the most part generalisable to others, but this should not be taken for granted.

Selection of participating centres and clinicians

Selection of participating centres from secondary care versus primary care has obvious implications for external validity, but RCTs of interventions that are confined to secondary care may also be undermined if they are restricted to specialist units.[67, 68] In one systematic review of laparoscopic cholecystectomy, for example, all 15 RCTs were based solely in university hospitals.[68] Problems also arise if participating clinicians are chosen because of their track record. For example, the Asymptomatic Carotid Atherosclerosis Study Group (ACAS) trial showed that endarterectomy for asymptomatic carotid stenosis reduced the 5-year absolute risk of stroke by about 5%.[69] However, ACAS only accepted surgeons with an excellent safety record, rejecting 40% of applicants initially,[70] and subsequently barring from further participation those who had adverse operative outcomes in the trial. The benefit from surgery in ACAS was due in major part to the consequently low operative risk.[69] Figure 3.3 compares the ACAS risks with the results of a meta-analysis of the 46 surgical case series that published operative risks during the 5 years after ACAS.[71] Operative mortality was eight times higher than in ACAS

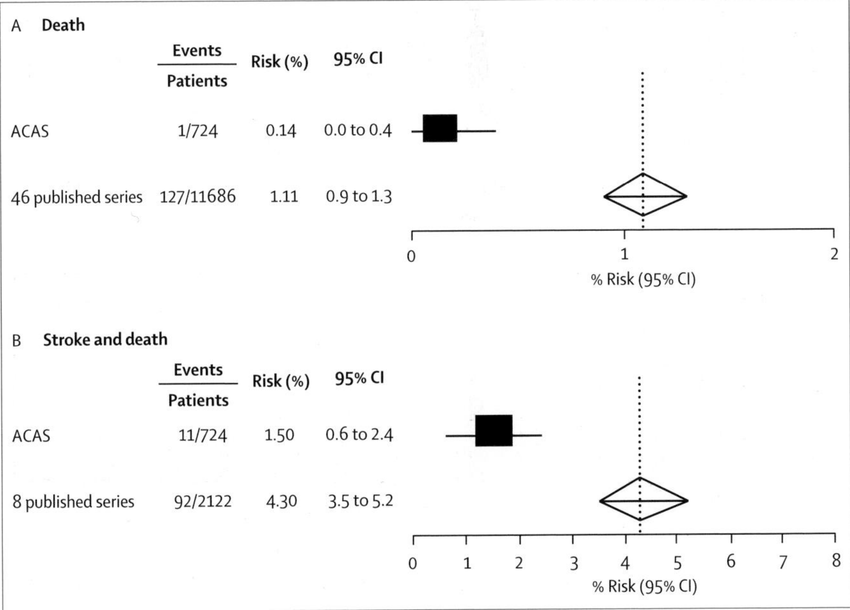

Figure 3.3: The overall results of a meta-analysis of (A) the operative risk of death and (B) stroke and death from all studies published between 1990 and 2000 inclusive that reported risks due to carotid endarterectomy for asymptomatic stenosis[71] compared with the same risks in the ACAS trial.[69] (Reprinted from Rothwell,[146] copyright 2005, with permission from Elsevier.)

(1.11% versus 0.14%, $p = 0.01$) and the risk of stroke and death was about three times higher in comparable studies in which outcome was also assessed by a neurologist (4.3% versus 1.5%, $p < 0.001$). Trials should not include centres that do not have the competence to treat patients safely but selection should not be so exclusive that the results cannot be generalised to clinical practice. It is unlikely, for example, that those surgeons rejected by ACAS ceased operating outside the trial.

Selection of patients

Only a small proportion of the patients with a condition get into a trial. At the national level only about one in every 200–300 patients undergoing carotid endarterectomy in North America at the time got into the large multicentre RCTs,[72] and similar proportions have been reported in breast cancer trials.[73] While these low rates mean that trials take many years to recruit, this is not a problem for external validity as long as the patients randomised in the participating centres are representative of the whole. However, as outlined below this is not always the case.

Selection prior to consideration of eligibility

Concern is often expressed about highly selective trial eligibility criteria, but there are several earlier stages of selection that can be more problematic. Figure 3.4 shows that the proportion of patients with a particular condition in the local community served by a participating centre who are considered for recruitment into a trial will often be well below 1%. For example, consider a trial of a new blood pressure lowering drug, which like most such trials is performed in a hospital clinic. Fewer than 10% of patients with hypertension are managed in hospital clinics, and this group will differ from those managed in primary care. Moreover, only one of the ten physicians who see hypertensive patients in this hospital is taking part in the trial, and this particular physician mainly sees cross-referrals of young patients with resistant hypertension. Thus, even before any consideration of eligibility or exclusion criteria, potential recruits are already highly unrepresentative of patients in the local community. Indeed, in judging external validity, an understanding of how patients were referred, investigated and diagnosed (i.e. their pathway to recruitment), as well as how they were subsequently selected and excluded, is often very much more informative than a list of baseline characteristics.

Selection by eligibility criteria

Patients are then further selected according to trial eligibility criteria (see figure 3.4). Some RCTs exclude women and many exclude the elderly.[74,75] One review of 214 drug trials in acute myocardial infarction (MI) found that over 60% excluded patients aged over 75 years.[74] Many RCTs also exclude patients with everyday comorbidty. For example, trials of antiplatelet drugs or non-steroidal anti-inflammatory drugs (NSAIDs) often bar recruitment of patients with any history of dyspepsia, even though this excludes over 50% of elderly patients in clinical practice.[76,77] Exclusion rates can be very high. In acute stroke, one study found that, of the small proportion of patients admitted to hospital sufficiently quickly to be suitable for thrombolysis,[78] 96% were ineligible based on the various other criteria of the relevant RCT.[79] A centre in another

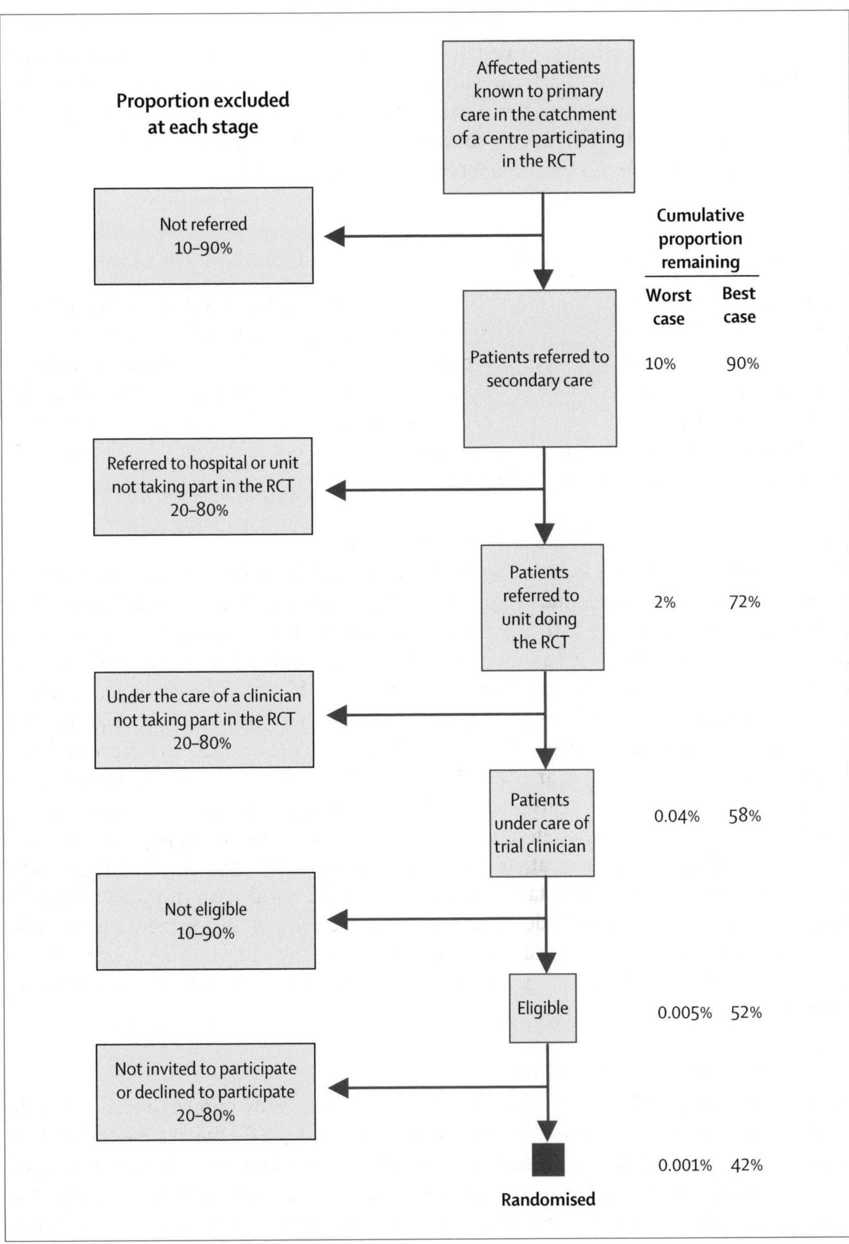

Figure 3.4: **The effect of the multiple stages of selection inherent in clinical practice on the proportion of patients in the catchment of a participating centre that are entered into an RCT performed in secondary care. The 'worst case' assumes that the proportion of patients excluded at each stage is at the top of the range quoted, and the 'best case' is based on the lowest proportion of patients excluded. (Reprinted from Rothwell,[146] copyright 2005, with permission from Elsevier.)**

acute stroke trial had to screen 192 patients over 2 years to find one eligible patient.[80] A review of 41 US National Institutes of Health RCTs found an average exclusion rate of 73%.[39]

Selection beyond the eligibility criteria

Strict eligibility criteria can limit the external validity of RCTs and result in lower rates of treatment in clinical practice,[81] but they are at least evident, or should be (see below). More difficult is the extent to which trials with seemingly reasonable eligibility criteria end up with highly selected populations. Recruitment of less than 10% of patients with the relevant condition in participating centres is common in pragmatic RCTs in all areas of medicine and surgery where the data have been collected.[24, 33, 82–87] These low rates of recruitment are partly due to additional selection by participating clinicians beyond that required by the eligibility criteria. Patients recruited into RCTs differ from those who are eligible but not recruited in terms of age, sex, race, severity of disease, educational status, social class and place of residence.[30, 34, 35, 37, 59, 74, 75, 88–90] The prognosis of patients included in RCTs is also usually better than those not in trials,[91] often markedly so.[6, 92] Yet, highly selective recruitment is not inevitable. The GISSI-1 trial of thrombolysis for acute MI, for example, recruited 90% of patients admitted within 12 hours of the event with a definite diagnosis and no contraindications.[93] As a consequence this study has excellent external validity and is one of only a very few RCTs in acute MI that had a control group mortality rate (13%) that was remotely consistent with routine clinical practice at the time.

Run-in periods

Pre-randomisation run-in periods are also often used to select or exclude patients.[94] In a placebo run-in, all eligible patients receive placebo and those who are poorly compliant are excluded.[95] There can be good reasons for doing this, but high rates of exclusion will reduce external validity of the study results. For example, one trial of the effect of salts on blood pressure excluded 93% of patients in a placebo run-in period.[96] Active treatment run-in periods in which patients who have adverse events or show signs that treatment may be ineffective are excluded are more likely to undermine external validity. For example, two RCTs of carvedilol, a vasodilatory beta-blocker, in chronic heart failure excluded 6% and 9% of eligible patients in treatment run-in periods,[97, 98] mainly because of worsening heart failure and other adverse events, some of which were fatal. In both trials, the complication rates in the subsequent randomised phase were much lower than in the run-in phase.[97, 98]

'Enrichment' strategies

Trials sometimes actively recruit patients who are likely to respond well to treatment.[99–101] For example, some trials of antipsychotic drugs have selectively recruited patients who had previously shown a good response to antipsychotic drugs.[102] Other trials have excluded non-responders in a run-in phase. One RCT of a cholinesterase inhibitor, tacrine, in Alzheimer's disease recruited 632 patients to a 6-week 'enrichment' phase in which they were randomised to different doses of tacrine versus placebo.[103] After a washout period, only the 215 (34%) patients who had a measured improvement on tacrine in the 'enrichment' phase were randomised to tacrine (at their best dose) versus placebo in the main phase of the trial. External validity is clearly undermined here.

Reporting of patient selection

The number of eligible non-randomised patients can be recorded, but is difficult to determine reliably, and underestimates selection because logs usually only cover patients referred to the participating clinician. Another useful index is the number of patients who are invited to participate and decline, but neither statistic is usually reported. However, inadequate reporting of trial eligibility criteria is a far greater barrier to the assessment of external validity.[104] The CONSORT guidelines[49] and the Uniform Requirements for Manuscripts Submitted to Biomedical Journals[105] require that all eligibility criteria should be reported, but a review of trials leading to clinical alerts by the US National Institutes of Health revealed that, of an average of 31 eligibility criteria, only 63% were published in the main trial report and only 19% in the clinical alert.[106] Inadequate reporting is a major problem in secondary publications, such as systematic reviews and clinical guidelines, where a lack of space and the need for a succinct message do not usually allow for detailed consideration of the eligibility and exclusion criteria of trials or other determinants of external validity. The same also applies to pharmaceutical marketing, although the motivation for concealing poor external validity may be different in this case.

Characteristics of randomised patients

Trial reports usually include the baseline clinical characteristics of randomised patients, and so it is argued that clinicians can assess external validity by comparison with their patient(s).[49, 50] This is clearly sensible, but baseline clinical characteristics can be misleading. The difficulty in extrapolating from baseline clinical characteristics is illustrated by the patients who were randomised to endarterectomy in the ECST[60] but did not have surgery because their surgeon and/or anaesthetist felt that they were too frail. Although this clinical impression was confirmed by a much worse outcome during follow-up compared with patients who were randomised to medical treatment (5-year risks: stroke 36% versus 18%, $p < 0.001$; stroke or death 52% versus 27%, $p < 0.0001$), their baseline clinical characteristics were no different (table 3.1).

A patient may also differ from the trial population in a way that seems unimportant, but which may have a major effect on external validity. For example, table 3.2 shows the baseline clinical characteristics of the patients randomised to warfarin in two RCTs of secondary prevention of stroke.[107–109] In one trial patients were in atrial fibrillation, and in the other they were in sinus rhythm. This difference might be expected to affect the risk of further ischaemic stroke, but would not be expected to affect the safety of warfarin. In fact, the risk of intracranial haemorrhage (ICH) on warfarin was 19 times higher ($p < 0.0001$) in Stroke Prevention in Reversible Ischaemia Trial (SPIRIT) (sinus rhythm) than in Atrial Fibrillation Trial (EAFT) (atrial fibrillation) after adjustment for differences in baseline clinical characteristics and the intensity of anticoagulation (see table 3.2).[109] Seemingly irrelevant differences between patients can have major effects on risks and benefits of treatment. This was further highlighted in SPIRIT by patients with leukoariosis on baseline brain imaging, who had a nine-fold greater risk of ICH on warfarin than did patients without leukoariosis.[107, 109]

There are many other factors related to patient characteristics that can influence the relevance of a trial to a particular patient, including the underlying pathology, the severity of disease, the stage in the natural history of the disease, comorbidity and the likely

Characteristic/outcome	Surgery (*n* = 1807)		No surgery (*n* = 1211)
	Not operated (*n* = 62)	Operated (*n* = 1745)	
Demography			
Male	36 (58%)	1263 (72%)	869 (72%)
Mean (SD) age (years)	64.1 (8.7)	62.5 (8.1)	62.3 (8.0)
Cerebrovascular events within past 6 months			
Hemispheric TIA or stroke	56 (90%)	1495 (85%)	1038 (86%)
Ocular event only	6 (10%)	250 (15%)	173 (14%)
Residual neurological signs	2 (3%)	106 (6%)	78 (7%)
Mean (SD) days since last symptoms	74 (56)	62 (53)	62 (52)
Other clinical data			
Previous stroke	2 (3%)	101 (6%)	78 (7%)
Mean (SD) systolic BP (mmHg)	154 (27.2)	151 (22.3)	150.2 (21.3)
Mean (SD) diastolic BP (mmHg)	89.0 (13.0)	86.2 (11.4)	86.3 (10.8)
Angina	15 (24%)	305 (18%)	190 (16%)
Previous myocardial infarction	7 (11%)	219 (13%)	136 (11%)
Previous coronary artery surgery	2 (3%)	47 (3%)	23 (2%)
Peripheral vascular disease	7 (11%)	292 (16%)	203 (17%)
Diabetes	8 (13%)	208 (12%)	145 (12%)
Current cigarette smoking	25 (44%)	844 (53%)	557 (52%)
Mean (SD) blood cholesterol (mmol/l)	6.4 (1.6)	6.4 (1.4)	6.4 (1.4)
Mean (SD) symptomatic carotid stenosis	60% (25)	62% (21)	59% (22)
Mean (SD) contralateral carotid stenosis	37% (26)	42% (26)	37% (27)

BP, blood pressure; TIA, transient ischaemic attack.

***Table** 3.1:* **Baseline clinical characteristics and outcomes of patients randomised in the ECST:[60] patients who were randomised to surgery but did not have the operation are compared with those who did and with patients who were randomised to medical treatment only**

absolute risk of a poor outcome without treatment. These issues are considered in detail in Chapter 9.

The intervention, control treatment, and pre-trial or non-trial management

External validity can also be affected if trials have protocols that differ from usual clinical practice. For example, prior to randomisation in the RCTs of endarterectomy for

Characteristic/outcome	SPIRIT (n = 651)	EAFT (*n* = 225)
Baseline clinical characteristics		
Male	66%	55%
Age > 65 years	47%	81%
Hypertension	39%	48%
Angina	9%	11%
Myocardial infarction	9%	7%
Diabetes	11%	12%
Leukoariosis on CT brain scan	7%	14%
Outcomes during trial		
Mean (SD) INR during trial	3.3 (1.1)	2.9 (0.7)
Patient-years of follow-up	735	507
Intracranial haemorrhage	27	0*
Extracranial haemorrhage	26	13
Adjusted hazard ratio (95% CI)*		
Intracranial haemorrhage	19.0 (2.4–250)	$p < 0.0001$
Extracranial haemorrhage	1.9 (0.8–4.7)	$p = 0.15$

CT, computed tomography; INR, international normalised ratio. *There were no proven intracranial haemorrhages, but no CT scan was performed in two strokes. For the purpose of calculation of the adjusted hazard ratio for haemorrhage, these two strokes were categorised as having been due to intracranial haemorrhage.

***Table* 3.2: Baseline clinical characteristics and outcomes of patients randomised to anticoagulation with warfarin in the EAFT[107] and the SPIRIT[108]**

symptomatic carotid stenosis, patients had to be diagnosed by a neurologist and have conventional arterial angiography,[110] neither of which are routine in many centres nowadays. The trial intervention itself may also differ from that used in current practice, such as in the formulation and bioavailability of a drug, or the type of anaesthetic used for an operation. The same can be true of the treatment in the control group in a trial, which may use a particularly low dose of the comparator drug, or fall short of best current practice in some other way. External validity can also be undermined by too stringent limitations on the use of non-trial treatments. For example, the effectiveness of antihypertensive drugs or drugs for the treatment of cardiac failure will be lower in elderly patients outside trials who are unable to stop their NSAIDs.[111] Any prohibition of non-trial treatments should be reported in the main trial publications along with details of relevant non-trial treatments that were used. The timing of many interventions is also critical, as is illustrated in figure 3.1 for endarterectomy for recently symptomatic carotid stenosis, and should be reported when relevant.

Outcome measures and follow-up

The external validity of an RCT also depends on whether the outcomes were clinically relevant. This can depend on subtle considerations, such as who actually measured the outcome, as illustrated by the lower operative risks of endarterectomy in studies where patients were assessed by surgeons rather than by neurologists,[112] but is more often dependent on what was measured and when.

Surrogate outcomes

Many trials use 'surrogate' outcomes, usually biological or imaging markers that are thought to be indirect measures of the effect of treatment on clinical outcomes. However, as well as being of questionable clinical relevance, surrogate outcomes are often misleading. Each of the treatments listed in table 3.3 had a major beneficial effect on a surrogate outcome, but even though each surrogate outcome had been shown to be correlated with a relevant clinical outcome in observational studies, the treatments proved to be ineffective or harmful in subsequent large RCTs that used these clinical outcomes.[113–125]

Scales

RCTs sometimes use complex scales, often made up of arbitrary combinations of symptoms and clinical signs.[126, 127] For example, a review of 196 RCTs of NSAIDs in rheumatoid arthritis identified more than 70 different outcome scales,[128] and a review of 2000 RCTs in schizophrenia identified 640 scales, many of which were devised for the particular RCT and had no supporting data on validity or reliability.[129] Interestingly, these unvalidated scales were more likely to show statistically significant treatment effects than were established scales.[130] However, the clinical meaning of apparent treatment effects (e.g. a 2.7 point mean reduction in a 100-point outcome scale made up of various symptoms and signs) is usually impossible to discern.

Treatment	Condition	Surrogate outcome	Clinical outcome
Fluoride	Osteoporosis	Increase in bone density[113]	Major increase in fractures[113]
Antiarrhythmic drugs	Post-MI	Reduction in ECG abnormalities[114]	Increased mortality[115]
β-Interferon	Multiple sclerosis	70% reduction in new lesions on brain MRI[116–119]	No convincing effect on disability[116–119]
Milrinone and epoprostanol	Heart failure	Improved exercise tolerance[120, 121]	Increased mortality[122, 123]
Ibopamine	Heart failure	Improved ejection fraction and heart rate variability[124]	Increased mortality[125]

ECG, electrocardiogram; MI, myocardial infarction.

***Table* 3.3: Examples where trials based on surrogate outcomes proved to be misleading predictors of the effect of treatment on clinical outcomes in subsequent trials**

Patient-centred outcomes

Simple clinical outcomes usually have most external validity, but only if they reflect the priorities of patients. For example, figure 3.5 shows the results of a study in which patients with multiple sclerosis and their clinicians were asked independently to select the three aspects of the disease that had the greatest influence on quality of life.[131] Clinicians focused mainly on the physical effects of the disease, whereas patients were more concerned about mental health, emotional well-being, general health and vitality, which are often not measured in RCTs. It is also important that clinical outcomes are expressed in a way that is most relevant to patients, even if this reduces the statistical power of the trial. For example, patients with epilepsy are much more interested in the proportion of patients rendered free of seizures in RCTs of anticonvulsants than they are in changes in mean seizure frequency.[132, 133]

Composite outcome measures

Many trials combine events in their primary outcome measure. This can produce a useful measure of the overall effect of treatment on all the relevant outcomes, and it usually affords greater statistical power, but there are problems. For example, the outcome that is most important to a particular patient may be affected differently by treatment than the combined outcome. Although the antiplatelet agent dipyridamole reduces the risk of the combined outcome of stroke, myocardial infarction and vascular death, it appears to have no effect on the risk of myocardial infarction alone[134] and

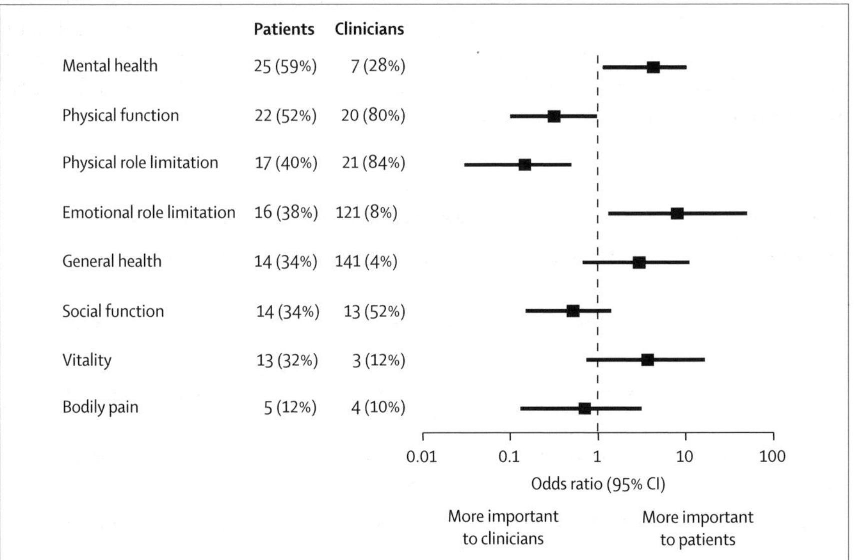

Figure 3.5: A comparison of the elements of quality of life that were of greatest concern to patients with multiple sclerosis (based on selecting the three of the eight aspects assessed in the Short Form-36 health-related quality of life measure that were most important) with those elements that their clinicians imagined were most important.[131] (Reprinted from Rothwell,[146] copyright 2005, with permission from Elsevier.)

would not be the optimal agent in a patient with unstable coronary artery disease. Composite outcomes also sometimes combine events of very different severity, and treatment effects can be driven by the least important outcome, which is often the most frequent. This is sometimes the case, for example, in trials of prevention of stroke that include transient ischaemic attacks in a composite outcome. An equally problematic composite outcome is the mixture of definite clinical events and episodes of 'hospitalisation'. The fact that a patient is in an RCT will probably affect the likelihood of hospitalisation, and likelihood of hospitalisation will certainly vary between different healthcare systems.

Length of treatment and follow-up

Another common problem for the external validity of RCTs is an inadequate duration of treatment and/or follow-up. For example, although patients with refractory epilepsy require treatment for many years, most RCTs of new drugs look at the effect of treatment for only a few weeks.[132, 133] Whether initial response is a good predictor of long-term benefit is unknown. The same problem has been identified in RCTs in schizophrenia, with fewer than 50% of trials having more than 6 weeks of follow-up and only 20% following patients for longer than 6 months.[33, 129] The contrast between beneficial effects of treatments in short-term RCTs and the less encouraging experience of long-term treatment in clinical practice has also been highlighted by clinicians treating patients with rheumatoid arthritis.[135]

Adverse effects of treatment

Reporting of adverse effects of treatment in RCTs and systematic reviews is often poor. In a review of 192 pharmaceutical trials, less then a third had adequate reporting of adverse clinical events or laboratory toxicology.[136] Treatment discontinuation rates provide some guide to tolerability, but pharmaceutical trials often use eligibility criteria and run-in periods to exclude patients who might be prone to adverse effects. Rates of discontinuation of treatment are therefore greater in clinical practice.[137, 138] Publication bias and inadequate reporting of adverse events in pharmaceutical industry RCTs is a longstanding and unresolved problem.[139, 140]

Clinicians are usually most concerned about the external validity of RCTs of potentially dangerous treatments, not least because iatrogenic complications are a leading cause of death in developed countries.[141] Risks can be overestimated in RCTs, particularly during the introduction of new treatments, when trials are often done in patients with very severe disease, but stringent selection of patients, confinement to specialist centres and intensive safety monitoring usually lead to lower risks than in routine clinical practice. RCTs of warfarin in non-rheumatic atrial fibrillation are a good example. All trials reported benefit with warfarin, but complication rates were much lower than in routine practice.[24, 142] Consequent doubts about external validity are partly to blame for major underprescribing of warfarin, particularly in patients over 75 years old,[24, 142, 143] who account for over 70% of cases of non-rheumatic atrial fibrillation,[24] and who are at highest risk without treatment.[24, 144]

Conclusion

Randomised trials and systematic reviews provide the most reliable data on the effects of treatment. However, although dogmatic refusal by clinicians to accept the results of RCTs is unacceptable, there is justifiable concern that external validity is often poor. This perception is leading to the underuse in routine practice of treatments that have been shown to be effective in trials. Some trials have excellent external validity[93, 145] but, as outlined above, many do not, particularly some of those performed by the pharmaceutical industry. Yet, researchers, funding agencies, ethics committees, medical journals, the pharmaceutical industry and their governmental regulators all neglect proper consideration of external validity. Judgement is left to clinicians, but reporting of the determinants of external validity in trial publications, and particularly in secondary reports and clinical guidelines, is rarely adequate. Some information is sometimes published in a preceding methods paper, but this is often 'buried' in an obscure journal not readily accessible to busy clinicians, and much relevant information is never published. RCTs and systematic reviews cannot be expected to produce results that are directly relevant to all patients and all settings, but to be externally valid they should at least be designed and reported in a way that allows patients and clinicians to judge to whom they can reasonably be applied. A consensus is required on how the design and reporting of trials could be improved in order to achieve this aim. Agreement on a list, along the lines of panel 3.2, of the most important issues that should be considered by clinicians and researchers would be a helpful first step.

References

1 Cochrane AL. *Effectiveness and Efficiency: Random Reflections on Health Services.* London: Nuffield Provincial Hospitals Trust, 1971.

2 Horton R. Common sense and figures: the rhetoric of validity in medicine. Bradford Hill Memorial Lecture 1999. *Stat Med* 2000; **19:** 3149–64.

3 Pocock SJ. *Clinical Trials: A Practical Approach.* Chichester: Wiley, 1983.

4 Friedman LM, Furberg CD, DeMets DL. *Fundamentals of Clinical Trials,* 3rd edn. New York: Springer, 1998.

5 Black D. The limitations of evidence. *J R Coll Physicians Lond* 1998; **32:** 23–26.

6 Hampton JR. Size isn't everything. *Stat Med* 2002; **21:** 2807–14.

7 Caplan LR. Evidence based medicine: concerns of a clinical neurologist. *J Neurol Neurosurg Psychiatry* 2001; **71:** 569–74.

8 Evans JG. Evidence-based and evidence-biased medicine. *Age Ageing* 1995; **24:** 461–63.

9 Charlton BG, Miles A. The rise and fall of EBM. *Q J Med* 1998; **91:** 371–74.

10 Naylor C. Grey zones in clinical practice: some limits to evidence-based medicine. *Lancet* 1995; **345:** 840–42.

11 Swales JD. Evidence-based medicine and hypertension. *J Hypertens* 1999; **17:** 1511–16.

12 Morgan WKC. On evidence, embellishment and efficacy. *J Eval Clin Pract* 1997; **3:** 117–22.

13 Feinstein AR, Horwitz RI. Problems in the 'evidence' of 'evidence-based medicine'. *Am J Med* 1997; **103:** 529–35.

14 Pashos CL, Normand ST, Garfinkle JB, et al. Trends in use of drug therapies in patients with acute myocardial infarction: 1988–1992. *J Am Coll Cardiol* 1994; **23:** 1023–30.

15 Garfield FB, Garfield JM. Clinical judgement and clinical practice guidelines. *Intl J Technol Assess Health Care* 2000; **16:** 1050–60.

16 Cabana MB, Rand CS, Powe NR, et al. Why don't clinicians follow clinical practice guidelines? A framework for improvement. *JAMA* 1999; **282:** 1458–65.

17 Davis DA, Taylor-Vaisey A. Translating guidelines into practice, a systematic review of theoretic concepts, practical experience and research evidence in the adoption of clinical practice guidelines. *Can Med Assoc J* 1997; **157:** 408–16.

18 Ford LG, Hunter CP, Diehr P, et al. Effect of patient management guidelines on physician practice patterns: the community hospital oncology program experience. *J Clin Oncol* 1987; **5:** 504–11.

19 Grol R, Dalhuijsen J, Thomas S, et al. Attributes of clinical guidelines that influence use of guidelines in general practice: observational study. *BMJ* 1998; **317**: 858–61.
20 Messerli FH. Antihypertensive therapy: Beta-blockers and diuretics – why do physicians not always follow guidelines? *Medscape Cardiology*, September 1999. Available at: http://www.medscape.com/cardiology/journals (accessed February 2007).
21 Sonis J, Doukas D, Klinkman M, et al. Applicability of clinical trial results to primary care. *JAMA* 1998; **280**: 1746.
22 Wilson S, Delaney BC, Roalfe A et al. Randomized controlled trials in primary care: case study. *BMJ* 2000; **321**: 24–27.
23 Sellors J, Cosby R, Trim K, et al., for the Seniors Medication Assessment Research Trial (SMART) Group. Recruiting family physicians and patients for a clinical trial: lessons learned. *Fam Pract* 2002; **19**: 99–104.
24 Oswald N, Bateman H. Applying research evidence to individuals in primary care: a study using non-rheumatic atrial fibrillation. *Fam Pract* 1999; **16**: 414–19.
25 Fahey T. Applying the results of clinical trials to patients in general practice: perceived problems, strengths, assumptions, and challenges for the future. *Br J Gen Pract* 1998; **48**: 1173–78.
26 Mant D. Can randomised trials inform clinical decisions about individual patients? *Lancet* 1999; **353**: 743–46.
27 Jacobson LD, Edwards AGK, Granier SK, Butler CC. Evidence-based medicine and general practice. *Br J Gen Pract* 1997; **47**: 449–52.
28 McCormick JS. The place of judgement in medicine. *Br J Gen Pract* 1994; **44**: 50–51.
29 Benech I, Wilson AE, Dowell AC. Evidence-based practice in primary care: past, present and future. *J Eval Clin Pract* 1996; **2**: 249–63.
30 Britton A, McKee M, Black N, et al. Threats to applicability of randomised trials: exclusions and selective participation. *J Health Serv Res Policy* 1999; **4**: 112–21.
31 Downs SH, Black N. The feasibility of creating a checklist for the assessment of the methodological quality both of randomised and non-randomised studies of health care interventions. *J Epidemiol Commun Health* 1998; **52**: 377–84.
32 Egglin TKP, Horwitz RI. The case for better research standards in peripheral thrombolysis: poor quality of randomised trials during the past decade. *Acad Radiol* 1996; **3**: 1–9.
33 Gilbody S, Wahlbeck K, Adams C. Randomized controlled trials in schizophrenia: a critical perspective on the literature. *Acta Psychiatr Scand* 2002; **105**: 243–51.
34 Licht RW, Gouliaev G, Vestergaard P, Frydenberg M. Generalisability of results of randomised drug trials. A trial on antimanic treatment. *Br J Psychiatry* 1997; **170**: 264–67.
35 Camm AJ. Clinical trials of arrhythmia management: methods or madness. *Control Clin Trials* 1996; **17**: 4s–16s.
36 Norris SL, Engelgau MM, Narayan KMV. Effectiveness of self-management training in type 2 diabetes: a systematic review of randomised controlled trials. *Diabetes Care* 2001; **24**: 561–87.
37 Moore DAJ, Goodall RL, Ives NJ, et al. How generalisable are the results of large randomised controlled trials of antiretroviral therapy. *HIV Med* 2000; **1**: 149–54.
38 Brown N, Melville M, Gray D, et al. Relevance of clinical trial results in myocardial infarction to medical practice: comparison of four year outcome in participants of a thrombolytic trial, patients receiving routine thrombolysis, and those deemed ineligible for thrombolysis. *Heart* 1999; **81**: 548–60.
39 Charleson ME, Horwitz RI. Applying results of randomised trials to clinical practice: impact of losses before randomisation. *BMJ* 1984; **289**: 1281–84.
40 Simon GE, Vonkorff M, Heilingenstein JH, et al. Initial antidepressant choice in primary care: effectiveness of fluoxetine vs. tricyclic antidepressants. *JAMA* 1996; **275**: 1897–902.
41 Davey Smith G, Egger M. Incommunicable knowledge? Interpreting and applying the results of clinical trials and meta-analyses. *J Clin Epidemiol* 1998; **51**: 289–95.
42 Hennen BK. Measuring complexity of clinical problems. *J Med Educ* 1984; **59**: 487–93.
43 Julian DG, Pocock SJ. Interpreting a trials report. In: Pitt B, Julian D, Pocock S, eds. *Clinical Trials in Cardiology*. London: WB Saunders, 1997; 33–42.
44 Idanpaan-Heikkila JE. WHO guidelines for good clinical practice (GCP) for trials on pharmaceutical products: responsibilities of the investigator. *Ann Med* 1994; **26**: 89–94.
45 Wermeling DP. Clinical research: regulatory issues. *Am J Health Syst Pharm* 1999; **56**: 252–56.
46 Medical Research Council. *MRC Guidelines for Good Clinical Practice in Clinical Trials*. London: MRC, 1998.
47 Medical Research Council. *Clinical Trials for Tomorrow*. London: MRC, 2003.
48 Department of Health. *Governance Arrangements for NHS Research Ethics Committees*. London: DoH, 2001. Available at: http://www.dh.gov.uk/PublicationsAndStatistics/Publications/PublicationsPolicyAndGuidance/PublicationsPolicyAndGuidanceArticle/fs/ en?CONTENT_ID=4005727&chk=CNcpyR (accessed February 2007).

49 Altman DG, Schulz KF, Moher D, et al., for the CONSORT Group. The revised CONSORT statement for reporting randomised trials: explanation and elaboration. *Ann Intern Med* 2001; **134:** 663–94.

50 Alderson P, Green S, Higgins JPT, eds. Cochrane Reviewers' Handbook 4.2.1 [updated December 2003]. In: *The Cochrane Library*, Issue 1, 2004. Chichester: Wiley.

51 LeBaron S, Reyher J, Stack JM. Paternalistic vs egalitarian physician styles: the treatment of patients in crisis. *J Fam Pract* 1985; **21:** 56–62.

52 Thomas KB. General practice consultations: is there any point in being positive? *BMJ* 1987; **294:** 1200–02.

53 Di Blasi Z, Harkness E, Ernst E, et al. Influence of context effects on health outcomes: a systematic review. *Lancet* 2001; **357:** 757–62.

54 Kleijnen J, de Craen AJM, van Everdingen J, Krol L. Placebo effect in double-blind clinical trials: a review of interactions with medications. *Lancet* 1994; **344:** 1347–49.

55 Kaptchuk TJ. Powerful placebo: the dark side of the randomised controlled trial. *Lancet* 1998; **351:** 1722–25.

56 Onel E, Hammond C, Wasson JH, et al. An assessment of the feasibility and impact of shared decision making in prostate cancer. *Urology* 1998; **51:** 63–66.

57 Benson J, Britten N. Patients' decisions about whether or not to take antihypertensive drugs: qualitative study. *BMJ* 2002; **325:** 873–76.

58 Redelmeier DA, Rozin P, Kahneman D. Understanding patients' decisions. *JAMA* 1993; **270:** 72–76.

59 Olschewski M, Schumacher M, Davis KB. Analysis of randomized and non-randomized patients in clinical trials using the comprehensive cohort follow-up study design. *Control Clin Trials* 1992; **13:** 226–39.

60 European Carotid Surgery Trialists' Collaborative Group. Randomised trial of endarterectomy for recently symptomatic carotid stenosis: final results of the MRC European Carotid Surgery Trial (ECST). *Lancet* 1998; **351:** 1379–87.

61 Lovett JK, Coull A, Rothwell PM, on behalf of the Oxford Vascular Study. Early risk of recurrent stroke by aetiological subtype: implications for stroke prevention. *Neurology* 2004; **62:** 569–74.

62 Masuhr F, Busch M, Einhaupl KM. Differences in medical and surgical therapy for stroke prevention between leading experts in North America and Western Europe. *Stroke* 1998; **29:** 339–345.

63 Sacco RL, Kargman DE, Gu Q, Zamanillo MC. Race-ethnicity and determinants of intracranial atherosclerotic cerebral infarction. The Northern Manhattan Stroke Study. *Stroke* 1995; **26:** 14–20.

64 Ricci S, Celani MG, Righetti E, Cantisani AT, for the International Stroke Trial Collaborative Group. Between country variations in the use of medical treatments for acute stroke: an update. *Cerebrovasc Dis* 1996; **6** (suppl 2): 133.

65 Bond R, Warlow CP, Naylor R, Rothwell PM. Variation in surgical and anaesthetic technique and associations with operative risk in the European Carotid Surgery Trial: implications for trials of ancillary techniques. *Eur J Vasc Endovasc Surg* 2002; **23:** 117–26.

66 Fine PEM. Variation in protection by BCG: implications of and for heterologous immunity. *Lancet* 1995; **346:** 1339–45.

67 Roberts C. The implications of variation in outcome between health professionals for the design and analysis of randomized controlled trials. *Stat Med* 1999; **18:** 2605–15.

68 Downs SH, Black NA, Devlin HB, et al. Systematic review of the effectiveness and safety of laparoscopic cholecystectomy. *Ann R Coll Surg England* 1996; **78:** 241–323.

69 Asymptomatic Carotid Atherosclerosis Study Group. Carotid endarterectomy for patients with asymptomatic internal carotid artery stenosis. *JAMA* 1995; **273:** 1421–28.

70 Moore WS, Young B, Baker WH, et al. Surgical results: a justification of the surgeon selection process for the ACAS trial. *J Vasc Surg* 1996; **23:** 323–38.

71 Bond R, Rerkasem K, Rothwell PM. High morbidity due to endarterectomy for asymptomatic carotid stenosis. *Cerebrovasc Dis* 2003; **16** (suppl 4): 65.

72 Barnett HJM., Barnes RW, Clagett GP, et al. Symptomatic carotid artery stenosis: a solvable problem. The NASCET trial. *Stroke* 1992; **23:** 1050–53.

73 De Vita VT. Breast cancer therapy; exercising all our options. *N Engl J Med* 1989; **320:** 527–29.

74 Gurwitz JH, Col NF, Avorn J. The exclusion of elderly and women from clinical trials in acute myocardial infarction. *JAMA* 1992; **268:** 1417–22.

75 Bungeja G, Kumar A, Banerjee AK. Exclusion of elderly people from clinical research: a descriptive study of published reports. *BMJ* 1997; **315:** 1059.

76 Jones R, Lydeard S. Prevalence of symptoms of dyspepsia in the community. *BMJ* 1989; **298:** 30–32.

77 Kay L. Prevalence, incidence and prognosis of gastrointestinal symptoms in a random sample of an elderly population. *Age Aging* 1994; **23:** 146–49.

78 Jorgensen HS, Nakayama H, Kammersgaard LP, et al. Predicted impact of intravenous thrombolysis on prognosis of general population of stroke patients: simulation model. *BMJ* 1999; **319:** 288–89.

79 National Institute of Neurological Disorders and Stroke rt-PA Stroke Study Group. Tissue plasminogen activator for acute ischaemic stroke. *N Engl J Med* 1995; **333:** 1581–87.

80 LaRue LJ, Alter M, Traven ND, et al. Acute stroke therapy trials: problems in patient accrual. *Stroke* 1988; **19:** 950–54.

81 Maynard C, Althouse R, Cerqueira M, et al. Underutilisation of thrombolytic therapy in eligible women with acute myocardial infarction. *Am J Cardiol* 1991; **68:** 529–30.

82 Steiner TJ, Clifford Rose F. Towards a model stroke trial. The single centre naftidrofuryl study. *Neuroepidemiology* 1986; **5:** 121–47.

83 Rovers MM, Zielhuis GA, Bennett K, Haggard M. Generalisability of clinical trials in otitis media with effusion. *Int J Pediatr Otorhinolaryngol* 2001; **20:** 29–40.

84 Califf RM, Pryor DB, Greenfield JC. Beyond randomised clinical trials: applying clinical experience in the treatment of patients with coronary artery disease. *Circulation* 1986; **74:** 1191–94.

85 Stroke Prevention in Atrial Fibrillation Investigators. Stroke Prevention in Atrial Fibrillation Study. *Circulation* 1991; **84:** 527–39.

86 Muller DWM. Selection of patients with acute myocardial infarction for thrombolytic therapy. *Ann Intern Med* 1990; **113:** 949–60.

87 Henderson RA, Raskino CL, Hampton JR. Variations in the use of coronary arteriography in the UK: the RITA trial coronary arteriogram register. *Q J Med* 1995; **88:** 167–73.

88 Bjorn M, Brendstrup C, Karlsen S, Carlsen JE. Consecutive screening and enrolment in clinical trials: the way to representative patient samples? *J Cardiac Failure* 1998; **4:** 225–30.

89 Bowen JT, Barnes TRE. The clinical characteristics of schizophrenic patients consenting or not consenting to a placebo controlled trial of antipsychotic medication. *Hum Psychopharmacol* 1994; **9:** 432–33.

90 Schmoor C, Olschewski M, Schumacher M. Randomized and non-randomized patients in clinical trials: experiences with comprehensive cohort studies. *Stat Med* 1996; **15:** 263–71.

91 Stiller CA. Centralised treatment, entry to trials and survival. *Br J Cancer* 1994; **70:** 352–62.

92 Woods KL, Ketley D. Intravenous beta blockade in acute myocardial infarction. Doubt exists about external validity of trials of intravenous beta-blockade. *BMJ* 1999; **318:** 328–29.

93 Gruppo Italiano per lo Studio della Streptochinasi nell'Infarto Miocardico (GISSI). Effectiveness of intravenous thrombolytic treatment in acute myocardial infarction. *Lancet* 1986; **1:** 397–402.

94 Pablos-Mendez A, Barr RG, Shea S. Run-in periods in randomised trials: implications for the application of results in clinical practice. *JAMA* 1998; **279:** 222–25.

95 Haynes RB, Dantes R. Patient compliance and the conduct and interpretation of therapeutic trials. *Control Clin Trials* 1987; **8:** 12–19.

96 Gomez-Marin O, Prineas RJ, Sinaiko AR. The sodium-potassium blood pressure trial in children: design, recruitment and randomisation. *Control Clin Trials* 1991; **12:** 408–23.

97 Australia-New Zealand Heart Failure Research Collaborative Group. Effects of carvedilol, a vasodilatory beta-blocker, in patients with congestive heart failure due to ischaemic heart disease. *Circulation* 1995; **92:** 212–18.

98 Packer M, Bristow MR, Cohn JN, et al., for the US Carvedilol Heart Failure Study Group. The effects of carvedilol on morbidity and mortality in patients with chronic heart failure. *N Engl J Med* 1996; **334:** 1349–55.

99 Amery W, Dony J. A clinical trial design avoiding undue placebo treatment. *J Clin Pharmacol* 1975; **15:** 674–79.

100 Quitkin FM, Rabkin JG. Methodological problems in studies of depressive disorder: utility of the discontinuation design. *J Clin Psychopharmacol* 1981; **1:** 283–88.

101 Hallstrom A, Verter J, Friedman L. Randomising responders. *Control Clin Trials* 1991; **12:** 486–503.

102 Leber PD, Davis CS. Threats to the validity of clinical trials employing enrichment strategies for sample selection. *Control Clin Trials* 1998; **19:** 178–87.

103 Davis KL, Thal LJ, Gamzu ER, et al., and the Tacrine Collaborative Study Group. A double-blind, placebo-controlled multicenter study of tacrine for Alzheimer's disease. *N Engl J Med* 1992; **321:** 406–12.

104 Hall JC, Mills B, Nguyen H, Hall JL. Methodologic standards in surgical trials. *Surgery* 1996; **119:** 466–72.

105 International Committee of Medical Journal Editors. *Uniform Requirements for Manuscripts Submitted to Biomedical Journals: Writing and Editing for Biomedical Publication.* February 2006. Available at: http://www.ICMJE.org (accessed February 2007).

106 Shapiro SH, Weijer C, Freedman B. Reporting the study populations of clinical trials. Clear transmission or static on the line? *J Clin Epidemiol* 2000; **53:** 973–79.

107 European Atrial Fibrillation Trial (EAFT) Study Group. Secondary prevention in non-rheumatic atrial fibrillation after transient ischaemic attack or minor stroke. *Lancet* 1993; **342:** 1255–62.

108 Algra A, Francke CL, Koehler PJJ, for the Stroke Prevention in Reversible Ischaemia Trial (SPIRIT) group. A randomized trial of anticoagulants versus aspirin after cerebral ischaemia of presumed arterial origin. *Ann Neurol* 1997; **42:** 857–65.
109 Gorter JW, for the Stroke Prevention in Reversible Ischaemia Trial (SPIRIT) and European Atrial Fibrillation Trial (EAFT) groups. Major bleeding during anticoagulation after cerebral ischaemia: patterns and risk factors. *Neurology* 1999; **53:** 1319–27.
110 Rothwell PM, Gutnikov SA, Eliasziw M, et al., for the Carotid Endarterectomy Trialists' Collaboration. Pooled analysis of individual patient data from randomised controlled trials of endarterectomy for symptomatic carotid stenosis. *Lancet* 2003; **361:** 107–16.
111 Merlo J, Broms K, Lindblad U, et al. Association of outpatient utilisation of non-steroidal anti-inflammatory drugs and hospitalised heart failure in the entire Swedish population. *Eur J Clin Pharmacol* 2001; **57:** 71–75.
112 Rothwell PM, Slattery J, Warlow CP. A systematic review of the risks of stroke and death due to carotid endarterectomy for symptomatic stenosis. *Stroke* 1996; **27:** 260–65.
113 Riggs BL, Hodgson SF, O'Fallon WM, et al. Effect of fluoride treatment on fracture rate in postmenopausal women with osteoporosis. *N Engl J Med* 1990; **322:** 802–09.
114 McAlistair FA, Teo KK. Antiarrhythmic therapies for the prevention of sudden cardiac death. *Drugs* 1997; **54:** 235–52.
115 The Cardiac Arrhythmia Suppression Trial (CAST) Investigators. Preliminary report: effect of encainide and flecainide on mortality in a randomized trial of arrhythmia suppression after myocardial infarction. *N Engl J Med* 1989; **321:** 406–12.
116 The IFNB Multiple Sclerosis Study Group. Interferon beta-1b is effective in relapsing–remitting multiple sclerosis. I. Clinical results of a multicenter, randomized, double-blind, placebo-controlled trial. *Neurology* 1993; **43:** 655–61.
117 The INFB Multiple Sclerosis Study Group and the University of British Columbia MS/MRI Analysis Group. Interferon beta-1b in the treatment of multiple sclerosis: final outcome of the randomized controlled trial. *Neurology* 1995; **45:** 1277–85.
118 Jacobs LD, Cookfair DL, Rudick AR, et al. Intramuscular interferon beta-1a for disease progression in relapsing multiple sclerosis. *Ann Neurol* 1996; **39:** 285–94.
119 Ebers GC for the PRISMS Study Group. Randomised double-blind placebo-controlled study of interferon beta-1a in relapsing-remitting multiple sclerosis. *Lancet* 1998; **352:** 1498–504.
120 Di Bianco R, Shabetai R, Kostuk W, et al. A comparison of oral milrinone, digoxin and their combination in the treatment of patients with chronic heart failure. *N Engl J Med* 1989; **320:** 677–83.
121 Sueta CA, Gheorghiade M, Adams KF, et al., and the Epoprostenol Multicentre Research Group. Safety and efficacy of epoprostenol in patients with severe congestive heart failure. *Am J Cardiol* 1995; **75:** 34A–43A.
122 Packer M, Carver JR, Rodeheffer RJ, et al., for the Promise Study Research Group. Effect of oral milrinone on mortality in severe chronic heart failure. *N Engl J Med* 1991; **325:** 1468–75.
123 Califf RM, Adams KF, McKenna WJ, et al. A randomized controlled trial of epoprostenol therapy for severe congestive heart failure. *Am Heart J* 1997; **134:** 44–54.
124 Yee KM, Struthers AD. Can drug effects on mortality in heart failure be predicted by any surrogate outcome measure? *Eur Heart J* 1997; **18:** 1860–64.
125 Hampton JR, van Veldhuisen DJ, Kleber FX, et al. Randomised study of ibopamine on survival in patients with advanced severe heart failure. *Lancet* 1997; **349:** 971–77.
126 Coste J, Fermanian J, Venot A. Methodological and statistical problems in the construction of composite measurement scales: a survey of six medical and epidemiological journals. *Stat Med* 1995; **14:** 331–45.
127 van Gijn J, Warlow C. Down with stroke scales. *Cerebrovasc Dis* 1992; **2:** 244–46.
128 Gøtzsche PC. Methodology and overt and hidden bias in reports of 196 double-blind trials of nonsteroidal antiinflammatory drugs in rheumatoid arthritis. *Control Clin Trials* 1989; **10:** 31–56.
129 Thornley B, Adams CE. Content and quality of 2000 controlled trials in schizophrenia over 50 years. *BMJ* 1998; **317:** 1181–84.
130 Marshall M, Lockwood A, Bradley C, et al. Unpublished rating scales – a major source of bias in randomised controlled trials of treatments for schizophrenia? *Br J Psychiatry* 2000; **176:** 249–52.
131 Rothwell PM, McDowell Z, Wong CK, Dorman P. Doctors and patients don't agree: cross sectional study of patients' and doctors' perceptions and assessments of disability in multiple sclerosis. *BMJ* 1997; **314:** 1580–83.
132 Binnie CD. Design of clinical antiepileptic drug trials. *Seizure* 1995; **4:** 187–92.
133 Walker MC, Sander JW. Difficulties in extrapolating from clinical trial data to clinical practice: the case of antiepileptic drugs. *Neurology* 1997; **49:** 333–37.
134 Diener HC, Cunha L, Forbes C, et al., for the European Stroke Prevention Study. 2. Dipyridamole and acetylsalicylic acid in the secondary prevention of stroke. *J Neurol Sci* 1996; **143:** 1–13.

3 Assessment of external validity of randomised trials

135 Pincus T. Rheumatoid arthritis: disappointing long-term outcomes despite successful short-term clinical trials. *J Clin Epidemiol* 1998; **41:** 1037–41.

136 Ioannidis JP, Contopoulos-Ioannidis DG. Reporting of safety data from randomised trials. *Lancet* 1998; **352:** 1752–53.

137 Jones J, Gorkin L, Lian J, et al. Discontinuation of and changes in treatment after start of new courses of antihypertensive drugs: a study of a United Kingdom population. *BMJ* 1995; **311:** 293–95.

138 Andrade SE, Walker AM, Gottlieb LK, et al. Discontinuation of antihyperlipidaemic drugs – do rates reported in clinical trials reflect rates in primary care settings. *N Engl J Med* 1995; **332:** 1125–31.

139 Hemminki E. Study of information submitted by drug companies to licensing authorities. *BMJ* 1980; **280:** 833–36.

140 McPherson K, Hemminki E. Synthesising licensing data to assess drug safety. *BMJ* 2004; **328:** 518–20.

141 Lazarou J, Pomeranz BH, Corey PN. Incidence of adverse drug reactions in hospitalised patients. *JAMA* 1998; **279:** 1200–05.

142 Landefeld CS, Beyth RJ. Anticoagulant-related bleeding: clinical epidemiology, prediction, and prevention. *Am J Med* 1993; **95:** 315–28.

143 Lip GH, Golding DJ, Masood N, et al. A survey of atrial fibrillation in general practice. *Br J Gen Pract* 1997; **47:** 285–89.

144 Antani MR, Beyth RJ, Covinsky KE, et al. Failure to prescribe warfarin to patients with non-rheumatic atrial fibrillation. *J Gen Intern Med* 1996; **11:** 713–20.

145 MRC/BHF Heart Protection Study of cholesterol lowering with simvastatin in 20,536 high-risk individuals: a randomised placebo-controlled trial. *Lancet* 2002; **360:** 7–22.

146 Rothwell PM. External validity of randomised controlled trials: 'to whom do the results of this trial apply?'. *Lancet* 2005; **365:** 82–93.

4

Applying results to treatment decisions in primary care

Paul Glasziou and David Mant

Introduction

> *All happy families are alike; all unhappy families are unhappy in their own way.* (Leo Tolstoy)

No two individuals have exactly the same 'disease'. The labels may be identical, but the host, the context and the process can all be subtlety or substantially different. Anyone who has seen an array of patients with 'stroke', 'depression' or 'osteoarthritis' knows how different these illnesses can be in different people. Given these, sometimes vast, differences in the nature of the illness and the person, the benefits and harms of treatment are also likely to differ. In turn, the balance of benefits and harms will differ. Hence we must always be on guard about relying on a diagnosis–treatment reflex. Instead we should ask the question: When do patients with this disease benefit from treatment? Patients in primary care may have the same label as those in secondary care but represent very different parts of the clinical spectrum, and hence require different treatment. For example, patients with diabetes are usually admitted to hospital when first-line treatment in primary care has failed – their illness is more severe and the primary goals of treatment focus on short-term physiology (e.g. blood pH and glucose levels) rather than long-term wellbeing (e.g. vascular disease risk factors).

While clinical trials in other settings provide us with important evidence about the effectiveness of available treatments, they leave general practitioners with a challenge in applying those results to patients in primary care. For the individual patient we will need to understand the nature and severity of their condition, their likely responsiveness to treatments, and their values and social context. This process is made easier when some trial and error is possible, such as with different options for symptom relief, and is most difficult with one-off irreversible decisions such as surgery. To understand better the elements of individualisation we will begin by looking at the additional evidence that has to be collected and applied to meet this challenge, the use of *n*-of-1 trials for chronic conditions, and then see how these elements can and cannot be applied to more difficult problems.

Is there a problem for primary care?

There are clear differences between patients in primary care and other settings, but it is less clear how often this impacts on treatment effects. For example, nicotine gum appeared equally effective in primary care and smoking clinics but less effective in hospital settings.[1] Conversely, a systematic review of mental health interventions for somatic symptoms[2] concluded that 'Treatment seems to be more effective in patients in secondary care than in primary care' but that there were several possible reasons '... because secondary care patients have more severe disease, they receive a different treatment regimen, or the intervention is more closely supervised'. A recent observational analysis of the outcome of pre-hospital penicillin in the treatment of children with meningococcal disease raises the possibility that treatment outside hospital (when facilities to manage cardiovascular collapse are not to hand) may increase rather than decrease mortality.[3] However, all these examples use indirect comparisons and hence are subject to confounding by many factors. Two studies that directly randomised patients to specialist or primary care showed no difference in impact. One showed similar outcomes for treatment of opiate addicts with buprenorphine,[4] and the other showed similar outcomes for follow-up of patients with breast cancer.[5] These trial results suggest that the key issue is usually not the setting in which the treatment is delivered but the spectrum of patients to whom it is delivered.

Since referral rates from primary care are around 10–15%, and the reasons for referral are related to morbidity, the spectrum in secondary and tertiary care is likely to comprise more severely ill patients. Hence deciding on treatment should involve more than merely applying a label: it should include an assessment of the severity (or baseline risk of the outcome) which that treatment might ameliorate or avoid, and the comorbidities and context of the patient. Sometimes this is simply a clinical assessment of severity, such as the degree of pain or dysfunction. At other times it may be measurement of a risk factor (such as blood pressure) or may involve formal calculation of a risk score.

To understand the issue of variation within a disease group, let us look at the example of cardiovascular risk. Figure 4.1, from the New Zealand tables, shows how risk factors can be combined to estimate overall risk. The risks can vary enormously across the same condition. For example, a total/high-density lipoprotein (HDL) cholesterol ratio of 7 in a 40-year-old male with no other risk factors is associated with a 5-year cardiovascular event rate of < 2.5% (the darkest grey squares on the chart in figure 4.1), while in contrast the event rate in a 70-year-old smoker with raised blood pressure is > 30% (the darkest green squares on the chart in figure 4.1). Hence the implications of the 'hypercholesterolaemia' are very different in these two patients (for a more detailed discussion of this issue see Chapter 16).

In the case of the 40 year old, the risk of disease is probably too low for this patient to opt for treatment – the number of patients who would need to be treated (NNT) for 1 year to prevent one case is about 80. In contrast, for the 70 year old, the NNT is < 10. In other words, the more precise is the individual estimate of the pretreatment risk (of the outcome the treatment is trying to avert), the easier it is to estimate precisely the individual benefit of treatment. Although the higher risk patients may be referred for secondary care, and enter trials, we need to individualise treatment over the full spectrum of risk.

As well as benefits, most treatments can do harm. To individualise treatment the risk of harm must also be estimated as precisely as possible. This is particularly obvious for treatments with life-threatening adverse effects, such as thrombosis with oral contraceptives or haemorrhage with anticlotting agents. Whichever oral contraceptive is used,

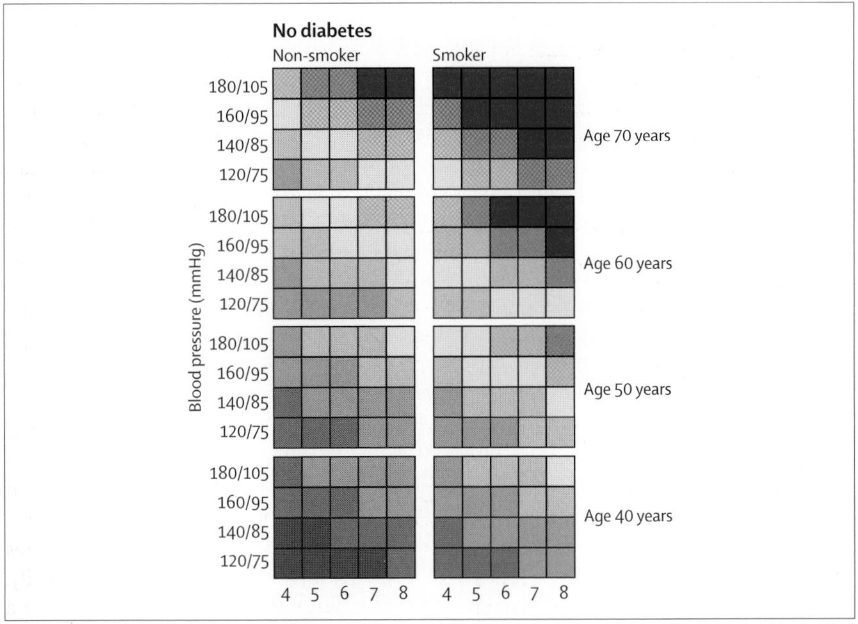

Figure 4.1: **Cardiovascular risk score based on five risk factors.**

pulmonary embolus is more likely in women who smoke or are > 35 years old. Whichever anticlotting treatment is used, serious haemorrhage is more likely in a patient with a history of peptic ulcer. Most of the trials of anticoagulant treatment for atrial fibrillation excluded patients with significant comorbidity or psychosocial problems associated with poor treatment compliance – this exclusion rate was over 90% in one trial.[6] This explains why the trials report considerably lower rates of haemorrhage than is reported from observational studies of warfarin use in the community.[7]

The above discussion suggests that, rather than a simple dichotomy of primary versus other care, we should examine the elements needed to achieve individualisation. To deal with the spectrum of patients, this examination needs to be done explicitly and accurately. It is illogical (if widely practised) to apply a meticulously, and often expensively, estimated relative risk of benefit or harm derived from a large clinical trial to a hopelessly crude back-of-the envelope individual assessment of prior risk without treatment. We now look at two approaches to assessing individual benefits and harms. First, sometimes we can try the direct approach of 'try it and see', where we monitor the (positive and negative) effects. Second, we can (and usually must) use an indirect approach, based on extrapolation from external evidence.

Direct assessment of effect in primary care: '*n*-of-1' trials

The individual effect of treatment in primary care can be assessed directly only when some trial and error is possible, such as with different options for symptom relief. Such an assessment is impossible with one-off irreversible decisions such as surgery. In managing chronic conditions in primary care it is common practice to try different doses or different drugs to see which helps and best suits a patient. When the initial treatment does not seem effective or appears to give adverse effects, then we might switch treatments.

Because of the dangers of bias in the trial-and-error approach, the 'ideal' method for assessing the treatment effect for an individual is the *n*-of-1 trial (for more details of this type of trial see Chapter 15). The *n*-of-1 trial allows a patient to try out a potential therapy by undergoing a sequence of periods on and off the therapy. For example, in osteoarthritis, does a non-steroidal anti-inflammatory drug (NSAID) provide sufficient additional relief compared to paracetamol such that it is worth the extra risks? In such patients we have offered *n*-of-1 trials in primary care which used three treatment–placebo pairs, that is three periods of one medication and three periods of the other (blinded by using a 'double dummy' placebo technique) (figure 4.2).[8] The response outcome assessed is the choice of the patient, who is then provided with the unblinded results and makes a decision about further treatment jointly with their doctor. By doing such an *n*-of-1 trial the patient can personally experience the effects of medication, both positive and negative, on them. This allows us and the patient to judge their personal responsiveness and personal adverse effects, and to make a more informed choice about whether the net effect is worthwhile to the patient. Thus the *n*-of-1 trial provides the 'gold standard' in informed patient choice.

Ideally then, patients should undergo well-conducted *n*-of-1 trials to individualise their therapy. This has led to a recent revision of the 'hierarchy of evidence' for interventions,

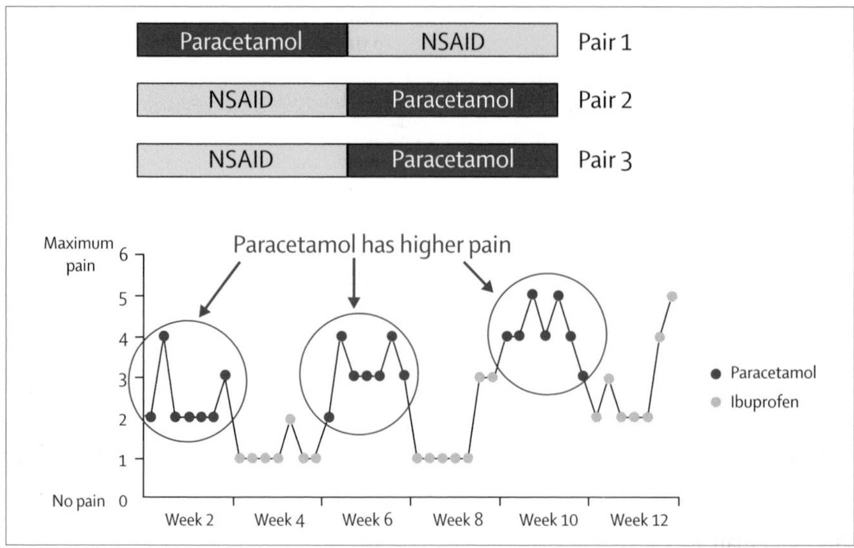

Figure 4.2: **Structure of an *n*-of-1 trial for osteoarthritis with six treatment periods randomised within three pairs.**

placing the *n*-of-1 trial at the top of the levels of evidence. These trials provide the best possible evidence for an individual patient, whereas standard randomised trials only tell us what works on average.[9]

However, the use of *n*-of-1 trials is very limited. They can be used only for chronic conditions where treatment has a reversible, symptomatic, short-term (hours to weeks) effect, and there is variation in individual responsiveness. The trials are often logistically difficult to set up and use. Thus *n*-of-1 trials cannot be done for treatments aimed at preventing future events (e.g. blood pressure reduction or aspirin aimed at preventing stroke) or for treating acute conditions (e.g. acute otitis media). However, *n*-of-1 trials do provide an ideal to which to aspire for other types of conditions, and they should be done more often in routine clinical practice, particularly when patients may be committing to a lifetime's treatment.

Indirect estimation of effect: extrapolation to primary care from other settings

When we cannot undertake an *n*-of-1 trial, the best we can do is attempt to predict the benefits and harms of treatment on the basis of the 'average' effect for a group of patients derived from a standard clinical trial, which will usually not have been done in primary care. The extrapolation can be done by applying the estimate of relative effect from the trial to the individualised assessment of the likelihood of disease (and known treatment side-effects) in the absence of treatment. In epidemiological terms we extrapolate by assuming that:[10]

Likely effect of treatment on individual = absolute risk for individual without treatment × relative treatment effect

Or, putting in the standard epidemiological terms, this may be stated as:

Absolute risk reduction (ARR) = patient expected event rate (PEER) × relative risk reduction (RRR)

The above equations assume there is only one outcome and no adverse effects. However, clinical management is rarely so simple. So let us look at the next simplest situation: two outcomes. If both the benefit and harm of treatment can be measured by the same outcome scale (e.g. death), we can simply apply the relative benefit of treatment estimated by the trial to the prior risk of death of the individual without treatment. This provides the best estimate of the absolute benefit of treatment to the individual. However, the relative benefit estimated from a group trial is usually an amalgam of benefit and harm, whether or not these two factors can be measured by a common outcome. This is shown schematically by the 'benefit–harm' model in figure 4.3. The model suggests that the lower risk patients in primary care are more likely to fall below the threshold than are the higher risk patients in secondary care. However, again this is an average risk: some primary care patients may be at higher risk and some secondary care patients may be at lower risk.

If the relative benefit of treatment is constant across settings and risk levels, then the absolute benefit will increase in proportion to the patient's risk level. In contrast the harms (adverse effects) of treatment, although varying with individuals, are usually not so closely related to the level of risk without treatment. So this simple model allows us to predict the likely benefits and harms, and hence the threshold point at which benefits outweigh harms. However, in making a decision to treat, clinicians must ask themselves how well these two assumptions on which the model is based (that both the relative risk reduction and the absolute risk of harm remain constant across settings and all levels of baseline risk) fit the evidence. Sometimes, as in the warfarin example discussed above, a specific group of patients can be defined who are at particularly high risk of adverse outcome for reasons that are essentially independent of the baseline risk the treatment is trying to minimise. Often we have fewer trial data than we would like to answer the question. In everyday practice, there may also be multiple outcomes to consider that may have different utilities for the individual. We need to explore each of these issues separately.

Putting theory into practice: assessing the transferability of the evidence to primary care

What issues need to be considered in transferring trial results from one setting to another and, in particular, to primary care? The Cochrane Methods Group on Applicability & Recommendations has suggested a two-stage process in going from information from (systematic reviews of) randomised trials to individualised decision-making.[11] The first stage involves an assessment of the transferability of the trial evidence; the second deals with its application by the clinician to the individual. To assess the transferability of the evidence it is necessary first to identify the benefits and harms of

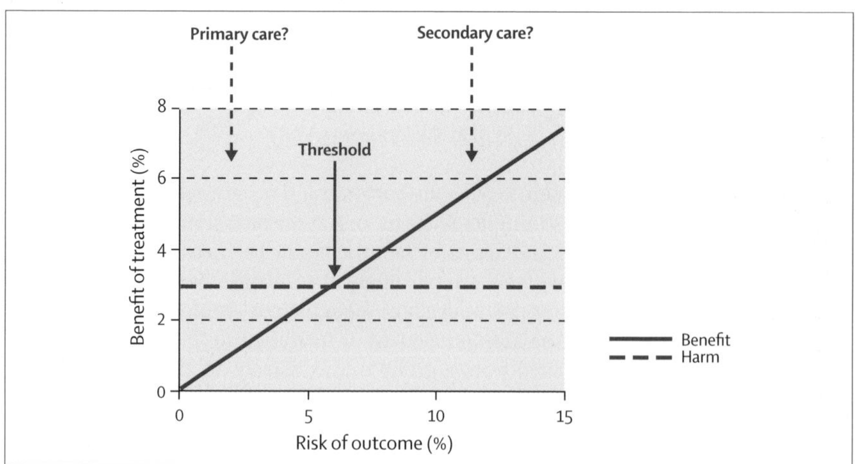

Figure 4.3: **The absolute effect of treatment generally increases with the risk of the outcome. Below the threshold, harms outweigh likely benefits. Above the threshold, the risk is high that the beneficial effect outweighs any potential harm.**

treatment, and then to decide whether they are likely to differ in primary compared to secondary care.

What are the benefits and harms?

The process of collating evidence on benefits and harms is perhaps best illustrated by a clinical example. At 5 p.m. on a Sunday afternoon a 2 year old, who is recovering from a cold, complains of severe pain in his left ear. The left ear drum is red and bulging, but the right one is normal, and he has no fever. How should he be treated, and in particular are antibiotics required? Responding to this clinical situation is impossible without prior homework. The clinician needs to have thought through the issues in advance of the consultation and to know how to access information that cannot easily be held in memory. The results can usefully be summarised in a 'summary of findings' table, which shows for each outcome the relative and absolute treatment effects, and the quality of evidence. The latter may vary across outcomes because of the way in which the outcome has been assessed and in the trials in which it was assessed.

A summary of findings table for the studies of antibiotics in children with otitis media is shown in Table 4.1. It is based on a Cochrane Systematic Review[12] which found nine randomised, placebo-controlled trials from a variety of settings. It shows that there is little impact of antibiotics in the first 24 hours, but that at 2–7 days there is a highly statistically significant relative reduction in symptoms of about one-third. We might easily say 'antibiotics work'. But that would ignore both the absolute benefit, as most children rapidly improve without treatment, and the harmful effects of antibiotics, such as adverse effects and antibiotic resistance.

So the summary table is an essential start, but it tells us only what the positive and negative effects are likely to be for an 'average' child. As no child is exactly average, we next need to consider how the effects may vary in different subgroups. We need to

Outcome	% in placebo group	RRR (%)	ARR/100	Comments
Beneficial effects				
Pain 2–7 days	14	28	5	Greater if fever, vomiting
Neutral or uncertain effects				
Pain < 1 day	38	0	0	No treatment effect found
Mastoiditis	0	?	–	1 case in 2250 (AB group)
'Glue ear' 3M	26	–	–	No treatment effect found
Adverse effects				
Vomiting, rash or diarrhoea	11	55	5	Vomiting, rash, diarrhoea

ARR, absolute risk reduction; RRR, relative risk reduction.

***Table** 4.1:* **Summary of findings from a systematic review of antibiotics for acute otitis media**

consider this in both relative and absolute terms. Once again, the data required for the next two steps are often limited within individual trials, and should usually be part of a systematic review process. The responsibility of the individual clinician is to be aware of the importance of this additional evidence and know how to access it.

Are the benefits or harms likely to be different in a primary care setting?

Does the setting in which the evidence was gathered suggest that the relative benefit for an individual in primary care will differ predictably from the average effect in the trial, and is this predictable from non-setting factors? A useful way to remember the variety of factors that may have an impact on the size of the effect is to use the mnemonic PICO used for question formulation in evidence-based medicine[13] (panel 4.1). The size of effect may vary by:

- the population
- the intervention and its intensity, dosage or timing
- the comparator or background therapy
- the outcome measurement method (e.g. the definition, instruments, and timing used).

Obviously the population differs between primary care and other settings, but the other three elements may also change (e.g. the delivery of the intervention or the comparison therapy used in primary care may be less intensive).

The four questions that must be addressed in undertaking PICO appraisal are set out in panel 4.1. The key thing to remember is that you are not assessing the generalisability of the absolute effect estimated by the trial but of the relative effect. For example, in applying the population question, many of the differences between the individual in front of you and the patients in the trial will influence their pretreatment risk of harm or benefit. This does not mean that they will necessarily influence the treatment effect itself. For example, this is likely to be the case for the two individuals with raised cholesterol levels mentioned above in the context of the New Zealand trial. The differences in age and co-risk factors make a huge difference to the likely real benefit from statin treatment (an NNT that is 10-fold different, being around 100 compared with < 10), although the relative benefit and harm of statin treatment is probably similar in both men.

Panel 4.1: Questions used to assess the generalisability of treatment effects

- Population: Is the individual in front of you sufficiently similar to trial participants to be likely to gain a similar *relative* benefit from treatment?
- Intervention: How similar will the treatment be to that given in the trial?
- Context: Are there specific contextual issues for the individual that are very different from the trial context and are likely to influence the outcome for the patient?
- Outcome: Are the outcomes assessed in the trial, and for which an indirect estimate of effect are available, the same outcomes that are important for this individual?

Common intervention issues include whether a relative effect holds for a class of drugs. A good recent example is the debate about the generalisability of class effects for beta-blockers, with the relative effect of atenolol in particular coming in for close scrutiny.[14] The question about context is more difficult. For example, when advising a patient whether he or she will benefit from knee surgery, issues such as the surgical expertise available at the local hospital, the infection rate at that hospital and the home circumstances of the individual may all mean that the relative effect reported from a trial may not be directly applicable to the individual's situation – but for different reasons, information on these factors may be difficult to obtain and quantification is often very difficult.

The approach to assessing individual benefit based on individual risk shown in figure 4.3 only works if the relative effect estimated from trials is stable (i.e. it does not vary much according to the individual's risk of disease or side-effects without treatment). In the case of otitis media, this appears to hold true for side-effects. The likelihood of adverse outcome from antibiotic treatment (i.e. diarrhoea, antibiotic resistance) does not appear to vary with baseline severity. The relative risk reduction does vary, but not substantially – in one of the randomised trials, a retrospective subgroup analysis suggested that children with high fever or vomiting benefited more than those without these symptoms,[15] but the difference in relative effect was modest (less than two-fold). Fortunately, this relative stability of effect estimates from group trials is not restricted to otitis media. The stability of relative effect has been observed in trials of interventions for many different conditions, and estimates of relative risk reduction are certainly more stable than estimates of absolute risk reduction. This was shown particularly clearly in the meta-meta-analysis done by Schmidt et al.[16] of over 115 group trials, which reported a variation in relative risk of less than half that in absolute risk (13% versus 31%).

However, it is wrong to imply that the relative effect is invariably constant across risk levels. For example, the risk factors for mastoiditis are not well understood and the trials of otitis media have not been powered to assess this rare outcome. If in future it becomes possible to define prior mastoiditis risk (e.g. on the basis of genetics or immunity), and to conduct a trial large enough to assess this outcome, the relative risk reduction achieved by antibiotics is unlikely to be constant. There are very good examples of trials in other disease areas where subgroup analysis has suggested that the relative effect of treatment will be substantially different between subgroups. Clearly empirical evidence would be useful, but often a clinical judgement will need to be used regarding this issue.

Applying the evidence to an individual patient in primary care

Assuming the answers to the PICO questions all suggest acceptable relevance to primary care, and the relative effect estimates from the trials seem to be stable, the final step in putting theory into practice is to apply the evidence assembled to make an assessment of absolute benefit of treatment for the individual patient in front of us. The theory behind this has already been set out in the section above on indirect assessment – the absolute risk reduction for an individual is obtained by applying the relative effect estimate to the individual's prior risk. However, this is only possible in clinical practice if the information on both relative effect and prior risk is to hand in a usable format. This is increasingly the case for some clinical conditions (e.g. most general practitioners in the UK now use coronary heart disease risk charts to assess the need for treatment of mild hypertension), but is certainly not the case for all.

The problem in applying trials from other settings to primary care is then that the spectrum may be different. But, as illustrated in figure 4.4, this is an average difference. In primary care, fewer patients may benefit from the intervention. However, in all settings we would prefer to understand which individual patients would have a net benefit. That may be a different proportion in different settings, but is dependent on the features of the individual, not the setting. However, to assess which patients would receive benefit requires appropriate predictive information to allow individualisation.

The information is available for cardiovascular disease because the treatment (prescribing medication) is the same in primary as secondary care, the relative effect estimates are fairly stable, and the key determinants of prior risk are easily characterised (by age, smoking status, cholesterol level and blood sugar). The lack of similar 'at hand' information for other conditions is more often due to lack of adequate characterisation of prior risk in primary care than to anxieties about the stability and transferability of the relative effect estimate. In addition, the lack of adequate evidence on prior risk often extends not only to the disease the treatment is trying to ameliorate but also to other potential adverse outcomes of treatment, particularly those associated with comorbidity.

Thus the problem of generalisability cannot be ignored but it is sometimes overestimated. It is not self-evident that trials undertaken in hospital are inapplicable to

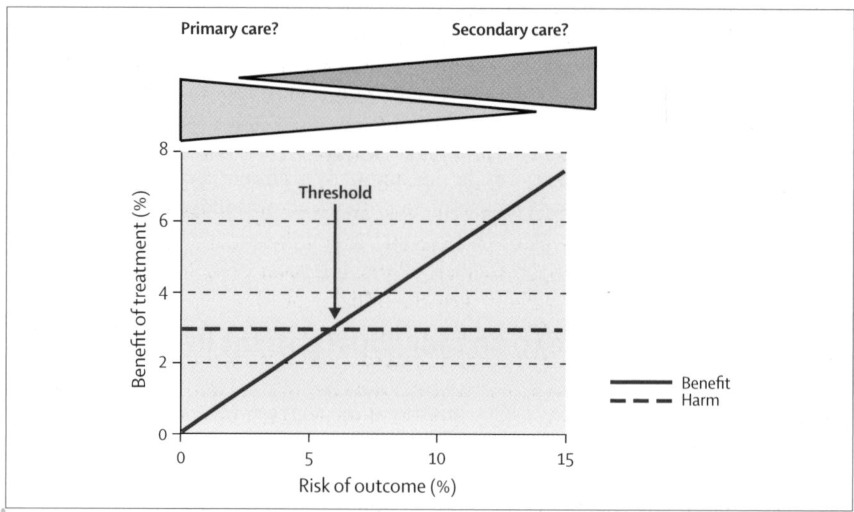

Figure 4.4: **As with figure 4.3, below the threshold harms outweigh likely benefits. The triangles above the plot show the possible differing spectrums of risk in primary and secondary care.**

primary care. The trial population is different, and the absolute group benefit of treatment will be lower in primary care because disease severity and the likelihood of adverse outcome is generally lower. However, this does not imply that the relative effect estimate will be different. What matters is how the circumstances of the trial compare with the context in which the patient is being treated, and this is best assessed by using the standard PICO appraisal already mentioned.

It is poor practice to prescribe a treatment without assembling the evidence to make this individual estimate of benefit and harm for the patient in front of you. However, we must stress again that, however perfect the model for estimating the trade-off between benefit and harm, the data on which the estimate is based will be imperfect. The estimate is just that – an estimate. When, whether for lack of evidence or fears about generalisability, the estimate is thought to be insecure, then a more direct measurement of benefit is necessary. At its simplest that is just what most clinicians do now – introduce the treatment cautiously and monitor the effect. But, whenever possible, particularly for life-long medications, clinicians should convince patients to make the effort to assess the trade-off formally using the *n*-of-1 trial paradigm.

Discussion

We have argued that there is little evidence of systematic differences in the relative effects of treatments between primary care and other settings. This is probably because the treatment itself is delivered in a similar way and to a similar standard in primary and secondary care. Nevertheless, having a good and stable estimate of relative effect is not enough while we still lack evidence of prior risk in primary care to apply the relative risk to allow us to assess the absolute benefit for the individual.

Moreover, we need to remain aware that group trials may mask important differences in individual response. As clinicians, we cannot distinguish between a treatment that improves everyone by 20% and one that makes some people worse and others better by 50%. A real example of this is the treatment of reflux, where most trials have shown that proton pump inhibitors such as omeprazole are, on average, more effective than H_2-receptor antagonists such as ranitidine. However, in a set of *n*-of-1 trials in 27 patients comparing these two drugs, Wolfe et al.[17] found that omeprazole was preferred by 14 patients but that ranitidine was preferred by six (with the remaining seven patients not showing a clear preference). This differential responsiveness was hidden within the standard trials. Similarly, work has been done in hypertension by rotating patients through the various possible initial drug choices, and thus enabling the patient and doctor to identify the most effective drug for that patient, and to assess any adverse effects. However, group trials remain important for making health policy decisions about which treatments to make available, and because *n*-of-1 trials are impossible for some interventions, group trials often provide the only reliable evidence of effect that we can obtain for the individual.

The other important constraint on generalisability of group trials is that, even if patients responded in the same way, we may not provide exactly the same therapy as the trials. The example of prehospital penicillin for meningococcal disease was cited at the beginning of this chapter – arguably penicillin given in general practice without the ability to provide circulatory support is not the same intervention as penicillin given in hospital with that facility at hand. A striking example of this problem from secondary care is carotid endarterectomy, where two important factors modify the effect. First, the degree of stenosis is important: as we might expect from the model shown in figure 4.3, those with more severe stenosis benefit more, and those at low risk may even by harmed by the surgery. Second, the timing of the procedure is important,[18] as the risk is highest soon after a transient ischaemic attack, and hence the organisation of care can modify the effect of treatment.

Finally, we have outlined a number of problems and traps in individualising treatment for patients in primary care. While there is no simple solution to many of these problems, a number of things may be done to improve our targeting of treatments. First, *n*-of-1 trials can often provide patients with a much more precise and reliable estimate of the benefit they are getting from their treatment, and such trials are feasible in everyday clinical practice. Second, while good clinical trials are important, we need to recognise the equal importance of good prognostic research in estimating individual risk without treatment. Third, systematic reviews should use their additional power to explore more carefully the possible modification of effect; and, particularly for important questions, the reviews should use individual patient data to do so. Finally, guidelines need to give much greater account of the need for individualisation. In particular, rather than simply provide 'one-size fits all' recommendations, guidelines should provide descriptions of the predictors of natural history and of the benefits and harms of treatment options, thus allowing the estimation of individual net benefits or harms. When this is too difficult, as a minimum guidelines should provide caveats about when harms may outweigh benefits, and some alternative treatment options. These steps would go some way to achieving the Hippocratic aim of firstly doing no (net) harm.

References

1 Silagy C, Lancaster T, Stead L, et al. Nicotine replacement therapy for smoking cessation. *The Cochrane Database of Systematic Reviews*, 2004, Issue 3. Art. No. CD000146 (DOI: 10.1002/14651858.CD000146.pub2).

2 Raine R, Haines A, Sensky T, et al. Systematic review of mental health interventions for patients with common somatic symptoms: can research evidence from secondary care be extrapolated to primary care? *BMJ* 2002; **325:** 1082.

3 Harnden A, Ninis N, Thompson M, et al. Pre-hospital parenteral penicillin for children with meningococcal disease: a case–control study. *BMJ* 2006; **332:** 1295–98.

4 Gibson AE, Doran CM, Bell JR, et al. A comparison of buprenorphine treatment in clinic and primary care settings: a randomised trial. *Med J Aust* 2003; **179:** 38–42.

5 Grunfeld E, Levine MN, Julian JA, et al. Randomized trial of long-term follow-up for early-stage breast cancer: a comparison of family physician versus specialist care. *J Clin Oncol* 2006; **24:** 848–55.

6 Sweeney KG, Gray DP, Steele R, Evans P. Use of warfarin in non-rheumatic atrial fibrillation: a commentary from general practice. *Br J Gen Pract* 1995; **45:** 153–58.

7 Fihn SD, Callahan CM, Martin DC, et al. The risk for and severity of bleeding complications in elderly patients treated with warfarin. The National Consortium of Anticoagulation Clinics. *Ann Intern Med* 1996; **124:** 970–79.

8 Nikles CJ, Yelland M, Glasziou PP, Del Mar C. Do individualized medication effectiveness tests (*n*-of-1 trials) change clinical decisions about which drugs to use for osteoarthritis and chronic pain? *Am J Ther* 2005; **12:** 92–97.

9 Guyatt GH, Haynes RB, Jaeschke RZ, et al. Users' guides to the medical literature: XXV. Evidence-based medicine: principles for applying the users' guides to patient care. Evidence-Based Medicine Working Group. *JAMA* 2000; **284:** 1290–96.

10 Glasziou PP, Irwig LM. An evidence based approach to individualising treatment. *BMJ* 1995; **311:** 1356–59.

11 Lubsen J, Tijssen JG. Large trials with simple protocols: indications and contraindications. *Control Clin Trials* 1989; **10** (suppl): 151S–60S.

12 Glaszioul PP, Sanders SL. Investigating causes of heterogeneity in systematic reviews. *Stat Med* 2002; **21:** 1503–11.

13 Glasziou PP, Hayem M, Del Mar CB. Antibiotics for acute otitis media in children. *The Cochrane Library*, 2000, Issue 3. Update Software: Oxford.

14 Lindholm LH, Carlberg B, Samuelsson O. Should beta blockers remain first choice in the treatment of primary hypertension? A meta-analysis. *Lancet* 2005; **366:** 1545–53.

15 Little P, Gould C, Moore M, et al. Predictors of poor outcome and benefits from antibiotics in children with acute otitis media: pragmatic randomised trial. *BMJ* 2002; **325:** 22.

16 Schmid CH, Lau J, McIntosh MW, Cappelleri JC. An empirical study of the effect of the control rate as a predictor of treatment efficacy in meta-analysis of clinical trials. *Stat Med* 1998; **17:** 1923–42.

17 Wolfe B, Del Rio E, Weiss SL, et al. Validation of a single-patient drug trial methodology for personalized management of gastroesophageal reflux disease. *J Manag Care Pharm* 2002; **8:** 459–68.

18 Rothwell PM. External validity of randomized controlled trials: 'To whom do the results of this trial apply?' *Lancet* 2005; **365:** 82–93.

5

The older patient

John Grimley Evans

Introduction

Older people are not well served by evidence-based medicine. As currently conceived, trials and systematic reviews tell clinicians what is likely to happen on average. But patients expect their doctors to do better than average, and older people show greater variability around their average than do younger people. There is a dearth of physiological information for a clinician to draw on in helping a particular patient with a particular pattern of illness. These problems can and must be solved, but for the present all one can do is to illustrate what clinicians dealing with older patients *need* to think about and what guideline writers and the evidence-based medicine industry *ought* to think about.

Ageing and being old

Ageing, in the sense of senescence, is characterised by a progressive loss of adaptability as time passes. The homoeostatic mechanisms on which constancy of the internal environment and survival depend become less sensitive, weaker, less accurate, and less well sustained. Sooner or later individual organisms meet a challenge from their external or internal environment, to which they can no longer mount an effective response and they die. A rise in mortality rates with age is therefore the hallmark of ageing. In the human species this rise in mortality first appears around the age of 11[1] and, apart from perturbations due to violent deaths in early adult life, is a continuous and approximately exponential process thereafter.

Ageing comes about through extrinsic factors in environment and lifestyle interacting with intrinsic factors determined by our genes. Under the influence of our genes and environments we start at different levels of functional ability and we age at different rates. Two broad characteristics that distinguish older people from younger people are, therefore, an average lower adaptability and a greater degree of heterogeneity. Although, on average, people of 80 years of age are weaker than people of 40 years of age, there are plenty of people aged 80 years who are fitter than many people aged 40 years.

A further influence on the well-being of older people is the deeply engrained ageist prejudice prevalent in western society. The prejudice arises culturally and is fostered by the media, as was racial prejudice before that became politically unfashionable. However, health economists have advanced arguments for older people having less claim than younger ones on the resources of society. These arguments are either specious or incompatible with the values of western society,[2] but comfort the prejudiced. Ageism contributes to the disregard of the needs of older people in the design, recruitment and implementation of clinical trials, while politicians and health service managers are keen to believe that older people do not benefit from treatment. The age-associated vulnerability of older people to illness is compounded by the way they are treated or, more commonly, not treated.

Ageing and risk/benefit ratios

Because of age-associated loss of adaptability, treatments that are physically or mentally challenging will on average give poorer results for older than for younger people in terms of fatality and complications. This does not necessarily eradicate the benefits of treatment but is likely to move the risk/benefit ratio adversely. Surgical interventions, for example, are typically more challenging than medical ones, although the newer types of minimally invasive surgery are increasingly applicable to frailer and poorer risk patients. The effects of age-associated vulnerability can be partly mitigated by more intensive care and monitoring than will suffice for younger people.[3, 4] The history of modern medicine glows with the achievements of concerned clinicians pushing the frontiers of applicability of new technologies to the benefit of ever more vulnerable patients. But this will not happen if, by managerial design or clinical neglect, vulnerable older people are excluded from the best of medical care and from the research that underpins such care.

In contrast with the rising risk of ill effects from challenging treatments, non-challenging treatments such as many medications can be more effective if given to older people than to younger ones. This is a particular case of the general principle that treatments will have an absolute effect proportional to the level of background risk. A treatment typically reduces the risk of an undesirable outcome from disease by a percentage that does not diminish with age. But, since the risk of an undesirable outcome of disease does increase with age, so, other things being equal, will the absolute benefit of treatment. This can be illustrated by the results of an early trial of beta-blockers[5] (table 5.1). Other interventions in which absolute benefits are demonstrably comparable with, or greater than, those for younger people include treatments for hypertension,[6] angiotensin converting enzyme (ACE) inhibitors for secondary prevention of cardiovascular disease,[7, 8] antiplatelet therapy for secondary stroke prevention,[9, 10] anticoagulants in atrial fibrillation[11] and statins for prevention of cardiovascular events.[12, 13]

Age	Control group	Timolol group	Reduction (%)	Lives saved per 1000
Cardiac deaths				
< 65	9.7	5.0	48.5	47
≥ 65	15.3	8.0	47.7	73
Reinfarctions				
< 65	13.0	9.2	29.2	38
≥ 65	17.9	9.4	47.5	85

Table 5.1: **Timolol after myocardial infarction[5]**

Not all medical – as distinct from surgical – treatments can be regarded as non-challenging for older people. Age-associated changes in pharmacokinetics, as in the case of benoxaprofen,[14] or in pharmacodynamics, as with benzodiazepines,[15] can result in treatments having a higher risk of severe adverse effects among older than among younger patients. For some other medications, notably the non-steroidal anti-inflammatory drugs (NSAIDs),[16] the mechanisms of an age-associated increase in risk of ill effects may relate more to comorbidity than to pharmacological issues. In some other instances, notably anticoagulant therapy, risks of haemorrhagic complication rise unnecessarily steeply with age because of inadequacies in treatment. Older patients commonly need smaller doses than those required for younger people, and general levels of supervision of therapy may not match the probability of the need for dose adjustment.[17]

There is a large literature on the clinical pharmacology of ageing[18] that can alert trialists to possible risks of adverse effects of drugs in older people. Protocols that insist on fixed doses of drugs are not always appropriate; there is often no reason why drugs should not be individually adjusted in trials to ensure maximum effectiveness. Impaired renal excretion of drugs such as digoxin or gentamycin has long been recognised as a clinical hazard in geriatric practice, but older people vary much more in the degree of renal impairment than was thought 20 years ago. The routine use of indirect methods of guessing the renal function of individuals, from the Galt formula for example, is unreliable and can result in both over- and underdosage. Reduced first-pass metabolism due to reduction in liver size and blood flow is another factor in the clinical pharmacology of ageing. There is, on average, an increased volume of distribution for lipophilic drugs, but age-associated changes in plasma protein binding of drugs are no longer thought to be as important as once assumed.[19] However, the striking feature of the clinical pharmacokinetics of ageing is not so much systematic change as increasing interindividual and intraindividual variability with age.[20] In terms of pharmacodynamics, drugs acting on the central nervous system including antiepileptics, sedatives and antidepressants may show enhanced effects in later life in association with changes in neurotransmitter systems[21] or perhaps changes in blood–brain permeability.

Pharmacological factors also affect the relevance of trial result to clinical practice. Surveys have suggested that age-associated changes in pharmacokinetics and pharmacodynamics may be only a minor cause of an increase with age in the incidence and severity of adverse drug reactions in clinical practice. Polypharmacy, careless prescribing and errors in compliance are perhaps of more importance in the community and hospital.[22] Certainly, the clinician implementing the results of evidence-based medicine needs to be aware that precision and supervision of prescribing and monitoring of compliance are likely to be less rigorous in 'real life' than in clinical trials.[23] This is a concern whatever the age of the patient, but the increased vulnerability of older patients, and the often poorer quality of the care they receive, reduce the margin for error.

Relevance of outcome measures

Trialists seem much possessed by death. Mortality provides an attractively hard endpoint for analysis, but morbidity may be more relevant clinically. There are fates worse than death, and for many older people disability and dependence hold greater dread. In clinical trials, morbidity and mortality may move together in treatment effects; revascularisation manoeuvres in acute myocardial infarction that reduce death rates are also likely to reduce infarct size and the risk of subsequent cardiac failure in survivors. In other contexts, such as heroic attempts to prolong the existence of people with inevitably fatal cancer, postponement of mortality may be associated with an increase in morbidity. But assessing the balance is a matter for the individual patient, whose values and personal life goals are extinguished in standardised measures of quality of life as used by trialists and imposed by regulators. What the clinician needs, and is so often not readily available, is a summary of the probabilities of the range of particular outcomes from treatment and non-treatment. The consequences of these in terms of symptoms and disability can then be matched against the values in an individualised quality-of-life assessment[24] drawn up with each patient. The matching may take place in a traditional clinical consultation or mediated by interactive video[25–27] or computer programmes. Matching treatment to preferences needs also to consider the issue of discounting, the way an individual values benefits and costs at different times in the future. People vary greatly in their general approach to this issue,[28] and many will have specific life goals and hopes that will influence their decisions about healthcare.

The duration of clinical trials is often too short to provide doctors and patients with the information they need for rational decision-making. Trials of cholinesterase inhibitors for Alzheimer's disease have been dominated by change over weeks rather than the months and years of impairment that sufferers and carers commonly have to face.[29] Trial duration is often too short to identify all the benefits and complications of treatment, many of which will also be missed in the processes of postmarketing surveillance. The probable association of sedatives and antidepressants with falls by older people is a case in point.[30]

Selection of older people into trials

It has long been recognised that older people are underrepresented in clinical trials, for example in treatments for cancer,[31, 32] cardiovascular disease[33] and Parkinson's disease.[34] The problem remains largely unsolved, despite efforts by bodies such as the British Medical Research Council[35] and others[36] to emphasise the need for research relevant to the world's ageing populations. None the less, the clinician has an ethical duty to assume that, until proved otherwise, a treatment shown to be effective for younger adults will also be effective for older ones. A recent review[37] suggests that underrepresentation of older people in trials distorts age-group differences in absolute risks more than relative risks. This is reassuring, but there remains a need for incentives or sanctions to encourage the inclusion of older people in trials, and more precise estimates of variation in treatment effects with age.

In addition to general underrepresentation of older people in clinical trials, those who do get enrolled may not be representative of the older people who will be subjected to the results. Typically, patients are selected for having only the target disease, uncomplicated by the comorbidity that so often complicates clinical practice among older people. Investigators want to avoid deaths or dropouts in their study group, and both requirements militate against older people, or others at risk of intercurrent illness. Participants are required to be able to give informed consent, or to have a principal carer who can give valid assent, and either by judgement or a formal run-in period are selected for ability to comply with the trial protocol. There will also be 'volunteer effects'; people agreeing to enter a trial are likely to be more intelligent and better educated than average, and to be favourably inclined to therapy. Harder to quantify will be the 'feel right' factors that determine whether a doctor tries to recruit a particular patient into a trial. This may include preconceptions about age as a risk factor for complications, or the appropriateness of treatment for a patient regarded by the doctor as having a poor quality of life. In an ideal world, randomised trials would be carried out in association with a simultaneous epidemiological study identifying and classifying all cases of the target condition arising within the same catchment area.[38] There can then be direct comparison of patients excluded from the trial with those enrolled.

The general trend of all these factors is for older patients enrolled in trials to be physically and mentally fitter, and socially better off, than the average for the patients to which trial results are to be generalised. Opinions differ on the magnitude and clinical significance of the non-explicit selection of patients into trials,[23, 39] and it may vary from one community to another.

Estimates of overall treatment effects in trials are often heavily weighted by results for the younger participants, who may differ clinically from their older colleagues. Older people tend to be relatively late and slow in presenting for diagnosis and treatment, and when they reach hospital will be later in the evolution of their illness than younger patients. There will be psychosocial reasons for this, especially a fear of hospitals or an unwillingness to 'make a fuss' or 'be a nuisance'. There are also relevant age-associated trends in the symptomatology of disease, including differences in pain perception, with reduced sensitivity to visceral and superficial pain[40] that can, for example, delay perception of heart attacks and heart failure.[41] A lower frequency of prodromal angina in older patients developing myocardial infarction has been shown to be associated with poorer results after treatment.[42] In meeting a trial protocol an assumed 'first attack' of an illness may be nothing of the sort, and important risk factors such as minor cerebrovascular disease may have been forgotten or misdiagnosed. Such factors may increase the risk of complications from treatment.

Changes in the clinical spectrum of disease in older people over time may make the results of trials out of date. Differences in health and social circumstances between successive cohorts of older people in changing societies can be surprisingly large. Over the last quarter century the influence of geriatric medicine has improved the standards of diagnosis applied to older people. Many instances of 'senile dementia', previously dismissed as 'normal ageing' and of no medical interest, are now recognised as potentially preventable or treatable Alzheimer's or vascular disease.[43, 44] Other diseases, such as motor neuron disease, transient global amnesia, epilepsy, progressive supranuclear palsy, once thought to be rare in old age are now recognised as not unusual. Changes in diagnostic criteria may affect detection; laboratory criteria suggest that myasthenia gravis may be more common in later life than is recognised clinically.[45]

5 The older patient

Improvement in diagnosis often comes about through better recognition of characteristic clinical patterns, and this means that only the more severe cases are recognised at first. Severity is likely to be associated with high risk of undesirable outcome and hence with greater absolute treatment effects; when trial results are later applied to milder cases the risk/benefit ratio may drift adversely. All these effects call for some form of continuous monitoring of treatment outcomes, since repetition of trials would be practically and ethically impossible.

Subgroup analysis

Subgroup analysis can reveal highly important information on the optimal targeting of treatment.[46] However, there are dangers of false-positive and false-negative results from post hoc analysis of clinical trials in a search for subgroups that differ in their response to treatment. The dangers are well known but possibly underestimated.[47] Spurious findings are more likely if subgroup-specific analyses are undertaken rather than a modelling search for interaction.[48–50] The practical danger lies not so much in finding apparent subgroup effects as in regarding them as anything more than hypothesis generating. Whether the hypothesis is worth pursuing in formal trials will depend on its biological plausibility and clinical implications, and whether there is support for it in observational data. Most new treatments are for diseases that increase in frequency with age, and there can be no reason for not prespecifying age as a variable to be pursued in subgroup analysis. The same issue applies to systematic reviews and meta-analyses. Ideally, one would wish to see trials designed to have sufficient power to detect clinically significant age effects, although this might require a considerable increase in trial size. Other approaches could include age-specific stopping rules in a trial to allow increased time for recruitment of older people.

Relative risks, even if similar across age groups, may not tell us all we need to know about age effects. Table 5.2 shows data on deaths from a review of trials of thrombolysis for acute myocardial infarction. There was a net gain from thrombolysis in terms of lives saved in all age groups, and the poorer result among patients aged over 75 years was not significantly different in statistical terms from the other age groups. To the clinician concerned with doing the best for each individual patient, the table suggests that, although thrombolysis prevents some later deaths among patients aged over

Age group	Benefit (SD) in deaths per 1000		
	Days 0–1	Days 2–35	Days 0–35
< 55	3 (2)	9 (2)	11 (3)
55–64	0 (3)	18 (3)	18 (4)
65–74	-3 (3)	31 (5)	27 (5)
≥ 75	-26 (8)	35 (11)	10 (13)

Table 5.2: **Fibrinolytic therapy in suspected acute myocardial infarction**[82]

75 years, it rapidly kills or brings forward the deaths of some others. A subsequent observational study of Medicare patients[51] suggested that this might indeed be true, and that in real life the elderly patients who do badly with thrombolysis are more numerous that they were in the trials. Subsequent debate[52, 53] missed the clinical point in focusing on overall mortality. Whatever the numerical balance between patients saved and patients killed, an individual will reasonably wish medical science to be able to say which group he or she is in before the treatment is applied.

Such situations call for case–control studies to generate hypotheses about causes and mechanisms to be tested in appropriate trials. There may also be reasonable prior hypotheses from other sources. The complications of thrombolytic therapy include myocardial rupture that may occur earlier following thrombolysis[54] and increases in risk with age and with delayed hospital admission.[55] The issue remains unresolved, and has been overtaken by further developments in revascularisation in acute myocardial infarction.[56] None the less it exemplifies both the need for a clinical perspective in interpreting results from clinical trials, and the relevance of observational studies from health services data.

A more rational and balanced approach to subgroup analysis to generate hypotheses for further and more refined evaluation may become more possible as funding agencies increasingly insist on the data from trials archived in the public domain. The traditional right enjoyed by researchers to hoard data and prevent access by other workers should be recognised and dealt with as an abuse.

The *n*-of-1 trial

The *n*-of-1 trial has a long history of use in psychological research[57] and is acknowledged as especially valuable as an aid for appropriate prescribing for some older patients with chronic and complex illness.[58] Indeed, as detailed in Chapter 15, it is surprising that *n*-of-1 trials are not used more often. Under double-blind conditions, the patient receives randomised periods of treatment or control, or, more commonly, sequences of paired treatment or control in randomised order. Symptom scores for each period are recorded and, after unblinding, treatment and control can be compared. The comparison may be between treatment and placebo[59] or between different treatments or different dosages. For patients taking several drugs, *n*-of-1 trials can be particularly useful in identifying which are effective or which are responsible for adverse effects.[60]

It has been proposed that hospital pharmacy services[58] or an academic department[60] might provide an '*n*-of-1 support service' of placebos and randomisation designs to enable clinicians to use *n*-of-1 trials in a more or less routine manner to refine their prescribing for individual patients. A similar service in general practice has been described.[61] The active involvement of patients in the evaluation and choice of their medications probably enhances the placebo component of treatment effects, and certainly improves the quality and effectiveness of the doctor–patient collaboration.

Although simple in principle, the design of an *n*-of-1 trial requires care. The outcomes of interest must be defined in advance, and an adequately reliable method of measurement identified and assessed for reliability and validity. A patient-rated scale of relevant symptoms will often answer the question of interest. The duration of each period of treatment or control will depend on the pharmacological properties of the treatments under evaluation, with due attention to ensuring adequate time for loading and wash-out, especially if there is a danger of undesirable interaction between the treatments being compared. Commonly, a trial of practical duration does not generate enough observations for formal statistical testing and a simple balance of scores or preferences may suffice.

Although designed to answer different questions from those needing conventional group trials,[62] *n*-of-1 trials can be combined to provide estimates of overall population effectiveness and prior probabilities of response for individual patients.[63] Conceivably, future information technology will allow for cumulative files of such data to guide clinicians and patients in their choice of treatment. With rising costs of effective drugs there is often hope that an *n*-of-1 trial will lead to the withdrawal of an ineffective drug or, if two treatments are indistinguishable in their effects, the continued prescription of the more cost-effective drug.[64] In practice, patients may resist the withdrawal of a drug, even if it is shown to be ineffective, unless this has been negotiated in advance of the trial being undertaken.[65]

Use of routine health service data

It is regrettable that the UK has fallen so far behind some other countries in the design and use of routine health service databases for research and evaluation. Forty years ago, the Oxford Record Linkage Study (ORLS) demonstrated the value of linking the different records generated by individuals.[66] The ORLS data were later used to show a link between prescriptions for minor tranquillisers and road traffic accidents.[67] Since then the potential for identifying adverse effects of drugs by linking prescription and routine morbidity records has been powerfully demonstrated in American data sets. A notable example is the association between prescriptions for certain types of drugs and subsequent falls by older people.[30] Given that clinical trials fail older people by being too small and too short, better systems of routine data collection could be a powerful complementary source of information. Unfortunately, particularly since the reforms of 1985, British health service data systems have been designed for the convenience of administrators and accountants rather than clinicians and medical scientists. This is a tragic waste of an opportunity. Routine data can complement trials and systematic reviews by assessing their relevance to 'real-life' clinical situations. They can monitor the 'roll-out' of new treatments, to audit their application and seek evidence that effects are compatible with the trial findings. With a longer term follow-up they can detect rare and indirect adverse effects more efficiently and reliably than conventional systems of postmarketing surveillance. They can be used to generate hypotheses about how best to deploy new treatments to groups and individuals.

Routine data systems complement, but cannot replace, randomised trials. As detailed in Chapter 1, there are pervasive and directly unquantifiable sources of bias in the application of treatments and in the selection of patients into different segments of healthcare systems. Standard methods of adjustment for case mix are unreliable,[68] a fact inadequately appreciated by creators of hospital star rating systems. The finding in health service data that older patients given beta-blockers after myocardial infarction fared better than those who were not, was compatible quantitatively with the advantage to be expected on the basis of clinical trials.[69] However, other evidence[70] indicated that older age and functional impairment were independently associated with the withholding of treatment from patients with no specific contraindications to beta-blockers. While this might partially explain the increased mortality in untreated patients, it does not imply that the withholding of treatment was appropriate. We see here perhaps another example of the well-known 'inverse care law'[71] that those people who most need treatment are the least likely to receive it – often because of good intentions with perverse effects.

An important function of a well-designed system of clinically orientated data would be as a substrate for specific studies, providing a sampling frame embodying basic demographic data, a diagnostic and therapeutic registry, and a ready-made structure into which study-specific data such as *n*-of-1 studies could be entered and their data accumulated.

Predictive equations

Although age commonly appears in lists of risk factors for diseases such as stroke or cancer, it would be a 'category error' to regard it as a cause or mechanism of disease in the same way as smoking for lung cancer or hypertension for stroke. Age is a numerical abstraction that cannot be a cause or mechanism for anything. It appears as a risk factor for disease because of the causes and mechanisms of disease with which it is statistically associated. If one aims at predicting the probability of disease in an individual, it is those causes and mechanisms that should be assessed, not age. Indeed, where sufficient is known about the aetiology and pathogenesis of a disease or other event, and provided that the other parameters are fed in first, age should 'drop off the end' of the predictive equation. The APACHE-III equation for predicting outcome from intensive care included 17 physiological variables that accounted for 47.2% of explanatory power; age accounted merely for an additional 3%.[72] Ethical as well as biological issues, not just statistical considerations, should determine the order in which variables are fed into predictive equations, especially if such equations are used as self-fulfilling prophecies rather than indicators of need for extra care.

The overall vulnerability of an elderly individual may not be adequately reflected in the sum of individual organ function. An overall 'frailty'[73] may determine the interactions between specific organ impairments. For decades geratologists have sought ways of recognising the 'biological age' of individuals as distinct from their chronological ages. Biological age is conceptualised in terms of the immediate probability of death and the remaining lifespan. Various attempts have been made to measure biological age as a function of age-associated changes,[74] but this epidemiological approach has recently been replaced by a search for 'biomarkers' of intrinsic ageing. On basic biological grounds it is to be expected that there are time-related processes in the body that affect all cells and tissues and will be manifested both as contributors to age-associated diseases and to the general vulnerability of frailty.[75] One process of possible relevance is the progressive shortening of chromosomal telomeres, with cell division leading to transcription errors and to ultimate failure of cell division. The mean length of peripheral blood cell telomeres is related to subsequent survival time,[76] and so qualifies as a potential biomarker. Future assessment of the appropriateness of medical interventions for individuals may include markers of generalised intrinsic ageing as well as measures of specific organ function.

Why is the older individual neglected?

Trials of new drugs, especially trials run for pharmaceutical companies, are concerned primarily with providing evidence of efficacy (Can it work in ideal situations?) rather than effectiveness (Does it do any good in real-life situations?).[77] Efficiency or cost-effectiveness (Is it cheaper than alternatives?) is a later matter of interest to both managers and clinicians, although they might differ over what constitutes an alternative. In particular, doing nothing is less acceptable in clinical practice than managers would wish.

Health service managers and their political masters are more content than they should be to ignore the needs of older people in the conduct of trials and reviews. Through ignorance or disingenuousness, politicians regard health services not as a means to help individuals attain personal life goals but as a branch of public health – maximising the fitness of the populace to serve the interest of the state. What a treatment does for individuals is, therefore, of little interest compared with what happens on average. It does not matter how many individuals a treatment kills as long as it is less than the number it saves. This philosophy is unaffected if the unit of measurement is quality-adjusted life years (QALYs) rather than individuals. QALYs, however, add a further dimension of ageism, since whatever benefits older individuals may obtain from treatments, their lower life expectancy means that they have fewer QALYs to offer the politician and health economist.[78] It is unfortunate that clinicians are not more powerful among the captains of the evidence-based medicine industry in resisting this 'collectivist' philosophy.[1] The size of trials and the statistical precision of their results enjoy too great a precedence over clinical relevance.

Western governments and insurers have been panicking over the rapid growth in healthcare costs. Attempts to control costs by regulation and rationing generate medical systems based on guidelines and protocols; these inevitably do less than best for a non-standard patient, even with a standard disease. But governments and insurers also have an interest in excluding older people from healthcare. Cross-sectional data show that average annual costs per person increase in old age. Contrary to popular misconception, this does not mean that ageing of a population will increase its healthcare costs. Health costs occur because people become ill, and will be incurred at whatever age that happens.[79, 80] In Western populations most illness is now delayed until our later years and is concerned mainly with improving quality, rather than duration, of life. This is surely as we would wish it, but the cross-sectional data allow unscrupulous politicians to imply that older people are responsible for rising healthcare costs and that much of health expenditure in later life is futile. This strengthens public prejudice and discourages researchers from trying harder to include older people in trials.

Conclusion

The challenge is not one that can be met by methodological tinkering. The rationale of the whole system of medical research and regulation needs radical change. While the randomised controlled trial remains a fundamental tool of medical progress, the need for and relevance of complementary and supplementary sources of evidence must be properly recognised. There needs to be a coherent structure of evaluation and subsidiary trials. The 'hierarchy of evidence', in which precedence is given to the form rather than the quality and relevance of data, should be consigned to the graveyard of human oversimplifications. However, the complementary and supplementary evidence from real life must be collected systematically and comprehensively in a form that can be readily accessed and interacted with by clinicians and patients. Clinical innovation and development should be encouraged and supported by adequate documentation and coordination.

Trialists and regulators should be required to draw clear distinction between the collectivist thinking appropriate to public health measures and the concern for individuals that should underpin clinical services. For the latter, the interaction between patient and clinician should guide the design and implementation of trials. Too little research is undertaken into individual predictors of response to treatment. In a rational world such research would follow automatically after the demonstration of the efficacy of a treatment. While the preoccupation of pharmaceutical companies and regulators with efficacy rather than effectiveness is largely to blame, funding agencies have also failed to develop a strategic vision focused on the needs of individual patients. Some agencies might be more enthused by biological rather than clinical approaches to the study of human ageing.[81]

While older patients have most to gain from a focus on the individual in health service research and practice, many of the issues discussed in this chapter apply also to women and members of ethnic minorities. But we are all more or less eccentric, and have a right to have our idiosyncrasies respected in the health services we pay for.

References

1 Grimley Evans J. A correct compassion. The medical response to an ageing society. *J R Coll Phys (London)* 1997; **31:** 674–84.

2 Grimley Evans J. Rationing health care by age. The case against. *BMJ* 1997; **314:** 11–12.

3 Scalea TM, Simon HM, Duncan AO, et al. Geriatric blunt multiple trauma: improved survival with early invasive monitoring. *J Trauma* 1990; **30:** 129–34.

4 Battistella FD, Din AM, Perez L. Trauma patients 75 years and older: long-term follow-up results justify aggressive management. *J Trauma* 1998; **44:** 618–23.

5 The Norwegian Multicenter Study Group. Timolol-induced reduction in mortality and reinfarction in patients surviving acute myocardial infarction. *N Engl J Med* 1981; **304:** 801–07.

6 MRC Working Party. Medical Research Council trial of treatment of hypertension in older adults: principal results. *BMJ* 1992; **304:** 405–12.

7 Flather MD, Yusuf S, Kober L, et al. Long-term ACE-inhibitor therapy in patients with heart failure or left-ventricular dysfunction: a systematic overview of data from individual patients. *Lancet* 2000; **355:** 1575–81.

8 The Heart Outcomes Prevention Evaluation Study Investigators. Effects of an angiotensin-converting-enzyme inhibitor, ramipril, on cardiovascular events in high-risk patients. *N Engl J Med* 2000; **342:** 145–53.

9 Antiplatelet Trialists' Collaboration. Collaborative overview of randomised trials of antiplatelet therapy – I: Prevention of death, myocardial infarction, and stroke by prolonged antiplatelet therapy in various categories of patients. *BMJ* 1994; **308:** 81–106.

10 Sivenius J, Riekkinen PJ, Laakso M. Antiplatelet treatment in elderly people with transient ischaemic attacks or ischaemic strokes. *BMJ* 1995; **310:** 25–26.

11 Atrial fibrillation investigators. Risk factors for stroke and efficacy of antithrombotic therapy in atrial fibrillation. *Arch Intern Med* 1994; **154:** 1449–57.

12 Hunt D, Young P, Simes J, et al. Benefits of pravastatin on cardiovascular events and mortality in older patients with coronary heart disease are equal to or exceed those seen in younger patients: results from the LIPID trial. *Ann Intern Med* 2001; **134:** 931–40.

13 Heart Protection Collaborative Group. MRC/BHF Heart Protection Study of cholesterol-lowering with simvastatin in 5963 people with diabetes: a randomised placebo-controlled trial. *Lancet* 2003; **361:** 2005–16.

14 Hamdy S, Aziz Q, Rothwell JC, et al. Explaining oropharyngeal dysphagia after unilateral hemplegic stroke. *Lancet* 1997; **350:** 686–92.

15 Grimley Evans J, Jarvis EH. Nitrazepam and the elderly. *BMJ* 1972; **4:** 487.

16 Hernández-Diáz S, Rodríguez LAG. Association between nonsteroidal anti-inflammatory drugs and upper gastrointestinal tract bleeding/perforation. An overview of epidemiologic studies published in the 1990s. *Arch Intern Med* 2000; **160:** 2093–99.

17 Garcia D, Regan S, Crowther M, et al. Warfarin maintenance dosing patterns in clinical practice: implications for safer anticoagulation in the elderly population. *Chest* 2005; **127:** 2049–56.

18 McLean AJ, Le Couteur DG. Aging biology and geriatric clinical pharmacology. *Pharmacol Rev* 2004; **56:** 163–84.

19 Benet LZ, Hoener B-A. Changes in plasma protein binding have little clinical significance. *Clin Pharmacol Ther* 2002; **71:** 115–21.

20 Perucca E, Berlowitz D, Birnbaum A, et al. Pharmacological and clinical aspects of antiepileptic drug use in the elderly. *Epilepsy Res* 200; **68:** 49–63.

21 Powers RE. Neurobiology of aging. In: Coffey CE, Cummings JL, eds. *Textbook of Geriatric Neuropsychiatry*. Washington, DC: American Psychiatric Press, 1994: 36–69.

22 Gurwitz JH, Avorn J. The ambiguous relation between aging and adverse drug reactions. *Ann Intern Med* 1991; **114:** 956–66.

23 Krumholz HM, Gross CP, Peterson ED, et al. Is there evidence of implicit exclusion criteria for elderly subjects in randomized trials? Evidence from the GUSTO-1 study. *Am Heart J* 2003; **146:** 839–47.

24 Mountain LA, Campbell SE, Seymour DG, et al. Assessment of individual quality of life using the SEIQoL-DW in older medical patients. *Q J Med* 2004; **97:** 519–24.

25 Murray E, Davis H, Tai SS, et al. Randomised controlled trial of an interactive multimedia decision aid on benign prostatic hypertrophy in primary care. *BMJ* 2001; **323:** 493–96.

26 Murray E, Davis H, Tai SS, et al. Randomised controlled trial of an interactive multimedia decision aid on hormone replacement therapy in primary care. *BMJ* 2001; **323:** 490–93.

27 Phelan EA, Deyo RA, Cherkin DC, et al. Helping patients decide about back surgery: a randomized trial of an interactive video program. *Spine* 2001; **26:** 206–11.

28 West RR, McNabb R, Thompson AGH, et al. Estimating implied rates of discount in healthcare decisions-making. *Health Technol Assess* 2003; **7**(38).

29 Grimley Evans J, Wilcock G, Birks J. Evidence-based pharmacotherapy of Alzheimer's disease. *Int J Neuropsychopharmacol* 2004; **7:** 351–69.

30 Grimley Evans J. Drugs and falls in later life. *Lancet* 2003; **361:** 448.

31 Trimble EL, Carter CL, Cain D, et al. Representation of older patients in cancer treatment trials. *Cancer* 1994; **74** (7 suppl): 2208–14.

32 Hutchins LF, Unger JM, Crowley JJ, et al. Underrepresentation of patients 65 years of age or older in cancer-treatment trials. *N Engl J Med* 2000; **341:** 2061–67.

33 Lee PY, Alexander KP, Hammill BG, et al. Representation of elderly persons and women in published randomized trials of acute coronary syndromes. *JAMA* 2001; **286:** 708–13.

34 Mitchell SL, Sullivan EA, Lipsitz LA. Exclusion of elderly subjects from clinical trials for Parkinson's disease. *Arch Neurol* 1997; **157:** 1393–98.

35 Medical Research Council. *The Health of the UK's Elderly People*. London: Medical Research Council, 1994.

36 Ferrucci L, Guralnik JM, Studenski S, et al. Designing randomized, controlled trials aimed at preventing or delaying functional decline and disability in frail, older persons: a consensus report. *J Am Geriatr Soc* 2004; **52:** 625–34.

37 Bartlett C, Doyal L, Ebrahim S, et al. The causes and effects of socio-demographic exclusions from clinical trials. *Health Technol Assess* 2005; **9:** 1–168.

38 Hornby R, Grimley Evans J, Vardon V. Operative or conservative treatment for trochanteric fractures of the femur: a randomised epidemiological trial. *J Bone Joint Surg* 1989; **71-B:** 619–23.

39 Jha P, Deboer D, Sykora K, Naylor CD. Characteristics and mortality outcomes of thrombolysis trial participants and nonparticipants: a population-based comparison. *J Am Coll Cardiol* 1996; **27:** 1335–42.

40 Gibson SJ, Farrell M. A review of age differences in the neurophysiology of nociception and the perceptual experience of pain. *Clin J Pain* 2004; **20:** 227–39.

41 Friedman MM. Older adults' symptoms and their duration before hospitalization for heart failure. *Heart Lung* 1997; **26:** 169–76.

42 Ishihara M, Sato H, Tateishi H, et al. Beneficial effect of prodromal angina pectoris is lost in elderly patients with acute myocardial infarction. *Am Heart J* 2000; **139:** 881–88.

43 Roth M, Tomlinson BE, Blessed G. Correlation between scores for dementia and counts of 'senile plaques' in cerebral grey matter of elderly subjects. *Nature* 1966; **209:** 109–10.

44 Neuropathology Group of the Medical Research Council Cognitive Function and Ageing Study (MRC CFAS). Pathological correlates of late-onset dementia in a multicentre, community-based population in England and Wales. *Lancet* 2001; **357:** 169–75.

45 Vincent A, Clover L, Buckley C, et al., and the UK Myasthenia Gravis Survey. Evidence of underdiagnosis of myasthenia gravis in older people. *J Neurol Neurosurg Psychiatry* 2003; **74:** 1105–08.

46 Rothwell PM. Subgroup analysis in randomised controlled trials: importance, indications and interpretation. *Lancet* 2005; **365:** 176–86.

47 Brookes ST, Whitley E, Peters TJ, et al. Subgroup analyses in randomised controlled trials: quantifying the risks of false-positives and false-negatives. *Health Technol Assess* 2001; **5**(33).

48 Davey Smith G, Egger M, Phillips AN. Meta-analysis: beyond the grand mean? *BMJ* 1997; **315:** 1610–04.

49 Thompson SG, Higgins JP. Treating individuals. 4: Can meta-analysis help target interventions at individuals most likely to benefit? *Lancet* 2005; **365:** 341–46.

50 Rothwell PM, Mehta Z, Howard SC, et al. Treating individuals 3: from subgroups to individuals: general principles and the example of carotid endarterectomy. *Lancet* 2005; **365:** 256–65.

51 Thiemann DR, Coresh J, Schulman SP, et al. Lack of benefit for intravenous thrombolysis in patients with myocardial infarction who are older than 75 years. *Circulation* 2000; **101:** 2239–46.

52 White HD. Thrombolytic therapy in the elderly. *Lancet* 2001; **356:** 2028–30.

53 Thiemann DR, Coresh J, Schulman SP, et al. Thrombolytic therapy and mortality. *Lancet* 2001; **357:** 1367.

54 Becker RC, Charlesworth A, Wilcox RG, et al. Cardiac rupture associated with thrombolytic therapy: impact of time to treatment in the Late Assessment of Thrombolytic Efficacy (LATE) study. *J Am Coll Cardiol* 1995; **25:** 1063–68.

55 Figueras J, Cortadellas J, Calvo F, Soler-Soler J. Relevance of delayed hospital admission on development of cardiac rupture during acute myocardial infarction: study in 225 patients with free wall, septal or papillary muscle rupture. *J Am Coll Cardiol* 1998; **32:** 135–39.

56 Mehta RH, Granger CB, Alexander KP, et al. Reperfusion strategies for acute myocardial infarction in the elderly: benefits and risks. *J Am Coll Cardiol* 2005; **45:** 471–78.

57 Martin M. Single subject designs for assessments of psychotropic drug effects in children. *Child Psychiatry Hum Dev* 1971; **2:** 102–15.

58 Price JD, Grimley Evans J. *N*-of-1 randomized controlled trials ('*N*-of-1 trials'): singularly useful in geriatric medicine. *Age Ageing* 2002; **31:** 227–32.

59 Price JD, Grimley Evans J. An *N*-of-1 randomized controlled trial ('*N*-of-1 trial') of donepezil in the treatment of non-progressive amnestic syndrome. *Age Ageing* 2002; **31:** 307–09.

60 Guyatt G, Sackett D, Taylor DW, et al. Determining optimal therapy – randomized trials in individual patients. *N Engl J Med* 1986; **314:** 889–92.

61 Nikles CJ, Clavarino AM, Del Mar CB. Using *n*-of-1 trials as a clinical tool to improve prescribing. *Br J Gen Pract* 2005; **55:** 175–80.

62 Spiegelhalter DJ. Statistical issues in studies of individual response. *Scand J Gastroenterol* 1988; **147** (suppl): 40–45.

63 Zucker DR, Schmid CH, McIntosh MW, et al. Combining single patient (*N*-of-1) trials to estimate population treatment effects and to evaluate individual patient responses to treatment. *J Clin Epidemiol* 2005; **50:** 401–10.

64 Karnon J, Qizilbash N. Economic evaluation alongside *n*-of-1 trials: getting closer to the margin. *Health Econ* 2001; **10:** 79–82.

65 Woodfield R, Goodyear-Smith F, Arroll B. *N*-of-1 trials of quinine efficacy in skeletal muscle cramps of the leg. *Br J Gen Pract* 2005; **55:** 181–85.

66 Acheson ED. Oxford Record Linkage Study. A central file of morbidity and mortality records for a pilot population. *Br J Prev Soc Med* 1964; **18:** 8–13.

67 Skegg DCG, Richards SM, Doll R. Minor tranquillizers and road accidents. *BMJ* 1979; **1:** 917–19.

68 Deeks JL, Dinnes J, D'Amico R, et al. Evaluating non-randomised intervention studies. *Health Technol Assess* 2003; **7**(27).

69 Soumerai SB, McLaughlin TJ, Spiegelman D, et al. Adverse outcomes of underuse of beta-blockers in elderly survivors of acute myocardial infarction. *JAMA* 1997; **277:** 115–21.

70 Vitagliano G, Curtis JP, Concato J, et al. Association between functional status and use and effectiveness of beta-blocker prophylaxis in elderly survivors of acute myocardial infarction. *J Am Geriatr Soc* 2004; **52:** 495–501.

71 Hart JT. The inverse care law. *Lancet* 2005; **1:** 405–12.

72 Knaus WA, Wagner DP, Lynn J. Short-term mortality predictions for critically ill hospitalized adults: science and ethics. *Science* 1991; **254:** 389–94.

73 Rockwood K, Hogan DB, MacKnight C. Conceptualisation and measurement of frailty in elderly people. *Drugs Aging* 2003; **17:** 295–302.

74 Comfort A. Test-battery to measure ageing-rate in man. *Lancet* 1969; **2:** 1411–14.

75 Kirkwood TB. The origins of human ageing. *Phil Trans R Soc (London), Ser B* 1997; **352:** 1765–72.

76 Cawthorn RM, Smith KR, O'Brien E, et al. Association between telomere length in blood and mortality in people aged 60 years or older. *Lancet* 2003; **361:** 393–95.

77 Haynes B. Can it work? Does it work? Is it worth it? The testing of healthcare interventions is evolving. *BMJ* 1999; **319:** 652–53.

78 Harris J. QALYfying the value of life. *J Med Ethics* 1987; **13:** 117–23.

79 Zweifel P, Felder S, Meiers M. Ageing of population and health care expenditure: a red herring? *Health Econ* 1999; **8:** 485–96.

80 Seshamani M, Gray A. Ageing and health-care expenditure: the red herring argument revisited. *Health Econ* 2004; **13:** 303–14.

81 House of Lords Science and Technology Committee. *Ageing: Scientific Aspects.* London: The Stationery Office, 2005.

82 Fibrinolytic Therapy Trialists' (FTT) Collaborative Group. Indications for fibrinolytic therapy in suspected acute myocardial infarction: collaborative overview of early mortality and major morbidity results from all randomised trials of more than 1000 patients. *Lancet* 1994; **343:** 311–22.

6

Applying results to treatment decisions in complex clinical situations

Louis R. Caplan

Treating individual patients

Caring for individual patients is complex. Care involves:

- understanding what is wrong with the patient
- understanding the patient's risks for disease
- understanding the patient – their background, genetics, socio-economic milieu, psychology, responsibilities, goals, etc.
- understanding the benefits and risks of potential therapeutic strategies to treat the patient's conditions and to prevent conditions that they are at risk of developing
- communicating with the patient – listening and conveying information, and teaching.

These functions are extensive and often difficult. They take time – a commodity now often jeopardised by large patient lists, managed care directives and the need to support oneself and one's family.

So-called evidence-based medicine relates to only one of these doctor functions – the understanding of the benefits and risks of potential therapeutic strategies. Of course, all treatment should be based on some evidence. It is hard to think of a polite word for treatment that has absolutely no evidential basis. Evidence is defined variously. Some devotees of evidence-based medicine limit evidence that they consider credible to that generated from randomised, double-blind, controlled trials (panel 6.1).[1] The almost

Panel 6.1: Levels of evidence and grading of recommendations for treatment[1]

Level of evidence

- Level 1: data from randomised trials with low false-positive (alpha) and low false-negative (beta) errors
- Level 2: data from randomised trials with high false-positive (alpha) or high false-negative (beta) errors
- Level 3: data from randomised concurrent cohort studies
- Level 4: data from randomised cohort studies that use historical controls
- Level 5: data from anecdotal case series

Strength of treatment recommendations

- Grade A: supported by level 1 evidence
- Grade B: supported by level 2 evidence
- Grade C : supported by level 3, 4 or 5 evidence

religious zeal for cloaking all decisions under the banner of 'evidence based' conceals the real problem – that is, what is the evidence? Does it apply to the individual patient being treated? What is the context in which the evidence was gathered and will be applied? Trials have theoretical and practical limitations. Herein I explore those limitations in relation to practical decisions that doctors must make every day. As a neurologist I will use as an example a patient with cerebrovascular disease, because this condition is most familiar to me.

Doctors often deal with complex decisions in patients with multiple problems. George Thibault[2] stated the issue in relation to patients quite well:

> *We then need to decide which approach in our large therapeutic armamentarium will be most appropriate in a particular patient, with a particular stage of disease and particular coexisting conditions, and at a particular age. Even when randomised clinical trials have been performed (which is true for only a small number of clinical problems), they will often not answer this question specifically for the patient sitting in front of us in the office or lying in the hospital bed.*[2]

Limitations of trials

To provide statistically valid results, randomised trials must contain large numbers of patients with sufficient end points for analysis. Enough end points must be obtained in a relatively short time. The condition studied must be acute and soon cause adverse end points or rapid improvement. Chronic conditions must be severe enough to cause definite definable end points within 1–5 years of follow-up. Many medical and neurological conditions are unsuitable for study by trials. Many conditions are not common enough to generate sufficient sample sizes. Patients who are too ill, too old, too young, female and 'of childbearing age', incapable of giving informed consent, too complex, or too full of coexisting illnesses are often not included in trials.

The major theoretical limitation of trials is the issue of numbers versus specificity.[3] For trials to yield statistically valid and important results, they must include many patients (numbers). For results to be useful to practising physicians, the data must be specifically applicable to individual patients who have the condition studied (specificity). To include large numbers of patients, the condition studied must be common, and usually multiple physicians at multiple centres must be used. A single doctor or centre would enrol too few patients or would take an unacceptably long time to accrue the number of patients needed. To achieve numbers, a 'lumping' strategy often predominates over 'splitting'. For example, to study agents that might effectively prevent stroke, trials have often lumped together patients who have had transient ischaemic attacks (TIAs), those with minor strokes, and even those at high risk of stroke but who have not yet had clinical brain ischaemia. The problem is that strokes have very heterogeneous causes, and one treatment strategy clearly cannot effectively treat all. Using this lumping strategy no single treatment has shown more than 30% effectiveness. Many of these trials have not required sufficient diagnostic testing so that clinicians could not identify the cause of the brain ischaemia in patients enrolled in the trial, and so could not determine the relevance of the results to their own specific patient with a known cause of brain ischaemia.

Inclusion and exclusion criteria are designed so that the patients entered will be 'pure breed', and it will be possible to follow them until study completion. Most severe co-existent diseases exclude patients, as do relative contraindications to the treatments studied. The many exclusions often make it difficult to recruit enough patients to meet sample size requirements. Estimates of the number of patients a centre believes it will recruit are usually at least 2–3 times more than the number actually entered once the trial starts. Trials studying the effectiveness of warfarin in preventing stroke in atrial fibrillation patients encountered this recruitment problem. The trials excluded patients already on warfarin and those in whom warfarin would be risky (e.g. patients with hypertension, peptic ulcer or past bleeding on warfarin). Severe intercurrent illness, such as alcoholism, cancer, liver and renal disease, are exclusions, as are cardiac lesions, other than atrial fibrillation, known to be potential sources of emboli. Physicians participating in these studies screened 15–25 atrial fibrillation patients to obtain each eligible patient.

Eligible patients are not always easy to enrol in trials. Many patients decline because they do not want to be 'guinea pigs' and view trials as something 'others' do. Some patients are put off by the acknowledged lack of a scientific basis for treatment and cannot accept that a 'flip of the coin' decides treatment. Some are disturbed that neither they nor their physicians will know what treatment they receive. Especially disconcerting to patients is the prospect that they might receive a placebo. They believe their problem is serious and warrants active treatment. With time and patience, some of these patients can be enrolled, but with much effort. Alas, some who have enrolled will be dissuaded later by their children, Aunt Tilly or an all-knowing friend, and will drop out. The medical profession must spend more time with public relations and the media to educate the public about trials and the need for participation. Trials are not at present well understood by the average person.

Some observations studied in a trial require clinical experience and judgement. All too often, important components of the examinations are delegated to house officers and young attending physicians. To document that all procedures have been followed and all necessary examinations and evaluations have been performed, most studies require mountains of paperwork. Forms take time to complete. Often, the actual filling out of forms is delegated to the most junior investigator or even a data-entry clerk. The validity of the data is thus jeopardised. The results are only valid if the data are reliable and accurate. Senior experienced clinicians should have seen all patients and personally reviewed the forms to ensure accuracy, but this is often not done.

The pace and clinical course of illness of some medical and neurological conditions are often variable and unpredictable. Stroke is an example of this variability. Different patients with the same vascular lesion (e.g. occlusion of the carotid artery in the neck) have widely different findings in terms of the size and location of infarction, and clinical course. The heterogeneity of outcomes dictates the necessity for using objective criteria, but criteria that are clinically important. The presence of a Babinski sign, exaggerated reflexes, slight facial weakness, slight dysarthria and minor subjective sensory findings do not affect disability. It is tempting to use brain imaging studies to quantitate strokes, but do imaging findings correlate with disability?

In order to compare the effectiveness of different treatments, outcomes must be measured and quantified. This is simple if large events such as death or new stroke are used, but are all strokes equal? In non-fatal diseases, other criteria (e.g. degree of neurological deficit, disability or other 'objective' measures) must be used. Especially in neurology, severity and disability scores are problematic. How can aphasia be compared with double vision, ataxia, facial numbness and limb weakness? How are weights assigned to various abnormalities? For some individuals, a hemianopia that makes reading difficult but does not affect daily living poses no major problem, but to a physician, editor or surveyor the same deficit would be devastating.

Some trials show statistically positive benefits of a treatment, but the amount of the benefit is small and may not be meaningful to most patients. For example, studies of anticholinergic medications in patients with Alzheimer's disease show a decreased pace in the increase in dementia over time, but do not show improvement in present functioning. Families do not see an improvement and cannot appreciate the delay in progressive dementia that might have developed without the drugs, especially if the medications have side-effects.

Meta-analysis and systematic evidence-based reviews are useful but are limited by the quality of the individual trials that are analysed and reviewed. The whole can only be the sum of its parts. Poor data, amalgamated or analysed even by the best statistical methodology, is still inferior data. Attempts to homogenise and summate disparate heterogeneous protocols and methodologies is a problem.

A clinical example

Having explored some theoretical and practical trial limitations, let us now turn to a real patient and see how information from trials is applied in the clinic.

I had a patient, a 59-year-old, Chinese woman, who had three attacks of brain ischaemia during the 4 weeks preceding her visit to me. During the first attack her right hand and face tingled for 5 minutes. During the second attack, which occurred 10 days later, her right arm and hand went weak and numb, and she could not move her fingers. She also could not recall words, and the words that she did use were sometimes incorrect. Her husband could not understand her. Eleven days later she had the third attack, during which she momentarily could not speak, and noticed numbness and tingling in her right face and hand, and she limped when she walked. This attack lasted only about 2 minutes. She had been told of high blood pressure 5 years ago but only took the medicine prescribed when she had a headache or felt poorly. She attended follow-up visits sporadically. She liberally used Chinese herbs and other alternative medical treatments.

Her blood pressure was 155/90, and her pulse was 80 beats/min and regular. General and neurological examinations were normal, except for slight cardiomegaly, and brisker reflexes in her right arm and leg. Ultrasound examinations of her neck and head showed high blood flow velocities in the left middle cerebral artery (MCA). Magnetic resonance imaging (MRI) of her brain showed a small parietal lobe cortical infarct and magnetic resonance angiography (MRA) showed severe (> 90% narrowing) stenosis of the left MCA. The right MCA had a minor degree of stenosis. The neck arteries were normal. The electrocardiogram (ECG) showed slight left ventricular enlargement. A transoesophageal echocardiogram was normal.

This patient had been having TIAs in the left cerebral hemisphere caused by severe stenosis of the left MCA. In addition, she had a small 'silent' infarct in the same vascular territory, although she gave no history of any persisting neurological deficit. Studies of patients from Boston's Chinatown area,[4] where this patient lives, and Hong Kong[5–7] showed that intracranial occlusive disease is common among Asians, especially women.

One of the stated aims of evidence-based medicine is to make it possible for physicians to search the literature to find the evidence base for the treatment of their patients. I searched trial data relevant to choosing treatment for this patient. We first looked at the results of trials of patients with TIAs and minor strokes who were treated with antiplatelet agents.[8–26] The data were clear that aspirin, aspirin with extended-release dipyridamole, ticlopidine and clopidogrel had been shown in trials, with low alpha and beta errors and with convincing meta-analysis data,[24–26] to be somewhat effective in patients with TIAs and minor strokes. Ticlopidine was slightly more effective than aspirin, but had more potential toxicity.[14, 15] Clopidogrel was as effective as ticlopidine and had less toxicity.[21] The combination of aspirin and clopidogrel was not more effective than clopidogrel alone, but caused more bleeding.[22] Aspirin with extended-release dipyridamole was at least as effective as other antiplatelet agents and might be superior.[19, 20] The evidence could be classified as grade A according to published criteria.[1] I explored these trials and meta-analyses further for their relevance to our patient. None of the trials included data on the vascular occlusive lesions that caused the brain ischaemia. There were no data in any of these analyses on patients with MCA stenosis, or on intracranial artery stenosis, or on Asian women. It was difficult to apply the data regarding antiplatelet agents to this patient with much certainty.

I next searched reports of patients with MCA disease, the condition my patient had.[4–7, 29–40] These series were descriptive and contained no prospective or randomised treatment data. There were some retrospective data suggesting that white patients with MCA disease often did well on warfarin-type anticoagulants. These data would be a low grade C at best. However, this retrospective data applied to white patients. Is it reasonable to extrapolate the data to Chinese individuals? The distribution of vascular disease is different in Asians and whites, and the pathology of the vascular disease in the MCAs may differ from disease of the internal carotid arteries (ICAs) in the neck, a disease predominantly of white men, wherein it has been studied more extensively.

I reviewed the published reports, and they indicated that blacks and Asians did not do as well on anticoagulant treatment as whites, and the clinical syndromes differed.

Asians had more deep striatocapsular infarcts, while whites had more surface infarcts, and whites had more TIAs, while Asians and blacks had more strokes. MCA disease was probably different in Asians than in whites. Asians and blacks are posited to have more disease of the vascular media and infarcts due to hypoperfusion distal to stenosis, while whites might have more intimal disease with luminal white and red thrombi causing distal intra-arterial embolisation.[5] I could not reliably extrapolate the results, anecdotal as they were, from treatment of white patients to the treatment of our Chinese woman. Some reports showed that Asian and white patients with severe MCA occlusive disease had a very high risk of stroke recurrence.[41, 42]

I next searched for randomised trials of anticoagulant treatment in stroke and TIA patients. Unfortunately, most of these studies were old, and none defined the causative vascular occlusive lesions. A Swedish study performed during the 1980s compared aspirin and anticoagulants in patients with carotid territory TIAs.[43] There was no difference in the frequency of recurrent ischaemia between the patients treated with aspirin and those treated with anticoagulants. The vascular lesions in this study were not defined, and there were probably no Asians studied.[43] A rather recent trial, the Warfarin–Aspirin Recurrent Stroke (WARS) study,[44] compared the effectiveness of aspirin and warfarin in patients with brain ischaemia. There was no superiority of either treatment, but there was a trend slightly in favour of aspirin. Vascular imaging was not mandated, and there were no data about patients with intracranial occlusive disease.[44] In a retrospective analysis of outcomes in patients with intracranial occlusive disease treated with warfarin and platelet antiaggregants, patients with intracranial stenosis, most commonly of the MCA, fared better on warfarin than on platelet antiaggregants.[45] This study included 97 white patients, 42 blacks and 12 'others'; 83 patients had intracranial anterior circulation vascular occlusive lesions, including 35 MCA stem and four MCA branch lesions.[45] The report did not analyse results by race, nor was it stated how many of the 'others' were Asians. The data favouring anticoagulant treatment in this study would rate, at best, a low grade C by published evidence-based criteria.[1]

A prospective trial (WASID) compared the effectiveness of 1300 mg/day aspirin with the effectiveness of warfarin in patients with intracranial artery occlusive disease (50–99% stenosis) shown by angiography.[46, 47] Warfarin resulted in better efficacy, but many more haemorrhages. Many patients were not maintained within the targeted therapeutic range for warfarin. When the data were analysed for those within the therapeutic range, warfarin was more effective than aspirin.[47] However, there were too few patients with MCA disease for a statistically meaningful analysis. The data could not be analysed for severity of stenosis within the wide 50–99% range. Very severe stenosis (recall that my patient had > 90% stenosis) would be a situation posited to be more likely to promote formation of red erythrocyte–fibrin thrombi, which would be better treated with anticoagulants than antiplatelets. There was no analysis by sex, and the number of Asians was not reported. Again, the trial did not report enough information relevant to my patient's situation to be very helpful.

An alternative treatment was angioplasty of the MCA lesion. Most reports of angioplasty and stenting involved the carotid arteries in the neck. Very few published reports concerned interventional treatment of intracranial disease, and there were no randomised trials.[48–54] I reviewed the experience of my colleagues and I at the New England Medical Center with patients with MCA stenosis treated with angioplasty.[54] Although most patients did well, impairment of flow in the lenticulostriate arteries was a problem in patients in whom the angioplasty involved the portion of the MCA from which the large perforating arterial branches originated. Angioplasty would entail a moderately high risk of stroke in this patient, who had no important clinical deficit and whose lesion involved the proximal MCA, including the lenticulostriate origins. Thus I would consider this treatment only if medical therapy failed.

Using these data, my own anecdotal experience, and information about the pathology and pathophysiology of brain ischaemia in general and in Asians, I decided that warfarin anticoagulation was probably the most effective medical treatment. However, there were specific problems with this treatment in this patient. She had hypertension and did not take hypertensive medications reliably. She used herbs, and some Chinese foods and herbs contain substances known to have anticoagulant properties. Furthermore, she had been non-compliant in the past and not reliable in coming to the clinic for follow-up. She spoke only Chinese, so that detailed explanations and discussions about anticoagulant treatment might be suboptimal.

I decided, despite the relative contraindications, to try anticoagulant treatment, because in my experience, and that reported in the literature, the likelihood of stroke without treatment was high. I explained the treatment in detail on a number of occasions to try to ensure compliance. Did I make the correct decision? Time will tell how she does. We received little guidance from trials in making our decision, so that our choice could not be considered evidence based. Would a managed-care protocol for this cerebrovascular disease patient dictate the use of platelet antiaggregants, as their use is evidence-based according to the criteria in panel 6.1? Would managed-care managers decline payment for vascular tests because the nature, location and severity of vascular lesions has not been unequivocally shown to effect response to treatment? Vascular lesions have not been shown to not effect treatment; rather, this issue has simply not been studied formally.

Conclusions

Courts continue to wrestle with the issue of the applicability of general laws and precedents from prior individual cases to the case being considered. Data from other sources is only relevant as evidence when it applies directly to the presently considered legal case. The medical profession should emulate this aspect of court procedures when it comes to evidence, for 'evidence' is really a legal term. Although there may be general evidence that a treatment has some effectiveness against a broadly characterised condition such as brain ischaemia, there may be no evidence that it is effective or ineffective for a given very specific vascular cause of brain ischaemia, unless it has been specifically tested for that disorder. Even when a treatment has been tested for that disorder, coexisting factors in that particular patient often complicate the decision about whether or not to use a particular agent in a particular patient at a particular time. Therapeutic decisions are sometimes very complex and require experienced physicians. Treatment decisions for individual patients cannot be made by protocols, rules or computer searches. Evidence from trials, past experience, and intimate detailed knowledge of the patient, the diseases and the wishes and desires of all concerned are required to make difficult therapeutic decisions.

Some envisage that the bulk of medical care in the future will be delivered by primary care physicians, who will spend much time at the computer reviewing evidence bases to guide therapeutic decisions. I suggest that what is also desperately needed is more time spent by general physicians and specialists at the bedside and in the clinic, finding out exactly what is wrong with each patient and getting to know each patient and their thoughts, fears, biases and wishes. Therapeutic decisions are made with, by and for complex individuals. They cannot be readily homogenised without losing the essence of what medical care is all about.

References

1 Cook DJ, Guyatt GH, Laupacis A, Sackett DL. Rules of evidence and clinical recommendations on the use of antithrombotic agents. *Chest* 1992; **102** (suppl 4): 305S–11S.

2 Thibault GE. Clinical problem solving: Too old for what? *N Engl J Med* 1993; **328:** 946–50.

3 Caplan LR. Evidence based medicine: concerns of a clinical neurologist (editorial). *J Neurol Neurosurg Psychiatry* 2001; **71:** 569–576.

4 Feldmann E, Daneault N, Kwan E, et al. Chinese–white differences in the distribution of occlusive cerebrovascular disease. *Neurology* 1990; **40:** 1541–45.

5 Huang YN, Gao S, Li SW, et al. Vascular lesions in Chinese patients with transient ischemic attacks. *Neurology* 1997; **48:** 524–25.

6 Wong KS, Huang YN, Gao S, et al. Intracranial stenosis in Chinese patients with acute stroke. *Neurology* 1998; **50:** 812–13.

7 Wong KS, Li H. Long-term mortality and recurrent stroke risk among Chinese stroke patients with predominant intracranial atherosclerosis. *Stroke* 2003; **34:** 2361–66.

8 Fields WS, LeMak NA, Frankowski RF, Hardy RJ. Controlled trial of aspirin in cerebral ischemia. *Stroke* 1977; **8:** 301–16.

9 Britton M, Helmers C, Samuelsson K. High dose acetylsalicylic acid after cerebral infarction: a Swedish co-operative study. *Stroke* 1987; **18:** 325–34.

10 UK–TIA Study Group. The United Kingdom Transient Ischaemic Attack (UK-TIA) Aspirin Trial: final results. *J Neurol Neurosurg Psychiatry* 1991; **54:** 1044–54.

11 The Dutch TIA Trial Study Group. A comparison of two doses of aspirin (30 mg vs 283 mg a day) in patients after a transient ischemic attack or minor ischemic stroke. *N Engl J Med* 1991; **325:** 1261–66.

12 The SALT Collaborative Group. Swedish aspirin low-dose trial (SALT) of 75 mg aspirin as secondary prophylaxis after cerebrovascular ischaemic events *Lancet* 1991; **338:** 1345–49.

13 Candelise L, Landi G, Perrone P, et al. A randomized trial of aspirin and sulfinpyrazone in patients with TIA. *Stroke* 1982; **13:** 175–79.

14 The Canadian Cooperative Study Group: a randomized trial of aspirin and sulfinpyrazone in threatened stroke. *N Engl J Med* 1978; **299:** 53–59.

15 Gent M, Blakely JA, Easton JD, et al. The Canadian American Ticlopidine Study (CATS) in thromboembolic stroke. *Lancet* 1989; **1:** 1215–20.

16 Hass WK, Easton JD, Adams HP Jr, et al. A randomized trial comparing ticlopidine hydrochloride with aspirin for the prevention of stroke in high-risk patients. *N Engl J Med* 1989; **321:** 501–07.

17 The American-Canadian Cooperative Study Group. Persantine–aspirin trial in cerebral ischemia. Part II. Endpoint results. *Stroke* 1985; **16:** 406–15.

18 Bousser MG, Schwege E, Haguenau M, et al. 'A.I.C.L.A.' controlled trial of aspirin and dipyridamole in the secondary prevention of atherothrombotic cerebral ischemia. *Stroke* 1983; **14:** 5–14.

19 Matias-Guiu J, Davalos A, Pico M, Monasterio V, et al. Low dose acetylsalicylic acid (ASA) plus dipyridamole versus dipyridamole alone in the prevention of stroke in patients with reversible ischemic attacks. *Act Neurol Scand* 1987; **76:** 413–21.

20 European Stroke Prevention Study Group. ESPS: principal end points. *Lancet* 1987; **2:** 1351–54.

21 Diener HC, Cunha L, Forbes C, et al. European Stroke Prevention Study 2. Dipyridamole and acetylsalicylic acid in the secondary prevention of stroke. *J Neurol Sci* 1996; **143:** 1–13.

22 CAPRIE Steering Committee. A randomised, blinded, trial of clopidogrel versus aspirin in patients at risk of ischaemic events (CAPRIE), *Lancet* 1996; **348:** 1329–39.

23 Diener H-C, Bogousslavsky J, Brass LM, et al., on behalf of the MATCH Investigators. Aspirin and clopidogrel vs clopidogrel alone after recent ischemic stroke or transient ischemic attack in high-risk patients (MATCH): randomized, double-blind, placebo-controlled trial. *Lancet* 2004; **364:** 331–37.

24 Sze P, Reitman D, Pincus M, et al. Antiplatelet agents in the secondary prevention of stroke: meta-analysis of the randomized control trials. *Stroke* 1988; **19:** 436–42.

25 Antiplatelet Trialists' Collaboration. Secondary prevention of vascular disease by prolonged antiplatelet treatment. *BMJ* 1988; **296:** 320–31.

26 Antiplatelet Trialists' Collaboration. Collaborative overview of randomized trials of antiplatelet treatment. I. Prevention of death, myocardial infarction and stroke by prolonged antiplatelet therapy in various categories of patients. *BMJ* 1994; **308:** 81–106.

27 Lascelles RG, Burrows EH. Occlusion of the middle cerebral artery. *Brain* 1965; **88:** 85–96.

28 Schwarze JJ, Babikian V, DeWitt LD, et al. 1994. Longitudinal monitoring of intracranial arterial stenoses with transcranial Doppler ultrasonography. *J Neuroimaging* 1994; **4:** 182–87.

29 Caplan LR, Babikian V, Helgason C, et al. Occlusive disease of the middle cerebral artery. *Neurology* 1985; **35:** 975–82.

30 Lhermitte F, Gautier JC, Derouesne C. Nature of occlusion of the middle cerebral artery. *Neurology* 1970; **20:** 82–88.

31 Bogousslavsky J, Barnett HJM, Fox AJ, et al., for the EC/IC bypass Study Group. Atherosclerotic disease of the middle cerebral artery. *Stroke* 1986; **17:** 1112–20.

32 Naritomi H, Sawada T, Kuriyama Y, et al. Effect of chronic middle cerebral artery stenosis on the local cerebral hemodynamics. *Stroke* 1985; **16:** 214–19.

33 Saito I, Segawa H, Shiokawa Y, et al. Middle cerebral artery occlusion: correlation of computed tomography and angiography with clinical outcome. *Stroke* 1987; **18:** 863–68.

34 Hinton R, Mohr JP, Ackerman R, et al. Symptomatic middle cerebral artery stenosis. *Ann Neurol* 1979; **5:** 152–57.

35 Corston RN, Kendall BE, Marshall J. Prognosis in middle cerebral artery stenosis. *Stroke* 1984; **15:** 237–41.

36 Moulin DE, Lo R, Chiang J, et al. Prognosis in middle cerebral artery occlusion. *Stroke* 1985; **16:** 282–84.

37 Feldmeyer JJ, Merendaz C, Regli F. Stenosis symptomatiques de l'artere cerebral moyenne. *Rev Neurol* 1983; **139:** 725–36.

38 Akins PT, Pilgram TK, Cross DT 3rd, Moran CJ. Natural history of stenosis from intracranial atherosclerosis by serial angiography. *Stroke* 1998; **29:** 433–38.

39 Allcock JM. Occlusion of the middle cerebral artery: serial angiography as a guide to conservative therapy. *J Neurosurg* 1967; **27:** 353–63.

40 Wong KS, Li H, Lam WW, et al. Progression of middle cerebral artery occlusive disease and its relationship with further vascular events after stroke. *Stroke* 2002; **33:** 532–36.

41 Wong KS, Li H. Long-term mortality and recurrent stroke risk among Chinese patients with predominant intracranial atherosclerosis. *Stroke* 2003; **34:** 2361–66.

42 Kern R, Steinke W, Daffertshofer M, et al. Stroke recurrences in patients with symptomatic vs asymptomatic middle cerebral artery disease. *Neurology* 2005; **65:** 859–64.

43 Garde A, Samuelsson K, Fahlgren H, et al. Treatment after transient ischemic attacks: a comparison between anticoagulant drug and inhibition of platelet aggregation. *Stroke* 1983; **14:** 677–81.

44 Mohr JP, Thompson JLP, Lazar RM, et al. A comparison of warfarin and aspirin for the prevention of recurrent ischemic stroke. *N Engl J Med* 2001; **345:** 1444–51.

45 Chimowitz MI, Kokkinos J, Strong J, et al. The Warfarin–Aspirin Symptomatic Intracranial Disease Study. *Neurology* 1995; **45:** 1488–93.

46 Chimowitz MI, Lynn MJ, Howlett-Smith H, et al. Comparison of warfarin and aspirin for symptomatic intracranial arterial stenosis. *N Engl J Med* 2005; **352:** 1305–16.

47 Koroshetz W. Warfarin, aspirin, and intracranial vascular disease. *N Engl J Med* 2005; **352:** 1368–70.

48 Higashida RT, Halbach W, Tsai. FY, et al. Interventional neurovascular technique for cerebral revascularization in the treatment of stroke. *AJR* 1994; **163:** 793–800.

49 Clark WM, Barnwell SL, Young LM, Coull BM. Safety and efficacy of angioplasty for intracranial atherosclerotic stenosis (abstract). *Stroke* 1994; **25:** 273.

50 Nakano S, Yokogami K, Ohta H, et al. Direct percutaneous transluminal angioplasty for acute middle cerebral artery occlusion. *AJNR* 1998; **19:** 767–72.

51 Suh DC, Sung K-B, Cho YS, et al. Transluminal angioplasty for middle cerebral artery stenosis in patients with acute ischemic stroke. *AJNR* 1999; **20:** 553–58.

52 The SSYLVIA Study Investigators. Stenting of Symptomatic Atherosclerotic Lesions in the Vertebral or Intracranial Arteries (SSYLVIA): study results. *Stroke* 2004; **35:** 1388–92.

53 Meyers PM, Schumacher HC, Higashida RT, et al. Use of stents to treat extracranial cerebrovascular disease. *Ann Rev Med* 2006; **57:** 437–54.

54 Takis C, Kwan E, Pessin MS, et al. Intracranial angioplasty, experience and complications. *AJNR* 1997; **18:** 1661–68.

7

External validity of pharmaceutical trials in neuropathic pain

C. Peter N. Watson

Introduction

There is a large and increasing number of placebo-controlled randomised controlled trials (RCTs) in neuropathic pain, yet we have lost direction in the advancement of oral pharmacotherapies for these conditions. RCTs are churned out, many by the pharamaceutical industry, showing an effect of a new drug over placebo, with no comparative data with a standard therapy or information regarding the clinical meaningfulness of the new agent in ordinary practice. There are many disorders of neuropathic pain in clinical practice, and they can be roughly divided into peripheral neuropathic pain and central pain. Peripheral neuropathic pain problems include a variety of painful, generalised neuropathies and also mononeuropathies such as traumatic injury due to accident or surgery, diabetic neuropathies, postherpetic neuralgia, phantom limb pain and others. The central pain problems include central post-stroke pain, spinal cord injury pain, syringomyelia and multiple sclerosis. The RCTs of different oral analgesics in these conditions can be mainly divided into antidepressants, anticonvulsants and opioids, and most trials have studied these drugs using painful diabetic neuropathy and postherpetic neuralgia as experimental models. This is because these conditions are relatively common, compared with other varieties of neuropathic pain, and are reasonably uniform and stable if subjects are appropriately recruited and carefully chosen. The extensive utilisation of these two disorders can, however, be a problem in terms of generalisability of study results to other less common types of nerve injury pain. Clinicians treating these patients know that, despite our best therapy, most patients are incompletely relieved and many are poorly or not palliated or do not tolerate the adverse effects of these drugs.

It is relatively easy for the pharmaceutical industry to meet the requirements for the approval of a new drug by submitting two RCTs showing a difference over placebo. Continuing this economically driven approach may simply continue to generate 'me too' drugs, as has occurred with the statins, triptans and many others, and is of limited help pragmatically for clinicians struggling with these patients who need to know if a new drug effect is clinically meaningful and any better than a standard therapy. The placebo-controlled trial also offers little from an explanatory point of view in terms of tailoring treatment to pathophysiological mechanisms, and addressing the question of whether the new drug works in a different group than the old drug. There are, therefore, significant problems with these trials, which provide barriers to better pain management. These problems include the lack of comparative studies (enabling us to determine if a new drug is any better than the standard therapy, and possibly whether it works in a different subgroup), the lack of data in these reports regarding clinical meaningfulness (how many patients obtain a satisfactory response and have tolerable side-effects) and whether these data, when reported, are relevant to office practice. It is the latter, that is the external validity of these trials, which will be analysed in this chapter.

7 External validity of pharmaceutical trials in neuropathic pain

Methods

A systematic review was carried out searching PubMed, Medline and the Cochrane Data Base for randomised controlled trials of analgesics (oral antidepressants, anticonvulsants and opioids) in neuropathic pain, and also searching using the terms 'postherpetic neuralgia' and 'painful diabetic neuropathy' (as these are the most common conditions used for clinical trials in neuropathic pain), as well as terms such as 'central pain', 'phantom limb pain' and other specific types of neuropathic pain. This review searched for trials on adults published in English from 1966 to 2005. The search excluded the neuropathic pain conditions of trigeminal neuralgia and complex regional pain syndrome type II (causalgia). In addition, the reference lists of retrieved articles were searched, and investigators in this area were contacted. Of particular interest were comparative trials within an analgesic class and of different analgesics in neuropathic pain. External validity was rated by the checklist published by Rothwell et al.[1] (see Chapter 3, panel 3.2). Trials were evaluated according to the quality criteria of Jadad et al.,[2] and to be included were required to score at least 3 out of 5 on their rating scale. A maximum score of 5 indicated that the RCT was randomised, double-blind, accounted for withdrawals, and described the methods of blinding and randomisation. Although we required that all trials fulfilled the first three criteria and scored 3, many scored 4 or 5. Trials were determined to be enriched if (a) previous treatment with the trial drug or a similar drug resulted in exclusion, or (b) patients having adverse events from the study drug prior to the treatment were excluded, or (c) non-responders to the drug were excluded. Measures of clinical meaningfulness, such as effect size, percentage of patients with 50% or greater improvement and number need to treat (NNT),[3,4] number needed to harm (NNH)[3,4] and number needed to quit (NNQ), were sought as a means of comparison of efficacy and safety.

Results

General

Forty-nine RCTs[5–53] (meeting the criteria described above) of antidepressants, anticonvulsants and opioids in peripheral and central neuropathic pain were identified. Six of the studies were comparative trials of different analgesics[10, 11, 23, 25, 26, 39] and six compared different antidepressants.[8, 9, 16, 19, 22, 31] Of the analgesics investigated in the trials, 26 studies were of antidepressants, 17 of anticonvulsants and nine of opioids (some RCTs involved more than one drug). Overall, 40/49 of the trials were carried out in postherpetic neuralgia, painful diabetic neuropathy or in both disorders. Forty-four of the 49 trials were favourable for the study drug. Of the antidepressant trials, seven were in postherpetic neuralgia,[5–11] 13 were in painful diabetic neuropathy[14–24] and seven were in other neuropathic pain[25–31] (HIV neuropathy, 2; 'neuropathic pain', 2; central pain, 1; spinal cord injury, 1; cisplatinum neuropathy, 1). Of the trials of anticonvulsants, seven involved gabapentin,[39–44] six involved pregabalin,[45–50] three involved lamotrigine[51–53] and one involved carbamazepine.[25] There were nine RCTs of opioids,[11, 32–39]with one trial using two different opioids (tramadol, 3; oxycodone, 3; methadone, 1; morphine, 2; levorphanol, 1).

Setting

The RCTs were carried out in 12 countries, including the USA (26), Denmark (8), Canada (6), two in each of Finland, Germany, Sweden and the UK, and one each in

Australia, India, Israel and Spain. Some trials were carried out in more than one country. Patients were recruited from advertisements or primary care in 16 trials, from a neurology or diabetic clinic population (secondary care) in 10, from a pain clinic (tertiary) in three, and from a mixed primary/secondary setting in eight. In 15 studies the source of patients was not stated.

Selection of patients

In 20 RCTs the diagnosis of neuropathic pain was not precisely determined and lacked description in the methods section; there was no documentation of pain in a nerve territory, of descriptors typical of neuropathic pain, of physical findings or of ancillary testing such as electromyography (EMG) or nerve conduction studies supporting nerve injury. A statement of only 'neuropathic pain' was not considered adequate. The number of eligibility criteria ranged from two to 19, with a median of four; in two studies the number of criteria was not stated. Exclusion criteria ranged from one to 19, with a median of seven, and in three cases the exclusion criteria were not stated. Run-ins with placebo or drug were used in two studies to select those to be included. Study enrichment was present if participants were excluded if they had an adverse event or were non-responsive to the study drug or previous use of the study drug or a closely related drug (e.g. gabapentin in pregabalin studies). Sixteen studies were determined to involve this form of selection. Nineteen studies stated the number of individuals screened, 23 stated the ratio of randomised to eligible subjects and 14 documented those who declined randomisation.

Clinical characteristics

The basic demographic details of the study population were stated in 49 trials, although racial subgroups were not stated in 32 trials. In 21 trials it was determined that the disorder studied lacked uniformity in that different types of neuropathic pain or different types of neuropathy within a category, such as painful diabetic neuropathy, were studied. In 34 trials the stage of the disorder in terms of pain was not clear because the duration of the pain was not characterised or was judged to be less than optimum (i.e. of 1 month duration or less). In 19 RCTs pain severity was not stated in the inclusion criteria, or was mild or was not described as being daily pain of moderate severity. Comorbidities were stated in three trials. The absolute risk in the control group was clear in 32 reports (the disorder was clearly chronic and severe because of the pain intensity and duration, and therefore unlikely to improve with time).

Differences between the trial protocol and routine practice

The trial intervention was deemed appropriate in 42 trials, and the timing of the treatment appeared satisfactory in 36. The control group was thought appropriate/relevant in 43 trials. Prohibition of non-trial treatments (e.g. of standard drugs used in neuropathic pain), often requiring pre-study drug withdrawal, occurred in 22 instances.

Outcome measures and follow-up

Surrogate outcomes were used in six instances, and were judged problematic because they included numbness, paraesthesia and sleep components, and there was not a clear pain rating scale. A clear statement of who measured outcomes was given in seven of the trial reports. Patient-centred outcomes were not found in any study. Clinic follow-up frequency was a median of 2 weeks (range 1–15 weeks), and did not include telephone contact. The median duration of the studies was 8 weeks (range 5–20 weeks). A measure of clinical meaningfulness was reported in 21 studies, most commonly as the NNT (nine studies) or as 50% or better pain relief (nine studies). Clinical meaningfulness was good to excellent (based on pain relief, satisfaction, adverse effect tolerability and satisfaction) in three studies, and there was a 30% improvement in one. The NNH and the NNQ were given in one RCT. An effect size was reported in one study. A quality of life measure was used in 21 studies (the most common measure was the SF-36), and satisfaction with pain relief was reported in three reports. Twenty-three reports stated that the study utilised an intention-to-treat analysis.

Adverse effects of treatment

The recording of adverse effects was done in 46/49 studies. Rates of discontinuation of treatment were reported in all studies, as this was a requirement of the RCT rating scale used (see above). The selection of the trial centre and clinicians was reported in three cases, although this information may have been inferred in many of the trials. Patients at risk of complications were excluded in 32 (see above: median number of exclusion criteria 7, range 1–19). No study excluded patients at risk of adverse effects occurring during a run-in period. Trial safety procedures were considered adequate in 43 trials. Open-ended recording of adverse effects was used in 33 studies and a checklist was used in three. Satisfaction with the tolerability of adverse effects was reported in two studies.

Discussion

Only six of the 49 trials were comparative trials of different analgesics, and these were non-industry-sponsored studies. It is important to do comparative trials with standard therapies to determine if a new drug is worthwhile, in terms of better pain relief and less side-effects, and to determine if some patients respond to one drug and not the other. Those who participate in industry-funded studies should argue for comparative trials, and if a study is done should insist on an independent data analysis and on its publication. Internet trial registries will help, but there is still no guarantee of the publication of unfavourable study results.

Postherpetic neuralgia and painful diabetic neuropathy were the subject of 40/49 (80%) of the studies, and thus it is unknown how effective antidepressants, anticonvulsants and opioids are in the many other nerve injury, painful conditions seen in clinical practice (it is a clinical impression that neuropathic conditions such as central post-stroke pain and incisional neuralgias after aortocoronary bypass and mastectomy are more intractable to pharmacotherapy). It appears important, therefore, to carry out trials in other neuropathic pain conditions to determine the generalisability of these results.

All the trials in postherpetic neuralgia and painful diabetic neuropathy had favourable outcomes, while 6/13 trials in the 'other' neuropathic pain category had negative outcomes. This raises the possibility that neuropathic pain conditions respond differently to oral analgesics. It may also be the case that only favourable trials were reported in the first two conditions. Therefore, these data argue for the study of a uniform population (which was the case in only approximately half of the studies), rather than a mixture of neuropathic pain conditions or of different neuropathic pain conditions, or of different neuropathies in the same condition, such as with diabetic neuropathy.

In terms of the setting, because over half of the patients were in secondary and tertiary healthcare settings, it is possible that in these patients the neuropathic pain was more intractable, which could result in a more intractable-pain population in some trials than is seen in primary care.

In approximately a quarter of the cases the diagnosis was not clear, and it was not clear that the condition was neuropathic pain.

Of the inclusion criteria, in approximately one-third of instances the pain severity that was included was mild, of short duration and not clearly on a daily basis.

In a third of trials there were more than six inclusion criteria, indicating that these trials probably involved quite highly selected groups of patients. This was particularly the case in the RCTs in painful diabetic neuropathy, and this selection of patients may make the study results less generalisable to the general population.

The number of exclusion criteria (median 7, range 1–19) argues for considerable selection in many of these studies. Clinically meaningful figures, such as the NNT and NNH, derived from RCTs with a large number of exclusion criteria will not be applicable to clinical practice, and the RCT results will not be as good as those from trials with fewer exclusion criteria. Excluding patients failing pre-study drug withdrawal might exclude poorly responsive subjects, and this together with the exclusion of patients previously treated with the study drug can 'enrich' trials, making them more salutary.

As a number of trials excluded patients previously treated with the study or similar drug, or patients not responding to the study drug, an enriched-enrolment type of population (i.e. patients who are more likely to respond) may have been entered into these trials. This was particularly true of the pregabalin and gabapentin trials. Gabapentin is a very similar drug to pregabalin, and had been available for some time prior to these trials. Thus excluding patients who had previously taken gabapentin could have resulted in considerable selection bias and, although this issue was mentioned, the numbers of patients were not given, making it impossible to determine the effect of this exclusion criterion.

A large number of trials did not state the number of patients excluded by being screened or who were deemed ineligible despite having the diagnosis, or were eligible but not entered into the trial, for reasons such as not agreeing to participate. This makes it difficult to know how representative the study population was of those patients actually seen in practice.

Clinical characteristics were stated in most trials, but notably absent was an indication of the proportion of different races. Attention to this may give some indication as to whether a drug would be more effective or have a different profile of adverse effects in one racial group than another.

7 External validity of pharmaceutical trials in neuropathic pain

In a significant proportion of trials it was unclear whether the disorder was a uniform condition, i.e. one type of neuropathic pain or one type of neuropathy in a pain condition such as diabetes (the subgroup of painful symmetrical distal sensory neuropathy rather than all diabetic neuropathies). It may be important to study uniform conditions rather than a variety of neuropathic pain conditions because of the possible variability in response to a drug. More data are needed in neuropathic pain conditions other than postherpetic neuralgia and painful diabetic neuropathy (central pain, such as post-stroke pain, multiple sclerosis and spinal cord injury; peripheral neuropathic pain, such as phantom pain; and postsurgical nerve injury pain after mastectomy, thoracotomy and coronary bypass surgery) in view of the negative results of trials or the lesser effect of drugs that appears in some neuropathic pain conditions.

In a proportion of trials, patients with mild pain were accepted, or it was not clear what the severity of pain was, whether the pain occurred daily or what the duration of the pain was. This can be problematic in RCTs, and it is important to choose patients with a fairly chronic stable pain state of moderate daily pain for at least 3 months duration in order to limit the number of patients needed in the trial. This is of special importance for crossover studies, where a period effect from natural resolution may be fatal to analysis as a crossover study.

Many trials (28/49 (57%)) did not give any indication of the clinical meaningfulness of the results, and very few (9/49 (18%)) used NNT data, with only one giving any indication of NNH or NNQ. A few studies indicated an effect size or some other means of conveying clinical meaningfulness.

More than 50% of trials prohibited other drugs known to relieve neuropathic pain. Unless patients on stable doses of these drugs, but with inadequate relief, are included in trials, it may not be possible to determine whether a synergistic or additive effect occurs with a new treatment. In clinical practice there is now a trend to treat many patients with polypharmacy, and trials of this approach are currently underway. Responsive patients may also be selected out if they cannot tolerate withdrawal of these agents during a run-in period.

A few studies used surrogate scales to rate pain, which included other symptoms and parameters. However, the majority did use reliable and valid pain rating scales and pain-relief rating scales.

Many trials (21/45 (57%)) did not include a quality-of-life outcome or use an intention-to-treat analysis (26/49 (53%)). Few used a satisfaction rating regarding pain relief, adverse effects or both. None utilised a patient-centred outcome measure.

All the trials were relatively short (weeks) and only two trials reported long-term follow-up. This extended follow-up should be possible with trial completers, and in this way adverse events that occur in the long term and long-term efficacy can be evaluated.

Adverse events were reported in most instances. The most common means of determining this was by using open-ended questions, a technique that carries a risk of underreporting of adverse events. It would seem reasonable that a modified checklist of the most common symptoms, with an additional category of 'other side-effects', should yield a more accurate assessment of adverse events. Furthermore, only two trials asked patients if they were satisfied with their treatment, and none specifically asked patients whether they were satisfied with the pain relief and the tolerability of the adverse effects.

Recommendations for future trials

Significant problems with RCTs in neuropathic pain were identified by this survey. The external validity of these studies may be improved by the following:

- More comparative trials of different analgesics.
- Further studies in neuropathic pain conditions other than postherpetic neuralgia and painful diabetic neuropathy.
- Publishing trials that find unfavourable (negative) results.
- The study of uniform neuropathic pain conditions.
- Generating subjects by advertising and from primary care, as they will more closely resemble patients seen in clinical practice than will patients sourced from secondary or tertiary care centres.
- Making the diagnostic criteria for a condition clear (it is inadequate to state 'postherpetic neuralgia' or 'diabetic neuropathy' without being more precise as to the definition).
- Making exclusion criteria reasonable and keeping them to a minimum.
- Discouraging the enrichment of studies.
- The recording of 'subjects screened', 'the correct diagnosis/ineligible' and 'eligible/declined' in a 'flow through the trial' figure.
- The recording of the racial origins of subjects.
- Including patients who have at least moderate pain on a daily basis for a period of 3 months or more.
- Having as an outcome a means for the clinician and regulatory body of determining clinical meaningfulness, such as the NNT, NNH or NNQ, as a part of every trial. This may be incorporated in a section entitled 'To whom do these results apply?'[1]
- Using rating scales that specifically evaluate pain and pain relief by a reliable and valid means, rather than using a surrogate or complex scale.
- Including as an outcome a quality-of-life measure to improve the determination of utility to clinical practice.
- Using an intention-to-treat analysis, as this more closely resembles clinical experience.
- Having an extended follow-up of study patients in order to determine the long-term adverse effect profile, the long-term drug efficacy, and the occurrence of late occurring, significant and/or unusual adverse events.
- The reporting of adverse events should include at least a limited checklist of the more common side-effects of the drug together with an 'other' category to pick up other side-effects, in order to evaluate safety more completely.
- It would seem reasonable to include a question asking patients if they are satisfied with the pain relief and the tolerability of the adverse events, if present.

- Those scientists participating with industry can improve external validity by arguing for comparative studies with a standard therapy, by insisting on a role in study design, by having access to and performing analysis of the data, and by writing an article arising from the research themselves, in order to avoid an industry 'spin' on the results. There should be an insistence on the publication of all studies, even if the results are unfavourable.

Acknowledgment
The author would like to thank Dr Jack Williams and Dr Judy Watt-Watson for their time and effort in reviewing this chapter.

References

1 Rothwell PM. Treating individuals. 1. External validity of randomized controlled trials: 'To whom do these results apply?' *Lancet* 2005; **365:** 82–93.
2 Jadad AR, Moore A, Carroll D et al., Assessing the reports of randomized clinical trials: Is blinding necessary? *Control Clin Trials* 2001; **17:** 1–12.
3 Laupacis A, Sackett DL, Robarts RS. An assessment of clinically useful measures of the consequences of treatment. *N Engl J Med* 1988; **318:** 1728–33.
4 Cook RJ, Sackett DL. The number needed to treat: a clinically useful measure of treatment effect. *BMJ* 1995; **310:** 452–54.
5 Watson CPN, Evans RJ, Reed K, et al. Amitriptyline versus placebo in postherpetic neuralgia. *Neurology* 1982; **32:** 671–73.
6 Max MB, Schafer SC, Culnane M, et al. Amitriptyline but not lorazepam relieves postherpetic neuralgia. *Neurology* 1988; **38:** 1427–37.
7 Kishore-Kumar R, Max MB, Schafer SC, et al. Desipramine relieves postherpetic neuralgia. *Clin Pharmacol Ther* 1990; **47:** 305–12.
8 Watson CPN, Chipman M, Reed K, et al. Amitriptyline versus maprotiline in postherpetic neuralgia: a randomized, double-blind, crossover trial. *Pain* 1992; **48:** 29–36.
9 Watson CPN, Chipman M, Reed K. Amitriptyline versus nortriptyline in postherpetic neuralgia. *Neurology* 1998; **51:** 1166–71.
10 Graff-Radford SB, Shaw LR, Naliboff BN. Amitriptyline and fluphenazine in postherpetic neuralgia. *Clin J Pain* 2000; **16:** 188–92.
11 Raja SJ, Haythornethwaite JA, Papagallo M, et al. Opioids versus antidepressants in postherpetic neuralgia: a placebo-controlled study. *Pain* 2002; **94:** 215–24.
12 Kvinesdal B, Molin J, Froland A, et al. Imipramine treatment of painful diabetic neuropathy. *JAMA* 1984; **251:** 1727–30.
13 Max MB, Culnane M, Schafter SC, et al. Amitriptyline relieves diabetic neuropathy pain in patients with normal or depressed mood. *Neurology* 1987; **37:** 589–96.
14 Sindrup SH, Ejlertsen B, Froland A, et al. Imipramine treatment in diabetic neuropathy: relief of subjective symptoms without changes in peripheral and autonomic nerve function. *Eur Clin Pharmacol* 1989; **37:** 151–53.
15 Sindrup SH, Gram LF, Brosen K, et al. The selective serotonin reuptake inhibitor paroxetine is effective in the treatment of diabetic neuropathy symptoms. *Pain* 1990; **42:** 135–44.
16 Sindrup SH, Gram L, Skjold T, et al. Clomipramine vs desipramine vs placebo in the treatment of diabetic neuropathy symptoms: a double-blind, crossover study. *Br J Clin Pharmacol* 1990; **30:** 683–91.
17 Sindrup SH, Grodun E, Gram LF, et al. Concentration-response relationship in paroxetine treatment of diabetic neuropathy symptoms: a patient-blinded dose escalation study. *Ther Drug Monitor* 1991; **13:** 408–14.
18 Max MB, Kishore-Kumar R, Schafter, et al. Efficacy of desipramine in painful diabetic neuropathy: a placebo-controlled trial. *Pain* 1991; **45:** 3–9.
19 Max MB, Lynch SA, Muir J, et al. Effects of desipramine, amitriptyline, and fluoxetine on pain in diabetic neuropathy. *N Engl J Med* 1992; **326:** 1250–56.
20 Sindrup SH, Bjerre U, Dejgaard A, et al. The selective serotonin reuptake inhibitor citalopram relieves the symptoms of diabetic neuropathy. *Clin Pharmacol Ther* 1992; **52:** 547–552.
21 Sindrup SH, Tuxen C, Gram LF. Lack of effect of mianserin on the symptoms of diabetic neuropathy. *Eur J Clin Pharmacol* 1992; **43:** 251–55.
22 Vrethem M, Boivie J, Arnqvist H, et al. A comparison of amitriptyline and maprotiline in the treatment of painful diabetic neuropathy in diabetics and nondiabetics. *Clin J Pain* 1997; **12:** 313–23.

23 Morello CM, Leckband SG, Stoner CP, et al. Randomized double-blind study comparing the efficacy of gabapentin with amitriptyline on diabetic peripheral neuropathy pain. *Arch Intern Med* 1999; **159:** 1931–37.

24 Rowbotham MC, Goli G, Kunz NR, Lei D. Venlafaxine extended release in the treatment of painful diabetic neuropathy: a double-blind, placebo-controlled study. *Pain* 2004; **110:** 697–706.

25 Leijon G, Boivie J. Central post-stroke pain: a controlled trial of amitriptyline and carbamazepine. *Pain* 1989; **36:** 27–36.

26 Kieburtz K, Simpson D, Yiannoutsos C, et al. A randomized trial of amitriptyline and mexiletine for painful neuropathy in HIV infection. AIDS Clinical Trial Group 242 Protocol Team. *Neurology* 1998; **51:** 1682–88.

27 Shlay JC, Chaloner K, Max MB, et al. Acupuncture and amitriptyline for pain due to HIV-related peripheral neuropathy: a randomized controlled trial. Terry Beirn Community Programs for Clinical Research on AIDS. *JAMA* 1998; **280:** 1590–95.

28 Semenchuk MR, Shennan S, Davis B. Double-blind, randomized trial of bupropion SR for the treatment of neuropathic pain. *Neurology* 2001; **57:** 1583–88.

29 Cardenas DD, Wanns CA, Turner JA, et al. Efficacy of amitriptyline for relief of pain in spinal cord injury: results of a randomized controlled trial. *Pain* 2002; **96:** 365–73.

30 Hammack JE, Michalak JC, Loprinzi CL, et al. Phase III evaluation of nortriptyline for alleviation of symptoms of cis-platinum-induced peripheral neuropathy. *Pain* 2002; **91:** 195–203.

31 Sindrup SH, Bach FW, Madsen C, et al. Venlafaxine versus imipramine in painful polyneuropathy: a randomized controlled trial. *Neurology* 2003; **60:** 1284–89.

32 Watson CPN, Babul N. Oxycodone relieves neuropathic pain: a randomized trial in postherpetic neuralgia. *Neurology* 1998; **50:** 1837–41.

33 Harati Y Gooch C, Swensen M, et al. Double blind randomized trial of tramadol for the treatment of the pain of diabetic neuropathy. *Neurology* 1998; **50:** 1842–46.

34 Sindrup SH, Andersen G, Madsen C, et al. Tramadol relieves pain and allodynia in polyneuropathy; a randomized, double-blind, controlled trial. *Pain* 1999; **83:** 85–90.

35 Watson CPN, Moulin D, Watt-Watson J, et al. Controlled-release oxycodone relieves neuropathic pain: a randomized controlled trial in painful diabetic neuropathy. *Pain* 2003; **105:** 71–78.

36 Rowbotham MC, Twilling L, Davies PS, et al. Oral opioid therapy for chronic peripheral and central neuropathic pain. *N Engl J Med* 2003; **13:** 1223–32.

37 Gimbel JS, Richards P, Portenoy RK. Controlled-release oxycodone for pain in diabetic neuropathy: a randomized controlled trial. *Neurology* 2003; **60:** 927–34.

38 Boureau F, Legallicier P, Kabir-Ahmadi M. Tramadol in postherpetic neuralgia: a randomized, double-blind, placebo-controlled trial. *Pain* 2003; **104:** 323–31.

39 Gilron I, Bailey JM, Dongshen T, et al. Morphine, gabapentin or their combination for neuropathic pain. *N Engl J Med* 2005; **352:** 1324–34.

40 Rowbotham M, Harden N, Stacey B, et al. Gabapentin for the treatment of postherpetic neuralgia: a randomized controlled trial. *JAMA* 1998; **280:** 1837–42.

41 Backonja M, Beydoun A, Edwards KR. Gabapentin for the symptomatic treatment of painful neuropathy in patients with diabetes mellitus. *JAMA* 1998; **280:** 1831–36.

42 Rice ASC, Maton S, and the Postherpetic Neuralgia Study Group. Gabapentin in postherpetic neuralgia: a randomized, double blind, placebo controlled trial. *Pain* 2001; **94:** 215–24.

43 Bone M, Critchley P, Buggy DJ, et al. Gabapentin in post-amputation phantom limb pain: a randomized, double-blind, cross-over study. *Regional Anaesth Pain Med* 2002; **27:** 481–86.

44 Pandey CK, Bose N, Garg G. Gabapentin for the treatment of pain in Guillain Barré syndrome: a double-blind, placebo-controlled, cross-over study. *Anesth Analg* 2002; **95:** 1719–23.

45 Dworkin RH, Corbin AE, Young JP. Pregabalin for the treatment of postherpetic neuralgia. *Neurology* 2003; **60:** 1274–83.

46 Sabatowski R, Galvez R, Cherry DA, et al. Pregabalin reduces pain and improves sleep and mood disturbances in patients with postherpetic neuralgia: results of a randomized, placebo-controlled clinical trial. *Pain* 2004; **109:** 26–35.

47 Lesser H, Sharma U, LaMoreaux L, et al. Pregabalin relieves symptoms of painful diabetic neuropathy a randomized controlled trial. *Neurology* 2004; **63:** 2104–19.

48 Rosenstock J, Tuchman M, Lamoreaux L, et al. Pregabalin for the treatment of painful diabetic peripheral neuropathy: a double-blind, placebo-controlled trial. *Pain* 2004; **110:** 628–38.

49 Freynhagen R, Strojek K, Griesing T, et al. Efficacy of pregabalin in neuropathic pain evaluated in a 12 week, randomized, double blind, multicentre, placebo-controlled trial of flexible and fixed-dose regimens. *Pain* 2005; **115:** 254–63.

50 Richter RW, Portenoy R, Sharma U, et al. Relief of painful diabetic peripheral neuropathy with pregabalin: a randomized, placebo-controlled trial. *J Pain* 2005; **6:** 253–60.

51 Eisenberg E, Lurie Y, Braker C, et al. Lamotrigine reduces painful diabetic neuropathy. *Neurology* 2001; **57:** 167–73.

52 Vestergard K, Andersen G, Gottrup H, et al. Lamotrigine for central post-stroke pain: a randomized controlled trial. *Neurology* 2001; **56:** 184–89.

53 Simpson DM, MacArthur JC, Olney R, et al. Lamotrigine for HIV associated painful sensory neuropathies; a placebo-controlled trial. *Neurology* 2003; **60:** 1508–14.

External validity of pharmaceutical trials in asthma and chronic obstructive pulmonary disease

Justin Travers, Suzanne Marsh, Philippa Shirtcliffe and Richard Beasley

The evidence derived from randomised controlled trials (RCTs) has become an increasingly important influence on the recommendations given in international guidelines and the medical care provided by clinicians. The evidence from RCTs may, however, be limited in the degree to which it applies to patients in routine clinical practice (i.e. its external validity). The external validity of an RCT can be difficult to assess, since the healthcare setting, subject baseline characteristics, disease states and proposed treatments may all differ between the RCT and the clinical setting.[1] Despite these difficulties, clinicians must attempt to assess the external validity of the RCT evidence to effectively inform individual patients of the likely benefits and risks of a proposed treatment.

In respiratory medicine, asthma and chronic obstructive pulmonary disease (COPD) are common conditions. Both manifest a wide range of clinical phenotypes.[2] Individuals with asthma differ in many ways, including in the age of onset of disease, the underlying atopic basis, response to different provoking factors, the clinical pattern and severity of disease, and the underlying inflammatory processes.[3] Individuals with COPD also differ in many ways, including the degree to which emphysema, chronic bronchitis, bronchospasm and small airways inflammation are present, as well as in the frequency and severity of exacerbations and the degree of dyspnoea.[4] This heterogeneity of disease states makes it particularly important that RCTs in asthma and COPD include a wide range of phenotypes, to allow the evidence to be generalised to the majority of individuals with these conditions. There is, however, evidence that RCTs in asthma and COPD may have highly selective eligibility criteria for which only a minority of individuals in the community with these conditions would be potentially eligible.[5, 6]

We recently conducted a random, community-based survey of respiratory health, giving a cross-sectional description of the characteristics of individuals with asthma and COPD in the community.[7] Data from these 'real-life' individuals were compared with the eligibility criteria for the major RCTs that inform clinical practice in asthma and COPD to determine what proportion of our individuals would meet trial inclusion criteria.[8, 9]

Consistent with accepted guidelines,[10] subjects in our study were identified as having current asthma if they:

- reported a doctor diagnosis of asthma and either symptoms of asthma or asthma medication use in the previous 12 months, and/or
- demonstrated an increase in the forced expiratory volume in one second (FEV_1) $\geq$ 15% compared to baseline after bronchodilator administration, and/or
- documented a diurnal peak flow variation $\geq$ 20% in any of the first 7 days of peak flow diary recordings.

A subject with current asthma was identified as having 'current asthma on treatment' if they reported use of asthma medication in the previous 12 months.

Subjects were identified as having COPD if the ratio of FEV_1 to forced vital capacity (FVC) was < 0.7 after the administration of a bronchodilator in the absence of specific pulmonary pathology, such as bronchiectasis or tuberculosis potentially causing the airflow obstruction.[11, 12] Subjects with COPD who were taking inhaled or oral steroids, or bronchodilators were identified as having COPD on treatment.

RCTs done in asthma and COPD patients were identified in a systematic manner.[13] To qualify as a trial forming the basis of consensus guidelines, a trial had to be cited as a reference accompanying a level A or B evidence-graded treatment recommendation in the Global Initiative for Asthma (GINA) workshop guideline *Global Strategy for Asthma Management and Prevention*,[10] or in the Global Initiative for Chronic Obstructive Lung Disease (GOLD) workshop guideline *Global Strategy for the Diagnosis, Management, and Prevention of Chronic Obstructive Pulmonary Disease*.[11]

The proportion of subjects with current asthma who met the eligibility criteria for the 17 RCTs included for analysis ranged from 0 to 36%, with a median of 4%. The proportion of subjects with current asthma on treatment who met the eligibility criteria for these trials ranged from 0 to 43%, with a median of 6%. Proportions of subjects with current asthma who did not meet common eligibility criteria are shown in table 8.1. The most selective criteria were bronchodilator reversibility and peak flow variability.

The proportion of subjects with COPD who met the eligibility criteria for the 18 RCTs included for analysis ranged from 0 to 20%, with a median of 5%. The proportion of subjects with COPD on treatment who met the eligibility criteria for these trials ranged from 0 to 9%, with a median of 5%. Proportions of subjects with COPD not meeting

Criterion	Subjects with current asthma excluded by criterion (%)
Bronchodilator reversibility ≥ 15%	76
Bronchodilator reversibility ≥ 12%	71
Peak flow variability ≥ 20%	66
FEV_1 ≥ 50% and < 80% of predicted	61
Inhaled corticosteroid use	48
Less than 10 pack-years of cigarette exposure	31
Active symptoms or use of rescue medication	20
FEV_1 ≥ 50% of predicted	12

FEV_1, forced expiratory volume in one second.

***Table 8.1:* Selectivity of eligibility criteria for asthma trials**

common eligibility criteria are shown in table 8.2. The most selective criteria were the requirement for a physician diagnosis of COPD, non-atopic status and a minimum 10 - pack-year smoking history.

These results are consistent with those of other investigators. Storms[6] reported that, amongst asthma patients attending a hospital specialist clinic, only 15% qualified for asthma clinical trials. In a Scandinavian study, Herland et al.[5] categorised subjects with obstructive lung disease who attended a general practice or hospital specialist clinic as having asthma, COPD or mixed obstructive lung disease. The characteristics of subjects with 'pure' asthma and with 'pure' COPD were compared with the eligibility criteria of a hypothetical RCT. The eligibility criteria used for the hypothetical asthma trial were absence of comorbidity, FEV_1 50–85% of predicted, bronchodilator reversibility of 12% or more in the last year, and either non-smoking status or being an ex-smoker with less than 10 pack-years exposure. Only 5.4% of the asthma patients met these criteria. The criteria used for their hypothetical COPD RCT were a $FEV_1 < 70\%$ of predicted normal, significant smoking history (> 15 pack-years) and absence of atopy. These criteria selected 17% of the COPD patients. Thus, even in a clinic population from which subjects with mixed obstructive lung disease are specifically excluded, common RCT eligibility criteria exclude the large majority of individuals with asthma or COPD.

These findings indicate that the treatment recommendations of the major asthma and COPD guidelines are limited with respect to the external validity of the RCTs on which they are based. For example, the common criterion that asthma subjects must be non-smokers to avoid the presence of concomitant COPD may lead to the exclusion of around a third of subjects with current asthma. The importance of this limitation is evident from studies that have shown a markedly reduced efficacy of inhaled corticosteroids in smokers with asthma, studies which were not undertaken for over 25 years following the introduction of these drugs.[14, 15] This delay in acquiring knowledge is

Criterion	Subjects with COPD excluded by criterion (%)
Physician diagnosis compatible with COPD	86
No atopy*	57
$FEV_1 \geq 50\%$ and < 80% of predicted	57
At least 10 pack-years cigarette exposure	55
No asthma diagnosis	42
Bronchodilator reversibility < 15%	29
Age at least 40 years	9

COPD, chronic obstructive pulmonary disease; FEV_1, forced expiratory volume in one second. *No positive skin-prick test to any of several common allergens.

***Table** 8.2:* **Selectivity of eligibility criteria for COPD trials**

likely to have led to subtherapeutic treatment with inhaled corticosteroids of smokers with asthma. Conversely, in smokers with asthma who have developed a significant irreversible component, the recommended adjustment of asthma therapy using peak flow targets can lead to overtreatment with inhaled and/or oral corticosteroids.[16]

Likewise, the common criteria that patients with asthma or significant bronchodilator reversibility are not eligible for COPD RCTs may lead to the exclusion of about half of all COPD subjects. While this has the advantage of avoiding the criticism that a demonstrated beneficial treatment effect was merely due to effective treatment of the asthma component of the subjects' disease, it is likely to reduce the efficacy of treatment amongst the broad population of COPD patients.

The highly selective eligibility criteria are only one of many factors affecting the external validity of these trials. The effects of trials having different healthcare settings, subject baseline characteristics and interventions may be more difficult to assess than eligibility criteria, but may also limit external validity.[1]

While recognising these limitations, it is also important to acknowledge that an RCT with highly selective eligibility criteria does have several advantages. It ensures a relatively homogenous population, thus reducing or eliminating the need for subgroup analyses and hence the number of subjects needed to be recruited into the trial. It may increase the likelihood of demonstrating a treatment effect by excluding subjects with diagnostic doubt, subjects with disease too mild or too severe to benefit from treatment and, in the case of asthma, subjects with relatively fixed reversible airflow obstruction.

Summary

These studies demonstrate that most subjects with asthma or COPD on treatment in the community are taking medication on the basis of RCTs for which they would not have been eligible. The degree to which the RCT evidence applies to these patients cannot be assessed directly, and the clinician should not necessarily assume that their patient will respond to a medication in the same way as trial subjects. As a result, clinicians should consider the treatment recommendations of major asthma and COPD guidelines to be limited with respect to the external validity of the RCTs on which they are based. We encourage the inclusion of a wider range of subjects with asthma and COPD in future clinical trials.

References

1 Rothwell PM. External validity of randomised controlled trials: 'To whom do the results of this trial apply?'. *Lancet* 2005; **365**: 82–93.

2 Wardlaw AJ, Silverman M, Siva R, et al. Multi-dimensional phenotyping: towards a new taxonomy for airway disease. *Clin Exp Allergy* 2005; **35**: 1254–62.

3 Bel EH. Clinical phenotypes of asthma. *Curr Opin Pulmon Med* 2004; **10**: 44–50.

4 Mannino DM, Watt G, Hole D, et al. The natural history of chronic obstructive pulmonary disease. *Eur Respir J* 2006; **27**: 627–43.

5 Herland K, Akselsen JP, Skjonsberg OH, Bjermer L. How representative are clinical study patients with asthma or COPD for a larger 'real life' population of patients with obstructive lung disease? *Respir Med* 2005; **99**: 11–19.

6 Storms W. Clinical trials: are these your patients? *J Allergy Clin Immunol* 2003; **112** (5 suppl): S107–11.

7 Marsh S, Aldington S, Williams M, et al. Physiological associations of computerized tomography lung density: a factor analysis. *Int J COPD* 2006; **1:** 181–87.

8 Travers J, Marsh S, Williams M, et al. External validity of randomised controlled trials in asthma: to whom do the results of the trials apply? *Thorax* 2007; **62:** 219–23.

9 Travers J, Marsh S, Williams M, et al. External validity of randomised controlled trials in COPD. *Respir Med* 16 November 2006 (Epub).

10 Global Initiative for Asthma. *Global Strategy for Asthma Management and Prevention.* Revised 2006 from the 2004 document. Available at: http://www.ginasthma.org/Guidelineitem.asp??l1=2&l2=1&intId=60 (accessed February 2007).

11 Global Initiative for Chronic Obstructive Lung Disease. *Global Strategy for the Diagnosis, Management, and Prevention of Chronic Obstructive Pulmonary Disease.* Updated November 2006 (based on an April 1998 NHLBI/WHO Workshop). Available at: http://www.goldcopd.com/Guidelineitem.asp?l1=2&l2=1&intId=989 (accessed February 2007).

12 Celli BR, MacNee W. Standards for the diagnosis and treatment of patients with COPD: a summary of the ATS/ERS position paper. *Eur Respir J* 2004; **23:** 932–46.

13 Moher D, Cook DJ, Eastwood S, et al. Improving the quality of reports of meta-analyses of randomised controlled trials: the QUOROM statement. Quality of Reporting of Meta-analyses. *Lancet* 1999; **354:** 1896–900.

14 Chalmers GW, Macleod KJ, Little SA, et al. Influence of cigarette smoking on inhaled corticosteroid treatment in mild asthma. *Thorax* 2002; **57:** 226–30.

15 Chaudhuri R, Livingston E, McMahon AD, et al. Cigarette smoking impairs the therapeutic response to oral corticosteroids in chronic asthma. *Am J Respir Crit Care Med* 2003; **168:** 1308–11.

16 Douma WR, Kerstjens HA, Rooyackers JM, et al. Risk of overtreatment with current peak flow criteria in self-management plans. Dutch CNSLD Study Group. Chronic non-specific lung disease. *Eur Respir J* 1998; **12:** 848–52.

Section 3

Is the overall trial result sufficiently relevant to this patient?

9

When should we expect clinically important differences in response to treatment?

Peter M. Rothwell

Introduction

> *The essence of tradegy has been described as the destructive collision of two sets of protagonists, both of whom are correct. The statisticians are right in denouncing subgroups that are formed post hoc from exercises in pure data dredging. The clinicians are also right, however, in insisting that a subgroup is respectable and worthwhile when established a priori from pathophysiological principles.* (A. R. Feinstein 1998[1])

As reviewed in Section 1, randomised controlled trials (RCTs) and systematic reviews are the most reliable methods of determining the effects of treatments.[2–5] However, when trials were first developed for use in agriculture, researchers were presumably concerned about the effect of interventions on the overall size and quality of the crop rather than on the well-being of any individual plant. Clinicians have to make decisions about individuals, and how best to use results of RCTs and systematic reviews to do this has generated considerable debate.[6–22] Unfortunately, this debate has polarised, with statisticians and predominantly non-clinical (or non-practising) epidemiologists warning of the dangers of subgroup analysis and other attempts to target treatment, and clinicians warning of the dangers of applying the overall results of large trials to individual patients without consideration of pathophysiology or other determinants of individual response. This rift, described by Feinstein as a 'clinico-statistical tragedy',[1] was widened in recent years by some of the more enthusiastic proclamations on the extent to which the overall results of trials can properly inform decisions at the bedside or in the clinic.[23–25]

The results of small 'explanatory' trials with well-defined eligibility criteria should be easy to apply to future individuals but, as outlined in Section 2, generalisability is often undermined by highly selective recruitment, resulting in trial populations that are unrepresentative even of the few patients in routine practice who fit the eligibility criteria.[26] Recruitment of a higher proportion of eligible patients is a major strength of large pragmatic trials, but deliberately broad and sometimes ill-defined entry criteria mean that the overall result can be difficult to apply to particular groups,[27] and that subgroup analyses are necessary if heterogeneity of treatment effect is considered likely. This chapter reviews some of the arguments for and against going beyond the assumption that the overall results of trials or systematic reviews are generalisable, and considers the clinical situations in which we might reasonably expect clinically important differences in response to treatment. Illustrative examples are drawn mainly from treatments for cerebrovascular or cardiovascular disease, but the principles are relevant to all areas of medicine and surgery.

Arguments against attempts to target treatment

That qualitative heterogeneity of relative treatment effect (defined as the treatment effect being in a different direction in different groups of patients, i.e. benefit in one subgroup and harm in another) is 'extremely rare' is the main argument against attempts to target treatments in general and subgroup analysis in particular.[2–5] However, even if true, this observation is much less reassuring than it appears. First, it automatically excludes the majority of treatments because they do not have a significant risk of harm and can therefore only be effective or ineffective. Yet, use of an ineffective treatment can be highly detrimental if it prevents the use of a more effective alternative or if side-effects impair quality of life. Second, the observation refers only to 'unanticipated' heterogeneity.[2–5] As outlined below, there are many examples where qualitative heterogeneity of relative treatment effect has been correctly anticipated. Third, the observation only applies to single-outcome events – it is argued that subgroup analyses based on composite outcomes are inappropriate.[2–5, 28] However, since qualitative heterogeneity of relative treatment effect is only possible for treatments that have a risk of harm, and such treatments almost always require a composite outcome to express the balance of both risk and benefit, qualitative heterogeneity as defined will inevitably be rare – a 'Catch-22', in fact.

There are several other arguments against attempts to target treatment. First, it is said that clinicians already tend to undertreat patients,[29] and we should not risk effective treatments being further restricted. However, as discussed below, one of the main purposes of subgroup analysis is, in fact, to extend the use of treatments to subgroups that are not currently treated in routine practice. Subgroup analyses in epidemiological studies and trials often show that benefit from treatment is likely to be more universal than expected, and that current 'indications' for treatment in routine clinical practice are inappropriate, as is now clear, for example, with treatment thresholds for blood pressure lowering or lipid lowering.[30, 31] Second, it is argued that subgroup analyses are almost always underpowered,[32–37] but this is simply an argument for larger trials and for meta-analysis of individual patient data. Third, it is argued that false-positive subgroup effects will be more common than genuine heterogeneity,[2–5, 32–37] and that these false observations will harm patients – 'subgroups kill people'.[38] Subgroup analyses have certainly led to mistaken clinical recommendations (see Chapter 11, panel 11.1), but these analyses would not have satisfied the rules suggested in Chapter 11, panel 11.2. Moreover, not doing subgroup analysis can also be harmful. Properly powered subgroup analyses most commonly show that relative treatment effect is consistent across subgroups and/or that treatments should be used more extensively than is currently the case.[30, 39, 40] Without such evidence, unfounded clinical concerns about possible heterogeneity and/or inappropriately narrow indications for treatment would reduce the use of effective treatments in routine practice.[26] Not doing subgroup analyses has very probably killed more people.

Situations in which clinically important differences in response to treatment might be expected

As discussed in Chapter 3, the response to and/or compliance with a treatment can be influenced strongly by the doctor–patient relationship, placebo effects and patient preference, all of which are likely to vary from one individual to another, and each of which should be considered when deciding on treatments in routine clinical practice. However, there are many other factors that can also sometimes lead to clinically important differences in response to treatment. Broadly speaking, these factors can be divided into four groups (panel 9.1).

Heterogeneity related to risk

Clinically important heterogeneity of treatment effect is common when different groups of patients have very different absolute risks of a poor outcome with or without treatment. Differences in absolute risks without treatment are often seen when comparing different trials. For example, in the two trials of blood pressure lowering in figure 9.1, the elderly hypertensives in the STOP trial[41] were at a much higher risk of stroke without treatment than were the young hypertensives in the MRC trial.[42] It is important, therefore, when applying the overall result of an RCT or systematic review to a treatment decision in routine clinical practice to concentrate on the absolute risk reduction (ARR) with treatment in the relevant RCT or the number needed to treat to prevent an adverse

***Panel 9.1:* The four main causes of clinically important differences in absolute and/or relative treatment effect between groups and individuals.**

Potential heterogeneity of treatment effect related to risk
- Differences in risks of treatment
- Differences in risk without treatment

Potential heterogeneity of treatment effect related to pathophysiology
- Different pathologies underlying a clinical syndrome
- Differences in the biological response to a single pathology
- Genetic variation

Potential heterogeneity of treatment effect related to timing of intervention
- Does benefit differ with severity of disease?
- Does benefit differ with stage in the natural history of disease?
- Is benefit related to the timing of treatment after a clinical event?

Potential heterogeneity related to comorbidity

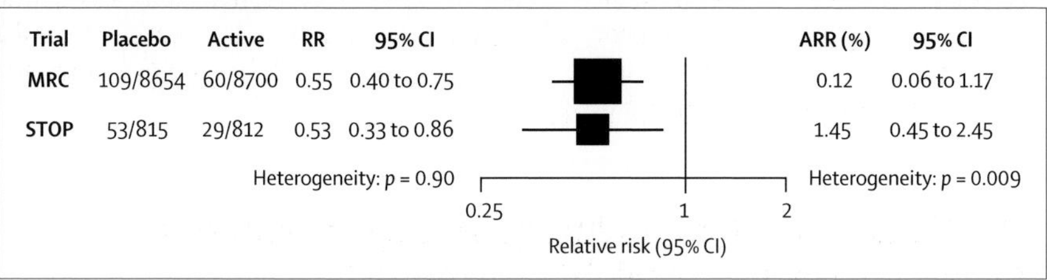

***Figure 9.1:* A comparison of the relative (RR) and absolute (ARR) reductions in the risk of stroke with treatment in two RCTs of blood pressure lowering in primary prevention.[41, 42]**

event (NNT).[43,44] An ARR tells us what chance an individual has of benefiting from treatment (i.e. an ARR of 25% indicates that there is a 1 in 4 chance of benefit; NNT = 4). In contrast, a particular relative risk reduction gives absolutely no information about the likelihood of individual benefit. As can be seen in figure 9.1, although the relative reductions in the risk of stroke with treatment were virtually identical in the two trials, there was a 12-fold difference in ARR. All other things being equal, 830 of the young hypertensives in the MRC trial would have to be treated for 1 year to prevent one stroke, compared with 69 of the elderly hypertensives in the STOP trial.

Differences in risk of a poor outcome without treatment can also lead to clinically important heterogeneity of treatment effect within individual trials. Trial populations are often skewed in terms of control group risk, with a few individuals contributing much of the overall observed risk,[45] and treatment may be ineffective or harmful in the low-risk majority. In vascular medicine, this is the case with endarterectomy for symptomatic carotid stenosis,[46] anticoagulation for uncomplicated non-valvular atrial fibrillation,[47] coronary artery bypass grafting[48] and antiarrhythmic drugs following myocardial infarction.[49] Clinically important heterogeneity of relative treatment effect by baseline risk has also been shown for blood pressure lowering,[50] aspirin[51] and lipid lowering[52] in primary prevention of vascular disease, and in treatment of acute coronary syndromes with clopidogrel,[53] and with enoxaparin versus unfractionated heparin.[54,55] There are many similar examples in other areas of medicine.[56,57]

The need for reliable data on risks and benefits in subgroups and individuals is greatest for potentially harmful interventions, such as warfarin or carotid endarterectomy, which are of overall benefit but which kill or disable a significant proportion of patients. Yet, evidence-based guidelines usually recommend these treatments in all cases similar to those in the relevant RCTs.[58–60] In considering this approach, it is useful to draw an analogy with the criminal justice system. Suppose that research showed that individuals charged by the police with certain crimes were usually guilty. Few would argue that they should therefore be sentenced without trial. Automatic sentencing would, on average, do 'more good than harm', with most criminals correctly convicted, but any avoidable miscarriages of justice are widely regarded as unacceptable. In contrast, relatively high rates of treatment-related death or disability ('miscarriages of treatment') are tolerated by the medical scientific community precisely on the basis that, on average, treatment will do 'more good than harm'. The analogy is only partial, but it holds to the extent that in both situations systems need to be in place to avoid doing harm. Yet, the contrast between the effort that is put into the defence of the accused in order to avoid wrongful conviction and the sometimes very limited efforts of the medical scientific community to identify patients at high risk of harm ('wrongful treatment') is stark. Admittedly, determination of guilt in a criminal trial is based on knowledge of past events, which can often be established with certainty, whereas likely benefit or harm from medical treatment depends on future events, which are usually less certain. However, the likely balance of risk and benefit in individual patients can be predicted to some extent with subgroup analysis and risk models, as has been shown, for example, with carotid endarterectomy.[61–63] Given that complications of treatment are now a leading cause of death in developed countries,[64] more effort is required to better target potentially harmful interventions.

Pathophysiological heterogeneity

Differences between groups of patients or individuals in underlying pathology, biology or genetics can each lead to clinically important heterogeneity of treatments effect. Some examples are given below, but increasing understanding of the molecular mechanisms of disease will probably lead to a substantial increase in the frequency with which this source of potential heterogeneity of treatment effect must be addressed.

Multiple underlying pathologies

Clinicians often have to treat patients with ill-defined clinical syndromes, which are likely to have multiple underlying pathologies, rather than single diseases. Primary generalised epilepsy is a typical example where the effects of treatment differ markedly between patients, probably in relation to the different underlying molecular pathologies. In vascular disease, clinically important heterogeneity of treatment effect in relation to underlying pathology is seen with thrombolysis for acute ischaemic stroke,[65,66] with aspirin in primary prevention of vascular disease, where benefit may be largely confined to men with elevated levels of C-reactive protein,[67] probably indicating underlying atherosclerosis, and with blood pressure lowering in secondary prevention of transient ischaemic attack (TIA) and stroke, where guidelines suggest that all patients be treated,[68–70] but there is clinical concern about patients with carotid stenosis or occlusion in whom cerebral perfusion is often severely impaired.[71,72] Table 9.1 shows stroke risk by systolic blood pressure (SBP) in patients with and without flow-limiting (≥ 70%) carotid stenosis who were randomised to medical treatment in RCTs of endarterectomy.[73] Major increases in stroke risk were seen in patients with flow-limiting stenosis, but only if the SBP is < 150 mmHg: the 5-year risk in patients with bilateral ≥ 70% stenosis is 64.3% versus 24.2% ($p = 0.002$) at higher blood pressures. This difference in risk was absent in patients who had been randomised to endarterectomy (13.4% versus 18.3%, $p = 0.6$), suggesting a causal effect and indicating that aggressive blood pressure lowering would very probably be harmful in patients with bilateral severe carotid disease in whom endarterectomy was not possible.

Stenosis group	Systolic blood pressure (mmHg)			
	< 130	130–149	150–169	≥ 170
Bilateral < 70%	1	1	1	1
Unilateral ≥ 70%	1.90 (1.24–2.89) $p = 0.02$	1.18 (0.92–1.51) $p = 0.30$	1.27 (0.99–1.64) $p = 0.13$	1.64 (1.15–2.33) $p = 0.03$
Bilateral ≥ 70%	5.97 (2.43–14.68) $p < 0.001$	2.54 (1.47–4.39) $p = 0.001$	0.97 (0.4–2.35) $p = 0.95$	1.13 (0.50–2.54) $p = 0.77$

*The hazard ratios are derived from a Cox proportional hazards model stratified by trial and adjusted for age, sex and previous coronary heart disease. Patients with bilateral < 70% stenosis are allocated a hazard of 1. Stenosis ≥ 70% is only consistently associated with an increase in the risk of stroke at lower levels of systolic blood pressure.

***Table 9.1:* Hazard ratios (95% CI) for the risk of stroke in patients categorised according to the severity of carotid disease within prespecified blood pressure groups[73] ***

Biological heterogeneity

Heterogeneity of relative treatment effect is also seen where there are predictable differences in the biological response to the underlying disease. For example, perioperative administration of antilymphocyte antibodies reduces rejection in cadaveric renal transplantation by 30%,[74,75] but is expensive and has serious adverse effects. Clinical concern that benefit might depend on pre-existing immune sensitisation prompted a meta-analysis of individual patient data from five RCTs. As predicted, treatment was found to be highly effective in the 15% of sensitised patients (hazard ratio (HR) for allograft failure at 5 years 0.20; 95% confidence interval (CI) 0.09 to 0.47), but was ineffective in the remaining 85% (HR 0.97; 95% CI 0.71 to 1.32).[75] The subgroup–treatment effect interaction was statistically significant ($p = 0.009$) (i.e. the effect of treatment was significantly different between the subgroups). A similar prespecified immunological subgroup analysis in a large trial of roxithromycin versus placebo after coronary angioplasty showed that treatment reduced re-stenosis and the need for revascularisation if the titre of *Chlamydia pneumoniae* antibody was high, but was ineffective or harmful if the titre was low (interaction: $p = 0.006$).[76]

Genetic heterogeneity

It has long been known that individuals respond differently to some drugs, and that this tendency can be inherited.[77,78] As reviewed in detail in Chapters 10 and 20, genotype is an important determinant of both the response to treatment and the susceptibility to adverse reactions for a wide range of drugs.[79,80] For example, it has recently been shown that the response to chemotherapy is dependent on gene expression in both colon cancer[81] and breast cancer,[82] and that the high-density lipoprotein (HDL) cholesterol response to oestrogen replacement therapy is highly dependent on sequence variants in the gene encoding oestrogen receptor alpha.[83] In each of these cases, statistically significant subgroup–treatment effect interactions have been reported. There is also great interest in genetic influences on the response to treatment in patients with human immunodeficiency virus type 1 (HIV-1).[84] However, subgroup analyses based on genotype do have particular methodological problems, as many genotypes may be studied and analyses will often be post hoc.

Heterogeneity related to stage of disease and timing of treatment

Even in situations where the pathophysiology of a disease is relatively uniform, there is often heterogeneity of treatment effect in relation to how and when interventions are used, such as at what stage of the disease is treatment most effective, or how soon after a clinical event is treatment sufficiently safe/most effective?

Severity or stage of disease

Treatment effects often depend on severity of disease. For example, in primary prevention of vascular disease, a pooled analysis of RCTs of pravastatin showed that the relative risk reduction (RRR) with treatment increased with baseline low-density lipoprotein (LDL) cholesterol (interaction: $p = 0.01$): RRR = 3% in the lowest quintile and RRR = 29% in the two highest quintles.[85] In stroke medicine, carotid endarterectomy is highly effective for $\geq 70\%$ recently symptomatic stenosis, modestly effective for 50–69% stenosis, but harmful for $< 50\%$ stenosis (interaction: $p < 0.0001$).[86] In cardiology, thrombolysis for acute myocardial infarction is ineffective or harmful in patients with

ST segment depression, but highly beneficial in patients with ST elevation (interaction: $p < 0.01$),[87] and early invasive treatment of unstable angina is of no benefit in patients with only minor ST segment change but of major benefit in patients with more marked changes (interaction: $p = 0.006$).[88] The stage of disease can also influence the effect of treatment of non-vascular disease, as is seen in cancer[89, 90] and in HIV/acquired immune deficiency syndrome (AIDS).[91–93]

Timing of treatment

Effect of treatment is often critically dependent on timing, as shown in figure 9.2 for benefit from endarterectomy for recently symptomatic carotid stenosis. The risk of a stroke on medical treatment is very high during the first few days and weeks after a TIA,[94] particularly in patients with carotid stenosis,[95] but falls rapidly with time, as therefore does benefit from endarterectomy.[63] Similar time dependence has been shown for benefit from thrombolysis for both acute myocardial infarction[87] and acute ischaemic stroke.[96]

Heterogeneity related to comorbidity

Treatment effects may also depend on comorbidity (i.e. conditions unrelated to the disease being treated), examples of which can be found in virtually all areas of medicine. In cardiovascular medicine, for example, angiotensin-converting enzyme (ACE)

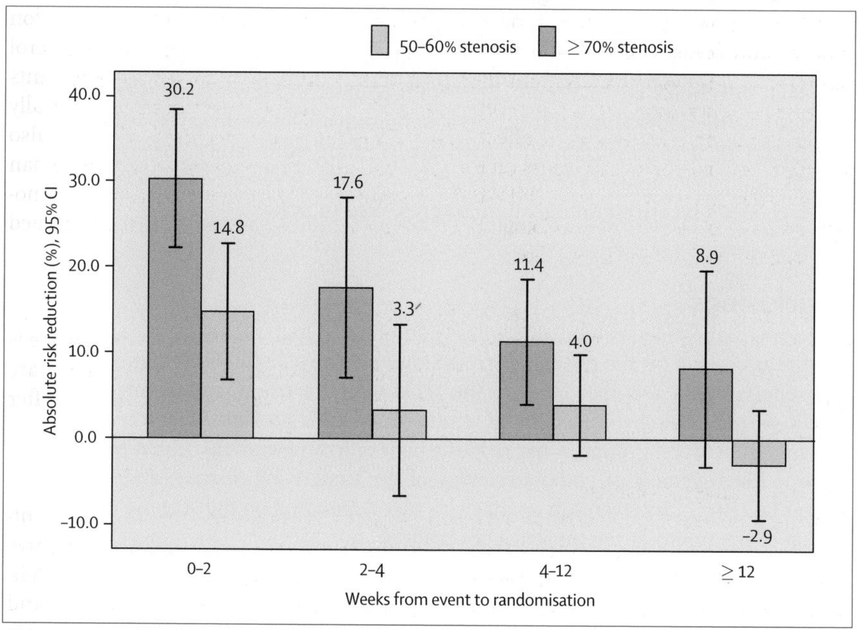

Figure 9.2: The effect of carotid endarterectomy in patients with 50–69% and ≥ 70% symptomatic stenosis in relation to the time from the last symptomatic ischaemic event to randomisation.[48] The numbers given above the error bars are the exact absolute risk reductions. (Reprinted from Rothwell,[99] copyright 2005,with permission from Elsevier.)

inhibitors and angiotensin II receptor blocking drugs are harmful in patients with renovascular disease but highly beneficial in other hypertensive patients,[97] and thiazide diuretics and beta-blockers can impair control of blood glucose in hypertensive patients with diabetes. Similarly, benefit from diltiazem after myocardial infarction may depend on the presence of heart failure because of the negative chronotropic and inotropic effects of the drug.[98]

Underuse of treatment in specific groups

Subgroup analysis and other methods of determining heterogeneity of treatment are justified, if appropriate methods are used (see Chapter 11), if there are good reasons to suspect clinically important differences in treatment effect. However, it is also important to understand that such analysis can also be very useful to clinicians when no differences are found, particularly where treatments are shown to be effective in groups of patients who tend to be undertreated in routine practice. For example, statins were not used in the elderly for many years until they were shown to be highly effective by subgroup analysis in the Heart Protection Study.[30] Proof of some benefit by subgroup analysis was also required to counter underuse in the elderly of thrombolysis for acute myocardial infarction,[87] and of endarterectomy for symptomatic carotid stenosis.[63] In each case, treatment had already been shown to be highly effective overall. Use of treatment in routine clinical practice is also often inappropriately limited to patients with measurements of physiological parameters above certain arbitrary cut-off points, such as treatment thresholds for blood pressure and total cholesterol in prevention of vascular disease. There is increasing evidence from subgroup analysis in large trials that such thresholds are inappropriate.[30, 68] Proof of lack of heterogeneity of treatment effect is also therefore a useful function of subgroup analysis. However, as highlighted in Chapter 11, it is important that such analyses are sufficiently powered to detect benefit, and pooled analyses of multiple trials will often be required for subgroups such as the elderly who are commonly underrepresented in trials.

Conclusions

Large pragmatic trials with broad eligibility criteria and high inclusion rates provide the most reliable data on the effects of treatments, but they should be designed, analysed and reported in a way that leads to the most effective use of treatments in routine practice. Predictable heterogeneity of treatment effect is possible when there are large differences between groups in the risk of a poor outcome with or without treatment, if there is heterogeneity of pathophysiology of the underlying disease, and if the risks and/or benefits of intervention are likely to vary depending on the stage of disease, the timing of treatment or the presence of comorbidity.

References

1 Feinstein AR. The problem of cogent subgroups: a clinicostatistical tragedy. *J Clin Epidemiol* 1998; **51:** 297–99.

2 Peto R. Statistics of cancer trials. In: Halan KE, ed. *Treatment of Cancer*. London: Chapman & Hall, 1981.

3 Collins R, Peto R, Gray R, Parish S. Large-scale randomised evidence: trials and overviews. In: Weatherall DJ, Ledingham JGG, Warrell DA, eds. *Oxford Textbook of Medicine*. Oxford: Oxford University Press, 1996.

4 Yusef S, Collins R, Peto R. Why do we need some large, simple randomized trials? *Stat Med* 1984; **3:** 409–20.

5 Collins R, MacMahon S. Reliable assessment of the effects of treatment on mortality and major morbidity, I: clinical trials. *Lancet* 2001; **357:** 373–80.

6 Bailey KR. Generalising the results of randomised clinical trials. *Control Clin Trials* 1994; **15:** 15–23.

7 Davey Smith G, Egger M, Phillips AN. Beyond the grand mean. *BMJ* 1997; **315:** 1610–14.

8 Wittes RE. Problems in the medical interpretation of overviews. *Stat Med* 1987; **6:** 269–76.

9 Lau J, Ionnidis JPA, Schmid CH. Summing up evidence: one answer is not always enough. *Lancet* 1998; **351:** 123–27.

10 Ionnidis JPA, Lau J. Uncontrolled pearls, controlled evidence, meta-analysis and the individual patient. *J Clin Epidemiol* 1998; **51:** 709–11.

11 Chalmers I. A patient's attitude to the use of research evidence for guiding individual choices and decisions in healthcare. *Clin Risk* 2000; **6:** 227–30.

12 Suillivan FM, MacNaughton RJ. Evidence in consultations: interpreted and individualised. *Lancet* 1996; **348:** 941–43.

13 Senn S. Applying results of randomised trials to patients. *BMJ* 1998; **317:** 537.

14 Oxman AD, Guyatt GH. A consumer's guide to subgroup analyses. *Ann Intern Med* 1992; **116:** 78–84.

15 Black D. The limitations of evidence. *J R Coll Phys (London)* 1998; **32:** 23–26.

16 Hampton JR. Size isn't everything. *Stat Med* 2002; **21:** 2807–14.

17 Caplan LR. Evidence based medicine: concerns of a clinical neurologist. *J Neurol Neurosurg Psychiatry* 2001; **71:** 569–74.

18 Evans JG. Evidence-based and evidence-biased medicine. *Age Ageing* 1995; **24:** 461–63.

19 Swales JD. Evidence-based medicine and hypertension. *J Hypertens* 1999; **17:** 1511–16.

20 Feinstein AR, Horwitz RI. Problems in the 'evidence' of 'evidence-based medicine'. *Am J Med* 1997; **103:** 529–35.

21 Fahey T. Applying the results of clinical trials to patients in general practice: perceived problems, strengths, assumptions, and challenges for the future. *Br J Gen Pract* 1998; **48:** 1173–78.

22 Mant D. Can randomised trials inform clinical decisions about individual patients? *Lancet* 1999; **353:** 743–46.

23 Sackett DL, Straus SE. Finding and applying evidence during clinical rounds: the 'evidence cart'. *JAMA* 1998; **280:** 1336–38.

24 Sackett DL. Applying overviews and meta-analyses at the bedside. *J Clin Epidemiol* 1995; **48:** 61–70.

25 Ellis J, Mulligan I, Rowe J, Sackett DL. Inpatient general medicine is evidence based. *Lancet* 1995; **346:** 407–10.

26 Rothwell PM. External validity of randomised controlled trials: 'To whom do the results of this trial apply?' *Lancet* 2003; **365:** 82–93.

27 Rothwell PM. Can overall results of clinical trials be applied to all patients? *Lancet* 1995; **345:** 1616–19.

28 Yusuf S, Wittes J, Probstfield J, Tyroler HA. Analysis and interpretation of treatment effects in subgroups of patients in randomised clinical trials. *JAMA* 1991; **266:** 93–98.

29 Rose G. High-risk and population strategies of prevention: ethical considerations. *Ann Med* 1989; **21:** 409–13.

30 Heart Protection Study Collaborative Group. MRC/BHF Heart Protection Study of cholesterol lowering with simvastatin in 20,536 high-risk individuals: a randomised placebo-controlled trial. *Lancet* 2002; **360:** 7–22.

31 Lewington S, Clarke R, Qizilbash N, et al. Age-specific relevance of usual blood pressure to vascular mortality: a meta-analysis of individual data for one million adults in 61 prospective studies. *Lancet* 2002; **360:** 1903–13.

32 Assmann SF, Pocock SJ, Enos LE, Kasten LE. Subgroup analysis and other (mis)uses of baseline data in clinical trials. *Lancet* 2000; **355:** 1064–69.

33 Stallones RA. The use and abuse of subgroup analysis in epidemiological research. *Prev Med* 1987; **16:** 183–94.

34 Pocock SJ, Hughes MD. Estimation issues in clinical trials and overviews. *Stat Med* 1990; **9:** 657–71.

35 Brookes ST, Whitley E, Peters TJ, et al. Subgroup analyses in randomised controlled trials: quantifying the risks of false-positives and false-negatives. *Health Technol Assess* 2001; **5**(33). Available at: http://www.ncchta.org (accessed February 2007).

36 Moreira ED, Stein Z, Susser E. Reporting on methods of subgroup analysis in clinical trials: a survey of four scientific journals. *Braz J Med Boil Res* 2001; **34:** 1441–46.

37 Cui L, Hung HNJ, Wang SJ, Tsong Y. Issues related to subgroup analysis in clinical trials. *J Biopharmaceut Stat* 2002; **12:** 347–58.

38 van Gijn J. Extrapolation of trial data into practice: where is the limit? *Cerebrovasc Dis* 1995; **5:** 159–62.

39 International Stroke Trial Collaborative Group. The International Stroke Trial (IST): a randomised trial of aspirin, subcutaneous heparin, both, or neither among 19435 patients with acute ischaemic stroke. *Lancet* 1997; **349:** 1569–81.

40 Fourth International Study of Infarct Survival Collaborative Group. ISIS-4: a randomised factorial trial assessing early oral captopril, oral mononitrate, and intravenous magnesium sulphate in 58,050 patients with suspected acute myocardial infarction. *Lancet* 1995; **345:** 669–85.

41 Dahlof B, Lindholm LH, Hansson L, et al. Morbidity and mortality in the Swedish trial in old patients with hypertension (STOP-hypertension). *Lancet* 1991; **338:** 1281–85.

42 Medical Research Council Working Party. MRC trial of treatment of mild hypertension: principal results. *BMJ* 1985; **291:** 97–104.

43 Ebrahim S, Davey Smith G. The 'number needed to treat': does it help clinical decision making? *J Hum Hypertens* 1999; **13:** 721–24.

44 Furukawa TA, Guyatt CH, Griffith LE. Can we individualize the 'number needed to treat'? An empirical study of summary effect measures in meta-analyses. *Int J Epidemiol* 2002; **31:** 72–76.

45 Ionnidis JPA, Lau J. The impact of high-risk patients on the results of clinical trials. *J Clin Epidemiol* 1997; **50:** 1089–98.

46 Rothwell PM, Warlow CP, on behalf of the ECST. Prediction of benefit from carotid endarterectomy in individual patients: a risk modeling study. *Lancet* 1999; **353:** 2105–10.

47 Laupacis A, Boysen G, Connolly S, et al. Risk factors for stroke and efficacy of antithrombotic therapy in atrial fibrillation. Analysis of pooled data from five randomised controlled trials. *Arch Intern Med* 1994; **154:** 1449–57.

48 Yusuf S, Zucker D, Peduzzi P, et al. Effect of coronary artery bypass graft surgery on survival: overview of 10-year results from randomised trials by the Coronary Artery Bypass Graft Surgery Trialists' Collaboration. *Lancet* 1994; **344:** 563–70.

49 Boissel JP, Collet JP, Lievre M, Girard P. An effect model for the assessment of drug benefit: example of antiarrhythmic drugs in postmyocardial infarction patients. *J Cardiovasc Pharmacol* 1993; **22:** 356–63.

50 Li W, Boissel JP, Girard P, et al. Identification and prediction of responders to a therapy: a model and its preliminary application to actual data. *J Epidemiol Biostat* 1998; **3:** 189–97.

51 Sanmuganathan PS, Ghahramani P, Jackson PR, et al. Aspirin for primary prevention of coronary heart disease: safety and absolute benefit related to coronary risk derived from meta-analysis of randomised trials. *Heart* 2001; **85:** 265–71.

52 West of Scotland Coronary Prevention Group. West of Scotland Coronary Prevention Study: identification of high-risk groups and comparison with other cardiovascular intervention trials. *Lancet* 1996; **348:** 1339–42.

53 Bundaj A, Yusuf S, Mehta SR, et al., for the Clopidogrel in Unstable angina to prevent Recurrent Events (CURE) Trial Investigators. Benefit of clopidogrel in patients with acute coronary syndromes without ST-segment elevation in various risk groups. *Circulation* 2002; **106:** 1622–26.

54 Antman EM, Cohen M, Bernink PJLM, et al. The TIMI risk score for unstable angina/non-ST elevation MI. A method for prognostication and therapeutic decision making. *JAMA* 2000; **284:** 835–42.

55 Cohen M, Demers C, Garfinkel EP, et al. A comparison of low molecular weight heparin with unfractionated heparin for unstable coronary artery disease. *N Engl J Med* 1997; **337:** 447–52.

56 Pagliaro L, D'Amico G, Soronson TIA, et al. Prevention of bleeding in cirrhosis. *Ann Intern Med* 1992; **117:** 59–70.

57 International Study of Unruptured Intracranial Aneurysms Investigators. Unruptured intracranial aneurysms – risks of rupture and risks of surgical intervention. *N Engl J Med* 1998; **339:** 1725–33.

58 Royal College of Physicians of London. *National Clinical Guidelines for Stroke*. London, RCP, 2000.

59 Biller J, Feinberg WM, Castaldo JE, et al. Guidelines for carotid endarterectomy: a statement for healthcare professionals from a Special Writing Group of the Stroke Council, American Heart Association. *Stroke* 1998; **29:** 554–62.

60 Pearson TA, Blair SN, Daniels SR, et al., for the American Heart Association Science Advisory and Coordinating Committee. AHA Guidelines for primary prevention of cardiovascular disease and stroke: 2002 Update: consensus panel guide to comprehensive risk reduction for adult patients without coronary or other atherosclerotic vascular diseases. *Circulation* 2002; **106:** 388–91.

61 Rothwell PM, Slattery J, Warlow CP. A systematic comparison of the risks of stroke and death due to carotid endarterectomy for symptomatic and asymptomatic stenosis. *Stroke* 1996; **27:** 266–69.

62 Bond R, Rerkasem K, Rothwell PM. A systematic review of the risks of carotid endarterectomy in relation to the clinical indication and the timing of surgery. *Stroke* 2003; **34:** 2290–301.

63 Rothwell PM, Eliasziw M, Gutnikov SA, et al., for the Carotid Endarterectomy Trialists' Collaboration. Effect of endarterectomy for recently symptomatic carotid stenosis in relation to clinical subgroups and the timing of surgery. *Lancet* 2004; **363:** 915–24.

64 Lazarou J, Pomeranz BH, Corey PN. Incidence of adverse drug reactions in hospitalised patients. *JAMA* 1998; **279:** 1200–05.

65 Alder SJ, Moody AR, Martel AL, et al. Limitations of clinical diagnosis in acute stroke. *Lancet* 1999; **354:** 1523.

66 Hacke W, Brott T, Caplan L. Thrombolysis in acute ischemic stroke: controlled trials and clinical experience. *Neurology* 1999; **53** (suppl 4): S3–14

67 Ridker PM, Cushman M, Stampfer MJ, et al. Inflammation, aspirin, and the risk of cardiovascular disease in apparently healthy men. *N Engl J Med* 1997; **336:** 973–79.

68 PROGRESS Collaborative Group. Randomised trial of a perindopril-based blood-pressure-lowering regimen among 6,105 individuals with previous stroke or transient ischaemic attack. *Lancet* 2001; **358:** 1033–41.

69 Anon. National clinical guidelines for stroke: a concise update. *Clin Med* 2002; **2:** 231–33.

70 McAlister FA, Zarnke KB, Campbell NR, et al., for the Canadian Hypertension Recommendations Working Group. The 2001 Canadian recommendations for the management of hypertension: Part two – Therapy. *Can J Cardiol* 2002; **18:** 625–41.

71 Van der Grond J, Balm R, Kappelle J, et al. Cerebral metabolism of patients with stenosis or occlusion of the internal carotid artery. *Stroke* 1995; **26:** 822–28.

72 Grubb RL, Derdeyn CP, Fritsch SM, et al. Importance of hemodynamic factors in the prognosis of symptomatic carotid occlusion. *JAMA* 1998; **280:** 1055–60.

73 Rothwell PM, Howard SC, Spence D. Relationship between blood pressure and stroke risk in patients with symptomatic carotid occlusive disease. *Stroke* 2003; **34:** 2583–90.

74 Szczech LA, Berlin JA, Aradhye S, et al. Effect of anti-lymphocyte induction therapy on renal allograft survival: a meta-analysis. *J Am Soc Nephrol* 1997; **8:** 1771–77.

75 Szczech LA, Berlin JA, Feldman HI. The effect of antilymphocyte induction therapy on renal allograft survival. A meta-analysis individual patient-level data. Anti-Lymphocyte Antibody Induction Therapy Study Group. *Ann Intern Med* 1998; **128:** 817–26.

76 Neumann F-J, Kastrati A, Miethke T, et al. Treatment of *Chlamydia pneumoniae* infection with roxithromycin and effect on neointima proliferation after coronary stent placement (ISAR-3): a randomised, double-blind, placebo-controlled trial. *Lancet* 2001; **357:** 2085–89.

77 Kalow W, Gunn DR. Some statistical data on atypical cholinesterase of human serum. *Ann Hum Genet* 1959; **23:** 239–50.

78 Price Evans DA, Manley KA, McKusick VA. Genetic control of isoniazid metabolism in man. *BMJ* 1960; **2:** 485–91.

79 Weinshilboum R. Inheritance and drug response. *N Engl J Med* 2003; **348:** 529–37.

80 Philips KA, Veenstra DL, Oren E, et al. Potential role of pharmacogenomics in reducing adverse drug reactions. *JAMA* 2001; **286:** 2270–79.

81 Barratt PL, Seymour MT, Stenning SP, et al. DNA markers predicting benefit from adjuvant fluorouracil in patients with colon cancer: a molecular study. *Lancet* 2002; **360:** 1381–91.

82 Chang JC, Wooten EC, Tsimelzon A, et al. Gene expression profiling for the prediction of therapeutic response to docetaxel in patients with breast cancer. *Lancet* 2003; **362:** 362–69.

83 Herrington DM, Howard TD, Hawkins GA, et al. Estrogen-receptor polymorphisms and effects of estrogen replacement on high-density lipoprotein cholesterol in women with coronary disease. *N Engl J Med* 2002; **346:** 967–74.

84 Telenti A, Aubert V, Spertini F. Individualising HIV treatment – pharmacogenetics and immunogenetics. *Lancet* 2002; **359:** 722–23.

85 Sacks FM, Tonkin AM, Shepherd J, et al., for the Prospective Pravastatin Pooling Project Investigators Group. Effect of pravastatin on coronary disease events in subgroups defined by coronary risk factors. *Circulation* 2000; **102:** 1893–900.

86 Rothwell PM, Gutnikov SA, Eliasziw M, et al., for the Carotid Endarterectomy Trialists' Collaboration. Pooled analysis of individual patient data from randomised controlled trials of endarterectomy for symptomatic carotid stenosis. *Lancet* 2003; **361:** 107–16.

87 Fibrinolytic Therapy Trialists' (FTT) Collaborative Group. Indications for fibrinolytic therapy in suspected acute myocardial infarction: collaborative overview of early mortality and major morbidity results from all randomised trials of more than 1000 patients. *Lancet* 1994; **343:** 311–22.

88 Holmvang L, Clemmensen P, Lindahl B, et al. Quantitative analysis of the admission electrocardiogram identifies patients with unstable coronary artery disease who benefit the most from early invasive treatment. *J Am Coll Cardiol* 2003; **41:** 905–15.

89 PORT Meta-analysis Trialists Group. Postoperative radiotherapy in non-small-cell lung cancer: systematic review and meta-analysis of individual patient data from nine randomised controlled trials. *Lancet* 1998; **352:** 257–63.

90 Gale RP, Horowitz MM. How best to analyse new strategies in bone marrow transplantation. *Bone Marrow Transpl* 1990; **6:** 357–59.

91 Fischl MA, Richman DD, Griego MH, et al. The efficacy of azidothymidine (AZT) in the treatment of patients with AIDS and AIDS-related complex. A double-blind, placebo-controlled trial. *N Engl J Med* 1987; **317:** 185–91.

92 Concorde Coordinating Committee. Concorde: MRC/ANRS randomised double-blind controlled trial of immediate and deferred zidovudine in symptom-free HIV infection. *Lancet* 1994; **343:** 871–81.

93 Egger M, Neaton JD, Phillips AN, Davey Smith G. Concorde trial of immediate versus deferred zidovudine. *Lancet* 1994; **343:** 1355.

94 Coull A, Lovett JK, Rothwell PM, on behalf of the Oxford Vascular Study. Early risk of stroke after a TIA or minor stroke in a population-based incidence study. *BMJ* 2004; **328:** 326–28.

95 Lovett JK, Coull A, Rothwell PM, on behalf of the Oxford Vascular Study. Early risk of recurrent stroke by aetiological subtype: implications for stroke prevention. *Neurology* 2004; **62:** 569–74.

96 Wardlaw JM, Warlow CP, Counsell C. Systematic review of evidence on thrombolytic therapy for acute ischaemic stroke. *Lancet* 1997; **350:** 607–14.

97 Brown MJ. Matching the right drug to the right patient in essential hypertension. *Heart* 2001; **86:** 113–20.

98 Multicentrer Diltiazem Postinfarction Trial Research Group. The effect of diltiazem on mortality and reinfarction after myocardial infarction. *N Engl J Med* 1988; **319:** 385–92.

99 Rothwell PM. Treating individuals 2. Subgroup analysis in randomised controlled trials: importance, indications, and interpretation. *Lancet* 2005; **365:** 176–86.

Genes and the individual response to treatment

Urs A. Meyer

Introduction

Physicians prescribe drugs on the basis of their knowledge of the clinical problem and on the statistical probability that a certain medication will be beneficial for the patient. However, interindividual, or person-to-person, differences in drug responses are common and decrease the predictability of therapeutic outcomes. The variation can range from therapeutic failure to adverse or even fatal drug reactions. In this chapter I use the example of pharmacological individuality and the attempts to improve its predictability to illustrate the importance of genetic variation in determining the individual response to treatment.

The epidemiology of adverse drug reactions (ADRs) has been analysed extensively in prospective studies of hospital admissions[1] or meta-analyses of studies of hospitalised patients.[2] ADRs account for approximately 5% of hospital admissions, and in about 7% of patients serious drug reactions occur during their hospital stay. The incidence of fatal drug reactions in all patients admitted to hospitals is approximately 0.15% (table 10.1). ADRs clearly prolong hospital stays and continue to be a considerable burden to patients and healthcare systems. They most prominently involve drugs with a narrow therapeutic index (i.e. if very small changes in the dose level can cause either subtherapeutic or toxic results, e.g. ciclosporin, valproic acid and warfarin).

Therapeutic failures or inefficacy of treatment because of interindividual variations in drug response are more difficult to assess. However, many of the major drug therapies (antidepressants, lipid-lowering agents, bronchodilators) are effective in only 25–60% of patients.[4] A striking example is the lack of an analgesic effect of codeine or tramadol in patients with a genetic deficiency of cytochrome P450 2D6 (CYP2D6), as described later in this chapter.

Impact	Patients (%)
Hospital admission	~ 5%[1]
Serious ADR while in hospital	~ 7%[2]
Fatal ADR	0.15–0.3%[1, 2] *
Average prolongation of hospital stay because of ADR	~ 2 days[3]

*Estimates are > 10 000/year in the UK; > 100 000/year in North-America.

Table 10.1: **Impact of adverse drug reactions (ADRs)**

Causes of interindividual variation in drug response

What determines an individual's risk of developing an ADR or of having no benefit from a particular drug treatment? How much of this variability is a constant characteristic of the individual, and therefore predictable (e.g. by clinical and laboratory tests)? How many of the ADRs and therapeutic failures can thereby be prevented?

An important fact is that individuality in drug response is caused by multiple factors, including the patient's sex, age and pre-existing diseases (e.g. impaired renal, hepatic or cardiac function, or allergies), but also factors such as compliance, environmental factors (e.g. diet, concomitantly administered drugs, smoking and alcohol) and genetic factors (panel 10.1). Numerous studies have documented that an important component of this variation is indeed inherited or due to the individual genetic make-up of the patient. In the last 50 years, a large number of genes that code for drug-metabolising enzymes, drug receptors, drug transporters, ion channels and other drug targets have been shown to carry mutations that alter the expression or function of these drug targets, and contribute to the individual variability in the efficacy and toxicity of drug treatments. The study of these inherited variations in drug response constitutes the field of pharmacogenetics (figure 10.1). More recently, with the human genome sequence completed, the term 'pharmacogenomics' has arisen for genome-wide approaches to elucidating the inherited differences between people in their response to drugs. Thus,

Panel 10.1: Determinants of individual responses to drugs

Host factors

- Gender
- Age
- Weight
- Disease (impaired kidney or liver function, inflammation, etc.)
- Compliance
- Placebo effects
- Socio-economic factors

Environmental factors

- Smoking
- Nutrition
- Other drug treatments (drug–drug interactions)
- Recreational drugs
- Chemical exposition

Genes (pharmacogenetics)

- Genetic variability of expression and function of genes for:
  - drug-metabolising enzymes
  - drug transporters
  - ion channels
  - receptors
  - transcription factors

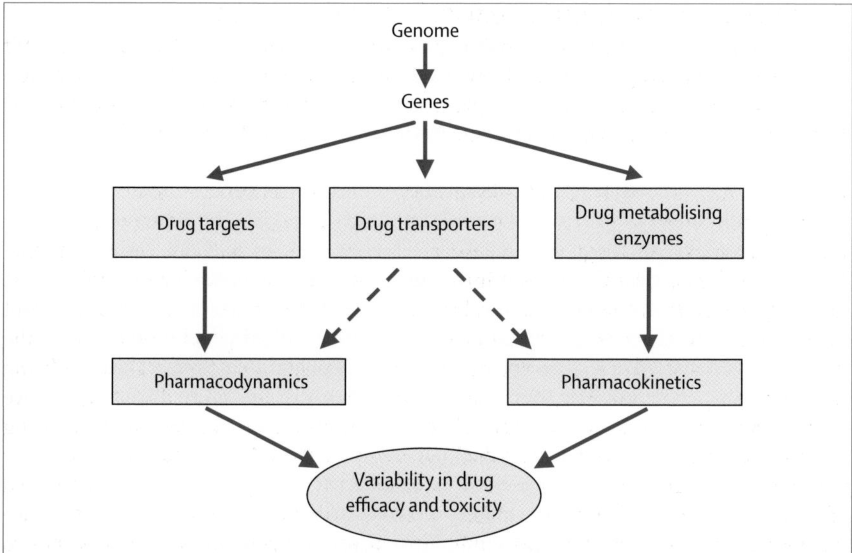

***Figure* 10.1: Principles of pharmacogenetics and pharmacogenomics.**

variability in drug response or individuality of drug effects are the result of contributions of host, environmental and genetic factors.

The individuality of genomes

Genomics, transcriptomics, proteomics and metabolomics are revolutionising the study of disease processes and the development of new drugs. These technologies increasingly enable medicine to make reliable assessments of the individual risk of acquiring a particular disease, raise the number and specificity of drug targets, and can explain some of the interindividual variation of the therapeutic effectiveness and toxicity of drugs. The ultimate promise of pharmacogenetics and pharmacogenomics is the expectation that knowledge of a patient's genome sequence in concert with clinical and laboratory tests might be used to individualise drug treatment to maximise efficacy, to target drugs only to those patients that are likely to respond and to prevent ADRs. For this to happen, we have to understand how the stable changes in the genome of an individual are translated into different transcripts and proteins and alter the function of drug targets.

How diverse are individual genomes? One of the striking observations from the analysis and resequencing of human genomes is the extent of DNA sequence similarity among individuals around the world. Any two unrelated humans are 99.9% identical in their DNA sequence. It is the 0.1% in sequence difference that constitutes the genetic variation between individuals and can cause inherited variations in drug response. The differences in sequence include single nucleotide polymorphisms (SNPs), various repetitive elements (micro- and mini-satellites) and small insertions, deletions, inversions and duplications.[5] However, more recently, an unexpectedly large extent of 'structural variation' between individual genomes has been reported, including large insertions, deletions, inversions and translocations. Of particular interest is the observation of gene copy number variants.[6] The combined differences in DNA sequence and structure constitute the genome of an individual. SNPs occur approximately once every 300–3000 base pairs if one compares the genomes of two unrelated individuals, and SNPs represent the majority of all variant DNA sites. It has been estimated that there are 11–15 million SNPs with a minor allele frequency of > 1%. Over 9 million SNPs are currently available in the public databases.[7,8] How can we use this information to predict drug responses? For clinical correlation studies in relatively small populations, SNPs that occur at frequencies of greater than 10% are most likely to be useful, but rare SNPs with a strong selection component and a more marked effect on phenotype are equally important. Once a large number of these SNPs and their frequencies in different populations are known, they can be used to correlate an individual's genetic 'fingerprint' with the probable individual drug response. It has been proposed that high-density maps of SNPs, or so-called haplotype blocks (sets of closely linked SNPs on a single chromosome, which tend to be inherited as a group[8]), in the human genome may allow the use of a limited number of SNPs as markers of xenobiotic responses, even if the target remains unknown, providing a 'drug-response profile' that is associated with contributions from multiple genes to a response phenotype. Current genetic microarray systems and other technologies can test thousands of SNPs. Moreover, new technologies may allow the sequencing of an entire human genome in a few hours in the near future. However, SNPs are not evenly distributed across the genome and differ between populations of different ethnic origin. In practice, therefore, and because of the complexities of defining disease phenotypes and clinical outcomes, the validity of this concept remains to be demonstrated.[9] Obviously, phenotyping methods will remain extremely important to assess the clinical relevance of genetic variations, as discussed below.

Some of the variations in DNA sequence occur at a relatively high frequency in particular populations and cause pharmacogenetic traits. If one gene locus, which comprises the corresponding genes on the chromosome pair (i.e. the one inherited from the mother and the one inherited from the father), codes for a drug-metabolising enzyme, a transporter protein or a drug receptor, mutations in these two genes (or variant alleles) may cause absence or functional impairment of this protein and result in an altered drug response (or drug response phenotype). If the incidence of the 'mutant allele' or gene variant is > 1% in the normal population, we call it a *genetic polymorphism* of drug response.

Monogenic causes or polymorphisms of drug response

The best studied examples of the effect of genes on individual drug responses are indeed polymorphisms of single genes with major effects on drug-metabolising enzymes, drug transporters, ion channels and receptors. An alternative situation is the occurrence of non-germline mutations of genes, for instance in cancer cells, which determine the presence or absence of a drug target.

Molecular studies in pharmacogenetics started with the initial cloning and characterisation of the drug-metabolising cytochrome P450 enzyme CYP2D6, and have now been extended to numerous human genes, including more than 30 drug-metabolising enzymes, several drug receptors, drug transporters and ion channels, as summarised in numerous reviews and websites.[10–16] Variants or alleles are different from the 'normal' gene by one or multiple mutations, but also include gene deletions and gene duplications or multiduplications. The mutations may have no effect on enzyme activity, or lead to enzymes with decreased or absent activity; duplications may lead to increased enzyme activity. The consequent categories of phenotypes are called *extensive metabolisers* (EM) for individuals homozygous or heterozygous for normal-activity enzymes, *intermediate metabolisers* (IM) or *poor metabolisers* (PM) for carriers of two decreased activity or loss of function alleles, and *ultrarapid metabolisers* (UM) for carriers of duplicated or multiduplicated active genes (figure 10.2). Although the number and complexity of the mutations may be large overall, only a small number of variant genes, usually 3–5 alleles, are common, and these account for most (usually over 95%) of mutant alleles. These variants can easily be detected by modern DNA methods, including DNA chip microarrays and mass spectrometry, and can assign most patients to a particular phenotype group.[17,18] But there also are limitations to genotyping. For instance, only around 20% of ultrarapid metaboliser phenotypes have CYP2D6 gene duplications, meaning that 80% of ultrarapid metabolisers are missed by present genotyping tests.[19]

The poor metaboliser phenotype for most of the polymorphic genes is inherited as an autosomal recessive trait, requiring the presence of two mutant alleles, whereas the ultrarapid metaboliser phenotype of CYP2D6 is inherited as a dominant trait. As already mentioned, these considerations apply only to monogenic traits, where one gene locus has a major effect on the phenotype and divides the population into two or three distinct groups. Approximately 45 monogenetic traits have been associated with an altered drug response in more than one clinical study. We have analysed these polymorphisms with regard to their possible clinical impact or the potential that they may considerably affect the choice and/or the dose of a drug. At this time this applies to only a few pharmacogenetic traits (table 10.2).

CYP2C9, VKORC1 and warfarin

Warfarin is a coumarin-based anticoagulant used worldwide that requires careful clinical management to balance the potentially lethal risks of overanticoagulation and bleeding with the equally daunting risks of underanticoagulation and clotting. In 2003, a total of 21 million prescriptions were written for warfarin in the USA alone. It is a legitimate target for a pharmacogenetic test because the surrogate for its clinical effect, the international normalised ratio (INR) of the prothrombin time, takes several days to reach its steady state, and improvements in both adverse outcomes and efficacy would be obtained if a pharmacogenetic test could more accurately predict dose.

Cytochrome P450 CYP2C9 is known to be the primary catalyst of the human metabolism of the (*S*)-enantiomer of warfarin.[20] Multiple retrospective studies from investigators all over the world have shown that variant alleles of the CYP2C9 gene encoding the

*2[Arg144Cys] and *3[Ile359Leu] alleles increase the anticoagulant effect of warfarin and decrease the mean daily dose required to maintain the INR of the prothrombin time within the target therapeutic range.[21] Aithal et al.,[22] the first group to report a clinical association between CYP2C9 genotype and warfarin dose, went on to study the contribution of other variables that affect the warfarin dose requirements, such as age, body size, and vitamin K and lipid status. Multiple linear regression models for warfarin dose indicated significant contributions from age and the CYP2C9 genotype.[23]

These data prompted Higashi et al.[24] to design a trial to test whether CYP2C9 genotyping could predict outcomes of patients on warfarin therapy. In this retrospective cohort

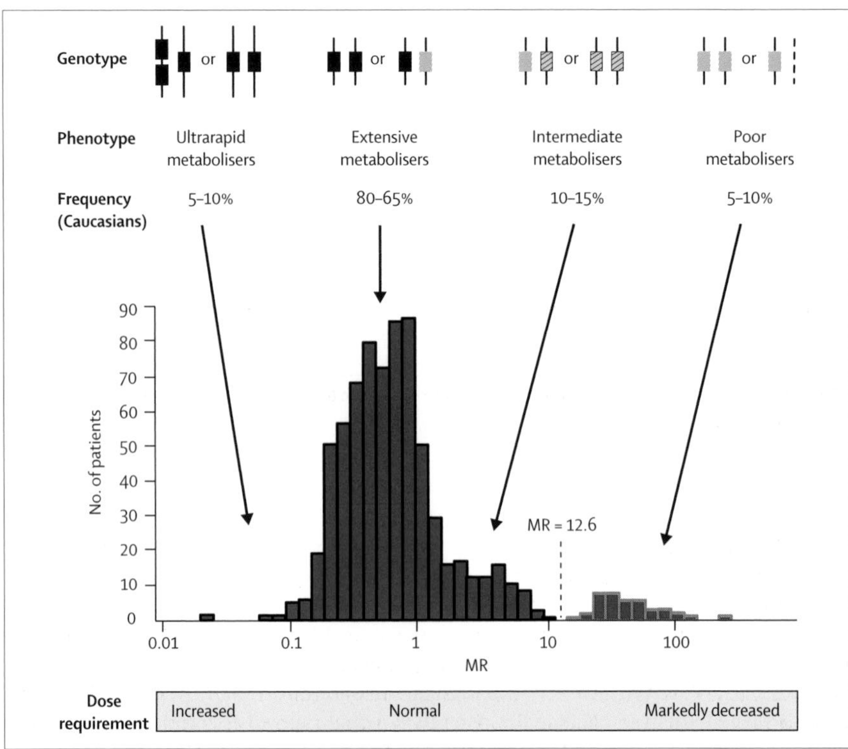

Figure 10.2: **Genotype–phenotype relationships of the CYP2D6 polymorphism. Null alleles of the CYP2D6 gene on chromosome 22 are indicated by green boxes, fully functional alleles by black boxes, decreased function alleles by hatched boxes, and deletion of the CYP2D6 gene by a dashed line. The associated phenotypes and their approximate frequencies in Caucasian populations are assigned to the subpopulations that have been determined by the urinary metabolic ratio (MR) of debrisoquine to 4-hydroxydebrisoquine. MR = 12.6 is the cut-off point between individuals with 'poor metabolism', as a result of decreased or absent CYP2D6 activity, and subjects with intermediate or extensive metabolism. To achieve the same plasma concentration of a drug, poor metabolisers require only a fraction of the dose of extensive metabolisers, and ultrarapid metabolisers need a higher dose. (Modified from Meyer,[15] Zanger et al.[44] and Kirchheiner et al.[49])**

Gene coding for enzyme/target	Drugs	Unwanted effect to be avoided
CYP2C9 and VKORC1	Warfarin, acenocoumarol	Haemorrhage, thromboembolic events
CYP2C19	Citalopram, escitalopram, sertraline, TCAs	ADRs in poor metabolisers
	Omeprazole, lansoprazole, rabeprazole	Decreased efficacy
CYP2D6	Antipsychotic drugs (e.g. thioridazine, risperidone)	Extrapyramidal symptoms, cardiotoxicity
	Antidepressants (e.g. venlafaxine, TCAs)	ADRs in poor metabolisers, lack of response in ultrarapid metabolisers
	Codeine, tramadol	Lack of analgesic effect
NAT2	Isoniazid	Hepatotoxicity
TPMT	Mercaptopurine, azathioprine	Myelosuppression, radiotherapy-related secondary tumours
UGT1A1	Irinotecan	Diarrhoea, myelosuppression
DPD	Fluorouracil	ADRs
HER2	Trastuzumab	Ineffective therapy

ADR, adverse drug reaction; TCA, tricyclic antidepressant

***Table 10.2:* Examples of genetic variations for which genetic tests may affect drug choice or dose and reduce adverse reactions**

study, 200 patients receiving long-term warfarin therapy for various indications underwent CYP2C9 genotyping and were evaluated by outcome measures, including anticoagulation status, measured by time to therapeutic INRs, rate of above-range INRs, and time to stable warfarin dosing or to serious or life-threatening bleeding events. Compared with patients with the wild-type genotype, patients with at least one variant allele of CYP2C9 (CYP2C9*2 or *3) had an increased risk of above-range INRs of 1.40 (95% confidence interval (CI) 1.03 to 1.90). The variant group also required more time to achieve stable dosing (odds ratio (OR) = 0.65; 95% CI 0.45 to 0.94), with a median difference of 95 days ($p = 0.004$). In addition, patients with a variant genotype had a significantly increased risk of a serious or life-threatening bleeding event (OR = 2.39; 95% CI 1.18 to 4.86). However, in spite of these results, and evidence that major bleeding or thromboembolic events could be reduced by genotyping by about 9%,[25] the benefit of DNA tests for CYP2C9 variants to adjust initial warfarin dose has been questioned because of the relatively small effect on warfarin dose and interethnic differences in the incidence of the CYP2C9 polymorphism.[26] Estimates are that the CYP2C9 polymorphism accounts for only 5–15% of variability in patient dose, and that other genetic factors and environmental factors are also important.

Warfarin exerts its anticoagulant effect by reducing the regeneration of vitamin K from vitamin K epoxide through inhibition of vitamin K epoxide reductase. This protein is encoded by the gene *VKORC1* for (vitamin K epoxide reductase complex subunit 1, the warfarin sensitive component of a large protein complex) of which rare mutations have been associated with warfarin resistance.[27] A number of recent studies now clearly establish that VKORC1 non-coding SNPs can be used to stratify patients into low-, intermediate- and high-dose warfarin groups.[28–32] Thus, the mean maintenance dose of warfarin differed significantly among different combinations of common (> 5%) non-coding SNPs, resulting in three haplotype groups. The maintenance doses were 2.7 ± 0.2 mg/day for A/A, 4.9 ± 0.2 mg for A/B and 6.2 ± 0.3 mg for B/B ($p < 0.001$) genotype groups.[29]

The haplotype distribution in the study proportions was closely linked to racial heritage or ethnicity, as is the incidence of the CYP2C9 polymorphism. The frequency of the AA genotype associated with warfarin sensitivity was much higher in Japanese and Chinese patients (0.83 and 0.82, respectively) than in Caucasians (0.14).[32] This can explain the reports that Chinese, Malay and Japanese patients usually require a 30–40% lower warfarin dose than do Caucasians.[33, 34]

In all these studies, the VKORC1 polymorphism alone could predict 25–30% of warfarin maintenance dose variability (panel 10.2). On the basis of these recent observations, new dosing algorithms for warfarin were developed.[31] Multivariate regression models that include the variables age, CYP2C9 and VKORC1 genotype, and height produced the best model, which predicts nearly 55% of the variability in the daily dose requirements of warfarin.

The therapeutic lesson for physicians is both obvious and subtle: Genotyping patients for CYP2C9 and VKORC1 in combination with host factors can save lives.

The main alternatives to warfarin, the coumarin derivatives acenocoumarol and phenoprocoumon, are widely or exclusively used in certain European countries.[35] Again, the

Panel 10.2: Mutlifactorial causes of individual variability in warfarin/acenocoumarol dose requirements

Host factors	Environmental factors	Genes
Sex	Dietary factors (vitamin K)?	CYP2C9 genotype
Age	Drug–drug interactions	VKORC1 genotype
Body surface		
Height		
Weight		
⬇		⬇
25–30% of predictable variability		~ 30–52% of predictable variability

(*S*)-enantiomers of these closely related chemicals are substrates of CYP2C9. The CYP2C9*3 allele is, therefore, related to low-dose requirements of racemic acenocoumarol, a higher frequency of overanticoagulation and an unstable anticoagulant response.[36–38] Bodin et al.[39] have demonstrated that the VKORC1 genotype explains 37% of the variability in response to acenocoumarol in healthy volunteers. The situation for the future dosing algorithms for acenocoumarol is, therefore, almost identical to warfarin. Phenoprocoumon is not significantly affected in its kinetics by the CYP2C9 polymorphism, and appears to be a clinically useful alternative to warfarin in patients carrying the CYP2C9*2 and *3 alleles.[40] The dependence of the maintenance dose of phenoprocoumon on the VKORC1 polymorphism has not yet been studied.

In spite of these recent developments demonstrating the potential of judiciously using host, environmental and genetic information to individualise therapeutic decisions, more than 40% of the variability in warfarin dose requirements may remain unaccounted for. Additional factors contributing to variability, for instance, are the vitamin K status. In some studies, plasma vitamin K concentration was indeed negatively correlated with the patient INR.[41] It also is highly likely that additional genetic factors are involved in causing interindividual variability in warfarin dose requirements. Candidates are polymorphisms of the apolipoprotein E (APOE) gene,[42] multidrug resistance 1 (MDR1) gene,[43] and possibly other genes encoding vitamin K-dependent clotting factors or additional components of the vitamin K epoxide reductase complex.

CYP2D6, antidepressants, antipsychotics and opioids

The clinical impact of the cytochrome P450 CYP2D6 polymorphism has been the subject of numerous reviews.[15, 44, 45] CYP2D6 metabolises a large number of drugs, including many drugs used in psychiatric patients, but also drugs used for the treatment of cardiovascular disease, pain, nausea, etc. In fact, the most commonly used drugs metabolised by CYP2D6 account for 189 million prescriptions, accounting for an estimated US $12.8 billion annual expenditure in the USA, or 5–10% of expenditures for outpatient prescription drugs.[46]

The CYP2D6 polymorphisms were discovered in the 1970s, and their molecular mechanisms were described in the late 1980s.[15, 44, 45] The most common mutations of the CYP2D6 gene on chromosome 22 were characterised and a genetic test for these mutations described in 1990.[47] At present, numerous alleles are known, including gene deletions and duplications, with over 70 distinct variants.[48] These variants lead to the four phenotype groups summarised in figure 10.2. Five to 10% of Caucasians are poor metabolisers, while 1–3% of Hispanics and African-Americans are estimated to be poor metabolisers. It also has been estimated that 5–10% of Caucasians are ultrarapid metabolisers.[45]

CYP2D6 affects the kinetics of a large number of drugs used in psychiatric patients, raising the question of how this information can be used by physicians to improve therapy in these patients.[49, 50]

CYP2D6 and antidepressants

The metabolism of the antidepressants amitriptyline, clomipramine, desipramine, doxepine, imipramine and nortriptyline, and of the tetracyclic compounds maprotiline and mianserin, is influenced by the CYP2D6 polymorphism to various degrees. For these agents, there are clearly two patient groups that may pose clinical problems. The poor metabolisers (and, to a lesser degree, the intermediate metabolisers) predictably have increased plasma concentrations on recommended doses of tricyclic antidepressants when given recommended doses of the drugs. The other group are the ultrarapid metabolisers, who are prone to therapeutic failures because the drug concentrations at normal doses are by far too low.[51] Five to 20% of patients may belong to one of these risk groups, depending on the population studied. Adverse effects clearly occur more frequently in poor metabolisers,[52, 53] and may be one of the causes of poor compliance. Moreover, toxic reactions may be misinterpreted as symptoms of depression, and lead to erroneous further increases in the dose. The metabolism of the recently introduced antidepressant drug venlafaxine is controlled by CYP2D6, but because the metabolites are equipotent antidepressants, the concentration of active drug is not changed much by the polymorphism. However, four patients admitted to hospital with arrhythmia were CYP2D6 poor metabolisers, suggesting a higher risk for cardiotoxicity in these individuals.[54] Another group of antidepressants are the selective serotonin reuptake inhibitors (SSRIs), which interact with CYP2D6 in three different ways. Paroxetine, fluvoxamine and fluoxetine are, in part, metabolised by CYP2D6. However, the phenotype differences in clearance or plasma levels are small in relation to the relatively large therapeutic index of these drugs. Of substantial importance is the effect of these agents to act as potent competitive inhibitors of CYP2D6 (paroxetine, fluoxetine). Such inhibition means that the elimination of other CYP2D6 substrates (e.g. of tricyclic antidepressants) is impaired, and these patients have an acquired poor metaboliser phenotype. Other competitive inhibitors of CYP2D6 are quinidine, buproprion and propafenone.

The therapeutic lessons from these studies are translated into clinical practice only very slowly, because the drug treatment of depression is a complex matter involving spontaneous remissions, placebo effects, difficult assessment of outcomes, etc. Moreover, the availability of genotyping tests is a recent event (see below), and there have been no prospective studies of the value of knowing the genotype for CYP2D6 and its cost–benefit ratio. Recommendations for dose adjustments for these drugs on the basis of kinetic data have been published.[49, 55] There is no doubt that CYP2D6 poor metabolisers have a poor tolerance to tricyclic antidepressants, and probably venlafaxine. At this time, it is justified to recommend that poor metabolisers should preferentially be treated with antidepressants that are not dependent on metabolism by CYP2D6 and do not inhibit CYP2D6, such as bupropion, citalopram, escitalopram, mirtazepine and sertraline.

The metabolism of several antidepressants is catalysed by another polymorphic CYP enzyme, CYP2C19, Thus, amitriptylin, clomipramin and imipramin are also metabolised by this enzyme. Moreover, the kinetics of citalopram and sertraline are variably affected by this polymorphism.[56, 57] Two to 4% of Caucasians and 10–25% of East Asians are poor metabolisers. The lack of prospective studies again suggest the pragmatic approach to preferentially use antidepressants not metabolised by CYP2C19 (e.g. bupropion, mirtazepin and paroxetin) in these patients.

CYP2D6 and antipsychotics

Several antipsychotic drugs are metabolised by CYP2D6. Increased ADRs after treatment with perphenazine, thioridazine and risperidone have been documented,[18] whereas data on the effect of the CYP2D6 polymorphism on haloperidol kinetics are conflicting. Antipsychotics not dependent on CYP2D6 for their metabolism are clozapine, olanzepine, quitiazepine and ziprasidone.

CYP2D6 and opioids

There are striking differences in the responses to opioids in association with the CYP2D6 polymorphism.[58] Dextromethorphan, codeine, hydrocodone, oxycodone, ethylmorphine and dihydrocodeine all are dealkylated by CYP2D6. The polymorphic *O*-demethylation of codeine is of clinical importance when this drug is given as an analgesic. About 5% of codeine is *O*-demethylated to morphine,[25] and this pathway is deficient in poor metabolisers. Poor metabolisers therefore experience little analgesic benefit from treatment with codeine. Similarly, respiratory, psychomotor and pupillary effects of codeine are decreased in poor metabolisers compared with extensive metabolisers. Codeine is frequently recommended as a drug of first choice for treatment of chronic severe pain. Physicians must appreciate that no analgesic effect is to be expected in the 5–10% of Caucasians who are of the poor metaboliser phenotype, or who are extensive metabolisers receiving concomitant treatment with a potent inhibitor of CYP2D6. Life-threatening opioid intoxication in a patient who was a CYP2D6 ultrarapid metaboliser treated with codeine was recently reported.[59] No morphine or morphine metabolites were detected in plasma when codeine was coadministered with quinidine.[60, 61] Although codeine may seem, on the surface, a poor candidate for a pharmacogenetic test, as the patient knows whether the medicine has worked or not, in fact there are many situations where analgesia is imperfect, and even in situations where a patient can tell that codeine is having no analgesic benefit his or her physician may not be aware, and self-reporting about pain is a notoriously variable and subjective phenomenon. It follows that the test may be valuable as a means of indicating which patients should not receive codeine as an analgesic, and who would most likely benefit from this drug.

N-Acetyltransferase and Isoniazid

One of the first pharmacogenetic traits to be recognised more than 50 years ago was the slow acetylation of the antituberculosis drug isoniazid, now known as the polymorphism of *N*-acetyltransferase 2 (NAT2) and inherited as an autosomal recessive trait.[62, 63]

Isoniazid is the treatment of choice for latent tuberculosis infection, and is included in most first-line therapy regimens in combination with rifampicin, ethambutol and pyrazinamide. However, acute or chronic hepatitis frequently develops in patients receiving these drugs, with an incidence of 1–36%, depending on different regimens and how one defines hepatic injury, from transient elevations of liver function tests to serious injury or even death.[64] Of the various drugs used in the combination therapy, isoniazid appears to be the most likely drug to induce hepatotoxicity.[65] Additional risk factors are alcohol consumption, advanced age and pre-existing chronic liver disease. In numerous studies, slow acetylators treated with isoniazid and rifampicin had a higher risk of hepatotoxicity than did rapid acetylators. Among patients with hepatotoxicity, slow acetylators had significantly higher serum aminotransferase levels.[64, 66] Additional genetic risk factors were a homozygous 'wild-type' genotype for CYP2E1 (CYP2E1c1/c1) conferring high activity to this enzyme.[65] In other studies, the acetylator genotype was a good predictor of isoniazid plasma levels and isoniazid-induced hepatotoxicity.[67] These data suggest that genotype-derived dosage regimens (e.g. 450, 300 and 150 mg/day for slow (homozygous for two defective alleles), intermediate (heterozygous) or rapid (homozygous for two active alleles) acetylators, respectively) should be considered in future prospective studies.

The resurgence of tuberculosis in many countries as a serious threat because of a growing prevalence of drug resistance and its association with high-risk patients, such as human immunodeficiency virus (HIV) seropositive individuals, convicts, homeless or drug users, has re-emphasised the role of genetic risk factors for the hepatotoxicity associated with antituberculous regimens.

The incidence of NAT2 slow acetylators can vary from 5% to 95%, depending on the geographic/ethnic origin of the population studied.[68] In addition to isoniazid, the NAT2 polymorphism affects the pharmacokinetics of a wide variety of arylamine and hydrazine drugs and chemical carcinogens. These include sulfonamides, such as salazosulfapyridine, the antiarrhythmic procainamide and the anticancer drug amonafide, for all of which dose adjustments according to the acetylator genotype or phenotype have been recommended, but are not part of common practice.

Pharmacogenomic strategies in cancer therapy: mercaptopurine, irinotecan and trastuzumab

The therapy of cancer almost always involves multiple drugs with considerable toxicity. In general, these strategies include variations in germline DNA (e.g. genetic polymorphisms), acquired somatic mutations in tumour cells (e.g. sensitising mutations in the tyrosine kinase domain of the EGFR gene) or variations in RNA expression. It is beyond the scope of this chapter to review the entire spectrum of the pharmacogenetics of cancer chemotherapy, but further details are given in Chapter 20.

The severe and potentially fatal bone marrow toxicity (acute leukopenia, anaemia and pancytopenia) in patients with thiopurine methyltransferase (TPMT) deficiency treated with standard doses of *mercaptopurine* and *azathioprine* is a rare (~1 in 300) event in the treatment of acute lymphoblastic leukaemia (ALL) in children. Patients with this deficiency can require up to a 15-fold reduction in mercaptopurin to prevent potentially fatal haemotoxicity.[69–71] Other pharmacogenetic examples of ADRs in cancer chemotherapy are the myelosuppression and neurotoxicity of *5-fluorouracil* in patients with a deficiency of dihydropyrimidine dehydrogenase (DPD), the myelosuppression and diarrhoea after the topoisomerase I inhibitor *irinotecan* in patients with an inherited deficiency in glucuronidation by a promoter polymorphism of UGT-glucuronosyltransferase UGT1A1, and the greater bone marrow toxicity of the topoisomerase II inhibitor *amonafide* in NAT2 rapid acetylators.[69, 70]

Another more recent aspect of the therapy of cancer is the targeting of signal-transduction pathways that control proliferation and metastasis of tumour cells. The epidermal growth factor receptor (EGFR, HER) family of transmembrane tyrosine kinases is such a target in solid tumours. One member of this family is HER2 (or ErbB2) and the gene for this receptor is amplified in up to 30% of breast cancers. In 1997, *trastuzumab (Herceptin)*, an antibody that blocks the action of HER2, was introduced. It is clear that trastuzumab should only be used in patients whose tumours have HER-2 protein overexpression. A similar situation is the treatment of chronic myeloid leukaemia with *imatinib (Gleevec)*, in which an aberrant gene (BCR-ABL) triggers a proliferation of white blood cells. Another tyrosine kinase of the HER family, HER1, is inhibited by the drug *gefitinib (Iressa)*. Gefinitib was active against non-small-cell lung cancer, but only in a small subgroup of patients who carried mutations of the tyrosine kinase intracellular domain. Several other antibodies and small molecules that target the EGFR are in clinical development.[72]

The lesson here is that the genetic instability of cancer cells leads to additional 'somatic' mutations and overexpression (or underexpression) of certain genes. These drugs should only be used in patients whose tumours have been tested for overexpression or mutations in these targets. RNA-microarray or protein expression analysis is, therefore, increasingly used as a 'biomarker' approach to identify the individual patients who will benefit from the treatment.[73] These pharmacogenomic tests are convincing examples of the concept of individualised medicine or of the matching of medicines with the genetic makeup of the individual and his or her disease.

Therapeutic lessons from pharmacogenetics and pharmacogenomics

Pharmacogenetics has provided a number of therapeutic lessons that make us understand clinical drug response and it has influenced the drug development process. Among the therapeutic lessons are that most drug effects vary considerably from person to person and that all drug effects are influenced by genes. But it has also been realised that most drug responses and toxicities are influenced by many genes interacting with environmental and behavioural factors. Genetic polymorphisms of single genes, including mutations in coding sequences, gene duplications, gene deletions and regulatory mutations, affect numerous drug-metabolising enzymes. Several cytochrome-P450 enzymes, NAT2 and several enzymes metabolising anticancer drugs are the examples discussed here. Individuals who possess these polymorphisms are at higher risk of experiencing ADRs or inefficacy of drugs at usual doses. Genetic polymorphisms of drug targets and drug transporters also are increasingly recognised (receptors, ion channels, growth factors) as causing variation in drug responses, but they have not been studied sufficiently with regard to their clinical importance to be able to indicate routine genotype-based dose adjustments, except for the VKORC1 polymorphism. Several targets of cancer therapy (e.g. the epidermal-growth-factor receptor) respond to treatment only in subgroups of patients who carry sensitising mutations of these targets. Finally, the frequency of variation of drug effects, whether multifactorial or genetic, varies considerably in populations of different ethnic origins.

One of the major challenges in the future is the interpretation of multigenic and multifactorial influences on drug responses. Indeed, as already discussed, most drug effects and treatment outcomes, or the individual risk for drug inefficacy or toxicity, are due to complex interactions between genes and the environment and host factors. Environmental variables include nutritional factors, concomitantly administered drugs, disease and many other factors, including lifestyle influences such as smoking and alcohol consumption. These factors act in concert with several individual genes that code for pharmacokinetic and pharmacodynamic determinants of drug effects. The challenge will be to define polygenic determinants of drug effects and to use a combination of genotyping and phenotyping tests to assess environmental influences. Applying dosing algorithms for warfarin and acenocoumarol considering these different influences at this time is one of the best examples of this approach.

The clinical potential of pharmacogenetics and pharmacogenomics

Why is pharmacogenetics so rarely applied in clinical practice, in spite of well-established genetic polymorphisms and available genotyping methods? Numerous reasons for the slow acceptance of pharmacogenetic principles have been put forward.[74–77] The lack of large prospective studies to evaluate the impact of genetic variation on drug therapy is one reason for the slow acceptance of these principles. On the other hand, pharmacogenetic information is increasingly included in product information or drug data sheets, alerting the physician to dosing problems. A recent search for pharmacogenetic information in the prescribing information available to practising physicians provided the following bleak results.[78] Information on increased risk for potentially life-threatening adverse effects or treatment failures with conditional recommendations for genetic evaluation were found for only four drugs, namely recombinant factor X, somatotropin, divalproex sodium and valproic acid. Only for one drug, thioridazine, did the information contain a contraindication for a genetic subgroup, namely CYP2D6 poor metabolisers, which may develop QTc (prolonged heart-rate-corrected QT interval) interval prolongation in the electrocardiogram and ventricular arrhythmia. Clearly, prescribing information sheets at present do not contain useful information for gene-guided dose adjustments or therapeutic decisions. In particular, there are no explicit recommendations for drug dosing in TPMT-deficient patients in the information for mercaptopurine or azathioprine, or for warfarin for patients with low activity alleles of CYP2C9 or mutations in VKORC1. Similarly, the prescription information for irinotecan does not contain information on the risk of patients with UGT1A1 deficiency. A major effort is underway in several countries to correct these obvious deficiencies in alerting physicians to potential problems, and this has included the first approval of a pharmacogenetic test: an oligonucleotide microarray test for CYP2D6 and CYP2C19 genotypes (figure 10.3). In the future, *not* performing a pharmacogenetic test may have obvious legal consequences.

Finally, pharmacogenomics and pharmacogenetics offer the potential to provide better healthcare through improved rational prescribing. I believe that their gradual acceptance in clinical practice will contribute to the education of healthcare professionals as

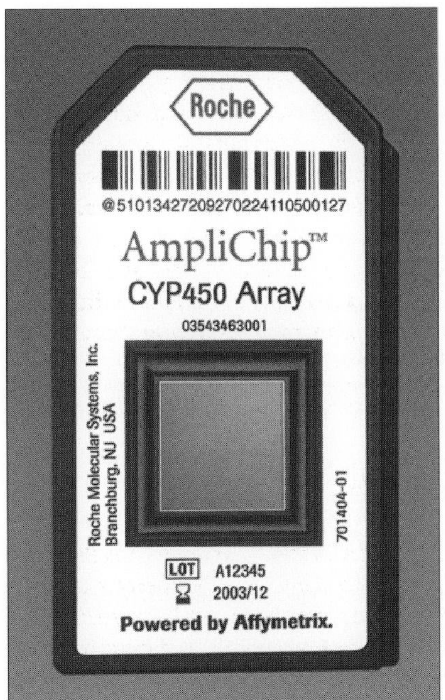

Figure 10.3: **The AmpliChip CYP450 array was recently approved as a test system for mutations of CYP2D6 and CYP2C19 in Europe and the USA.[79] (Courtesy of Roche Diagnostics (Switzerland) Ltd.)**

prescribers. In addition, we must recognise an increasingly important source of pressure to improve pharmacotherapy: increasingly, educated patients will come to expect the application of genomics and other technologies to drug selection and dosage when possible. The individualised medicine that many view as a new goal, is actually what physicians always intended, and is becoming what patients, and the regulatory bodies that protect them, expect (figure 10.4).

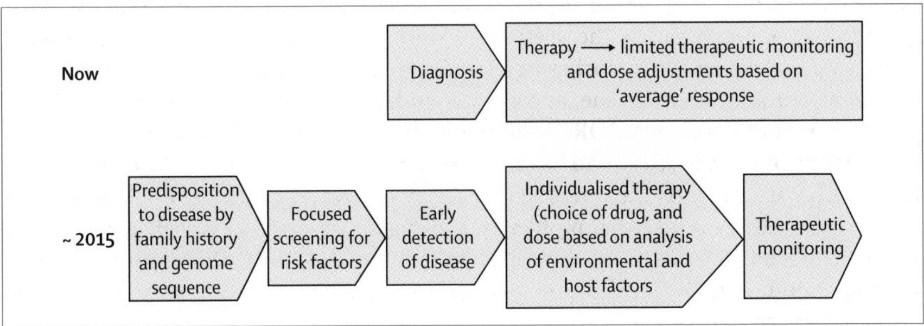

Figure 10.4: **The future of individualised medicine. Individualised drug therapy in the future will be based on early diagnosis and risk assessment driven by genetics/genomics, followed by targeted therapy and disease outcome monitoring by 'biomarkers'. This will replace the present paradigm of late-stage diagnosis and therapy. (Modified from Bell.[80])**

Acknowledgments
The author's research is supported by the Swiss National Research Foundation and the European Sixth Framework Program – Project 'Steroltalk'.

References

1 Pirmohamed M, James S, Meakin S, et al. Adverse drug reactions as cause of admission to hospital: prospective analysis of 18 820 patients. *BMJ* 2004; **329:** 15–19.
2 Lazarou J, Pomeranz BH, Corey PN. Incidence of adverse drug reactions in hospitalized patients: a meta-analysis of prospective studies. *JAMA* 1998; **279:** 1200–05.
3 Bates DW, Spell N, Cullen DJ, et al. The costs of adverse drug events in hospitalized patients. Adverse Drug Events Prevention Study Group. *JAMA* 1997; **277:** 307–11.
4 Spear BB, Heath-Chiozzi M, Huff J. Clinical application of pharmacogenetics. *Trends Mol Med* 2001; **7:** 201–04.
5 Wright AF. *Nature Encyclopedic of the Human Genome.* London: Nature Publishing, 2003: 959–68.
6 Feuk L, Carson AR, Scherer SW. Structural variation in the human genome. *Nat Rev Genet* 2006; **7:** 85–97.
7 Deloukas P, Bentley D. The HapMap project and its application to genetic studies of drug response. *Pharmacogenomics J* 2004; **4:** 88–90.
8 International HapMap Project. Available at: http://snp.cshl.org (accessed February 2007).
9 Roses AD. SNPs – where's the beef? *Pharmacogenomics J* 2002; **2:** 277–83.
10 Weinshilboum R. Inheritance and drug response. *N Engl J Med* 2003; **348:** 529–37.
11 Evans WE, McLeod HL. Pharmacogenomics – drug disposition, drug targets, and side effects. *N Engl J Med* 2003; **348:** 538–49.
12 Evans WE, Relling MV. Moving towards individualized medicine with pharmacogenomics. *Nature* 2004; **429:** 464–68.
13 Kalow W, Meyer UA, Tyndale RF. *Pharmacogenomics,* 2nd edn. Boca Raton, FL: Taylor & Francis, 2005.
14 Goldstein DB, Tate SK, Sisodiya SM. Pharmacogenetics goes genomic. *Nat Rev Genet* 2003; **4:** 937–47.
15 Meyer UA. Pharmacogenetics – five decades of therapeutic lessons from genetic diversity. *Nat Rev Genet* 2004; **5:** 669–76.
16 The Pharmacogenetics and Pharmacogenomics Knowledge Base. Available at: http://www.pharmgkb.org (accessed February 2007).
17 Daly AK. Development of analytical technology in pharmacogenetic research. *Naunyn Schmiedebergs Arch Pharmacol* 2004; **369:** 133–40.
18 de Leon J, Susce MT, Pan RM, et al. The CYP2D6 poor metabolizer phenotype may be associated with risperidone adverse drug reactions and discontinuation. *J Clin Psychiatry* 2005; **66:** 15–27.
19 Lovlie R, Daly AK, Matre GE, et al. Polymorphisms in CYP2D6 duplication-negative individuals with the ultrarapid metabolizer phenotype: a role for the CYP2D6*35 allele in ultrarapid metabolism? *Pharmacogenetics* 2001; **11:** 45–55.
20 Kunze KL, Wienkers LC, Thummel KE, Trager WF. Warfarin-fluconazole. I. Inhibition of the human cytochrome P450-dependent metabolism of warfarin by fluconazole: in vitro studies. *Drug Metab Dispos* 1996; **24:** 414–21.
21 Ablin J, Cabili S, Eldor A, et al. Warfarin therapy is feasible in CYP2C9*3 homozygous patients. *Eur J Intern Med* 2004; **15:** 22–27.
22 Aithal GP, Day CP, Kesteven PJ, Daly AK. Association of polymorphisms in the cytochrome P450 CYP2C9 with warfarin dose requirement and risk of bleeding complications. *Lancet* 1999; **353:** 717–19.
23 Kamali F, Khan TI, King BP, et al. Contribution of age, body size, and CYP2C9 genotype to anticoagulant response to warfarin. *Clin Pharmacol Ther* 2004; **75:** 204–12.
24 Higashi MK, Veenstra DL, Kondo LM, et al. Association between CYP2C9 genetic variants and anticoagulation-related outcomes during warfarin therapy. *JAMA* 2002; **287:** 1690–98.
25 Yue QY, Hasselstrom J, Svensson JO, Sawe J. Pharmacokinetics of codeine and its metabolites in Caucasian healthy volunteers: comparisons between extensive and poor hydroxylators of debrisoquine. *Br J Clin Pharmacol* 1991; **31:** 635–42.
26 Takahashi H, Wilkinson GR, Nutescu EA, et al. Different contributions of polymorphisms in VKORC1 and CYP2C9 to intra- and inter-population differences in maintenance dose of warfarin in Japanese, Caucasians and African-Americans. *Pharmacogenet Genomics* 2006; **16:** 101–10.
27 Rost S, Fregin A, Ivaskevicius V, et al. Mutations in VKORC1 cause warfarin resistance and multiple coagulation factor deficiency type 2. *Nature* 2004; **427:** 537–41.
28 D'Andrea G, D'Ambrosio RL, Di Perna P, et al. A polymorphism in the VKORC1 gene is associated with an interindividual variability in the dose-anticoagulant effect of warfarin. *Blood* 2005; **105:** 645–49.

29 Rieder MJ, Reiner AP, Gage BF, et al. Effect of VKORC1 haplotypes on transcriptional regulation and warfarin dose. *N Engl J Med* 2005; **352:** 2285–93.

30 Geisen C, Watzka M, Sittinger K, et al. VKORC1 haplotypes and their impact on the inter-individual and inter-ethnical variability of oral anticoagulation. *Thromb Haemost* 2005; **94:** 773–9.

31 Sconce EA, Khan TI, Wynne HA, et al. The impact of CYP2C9 and VKORC1 genetic polymorphism and patient characteristics upon warfarin dose requirements: proposal for a new dosing regimen. *Blood* 2005; **106:** 2329–33.

32 Mushiroda T, Ohnishi Y, Saito S, et al. Association of VKORC1 and CYP2C9 polymorphisms with warfarin dose requirements in Japanese patients. *J Human Genet* 2006; **51:** 249–53.

33 Takahashi H, Wilkinson GR, Caraco Y, et al. Population differences in *S*-warfarin metabolism between CYP2C9 genotype-matched Caucasian and Japanese patients. *Clin Pharmacol Ther* 2003; **73:** 253–63.

34 Zhao F, Loke C, Rankin SC, et al. Novel CYP2C9 genetic variants in Asian subjects and their influence on maintenance warfarin dose. *Clin Pharmacol Ther* 2004; **76:** 210–19.

35 Daly AK, King BP. Pharmacogenetics of oral anticoagulants. *Pharmacogenetics* 2003; **13:** 247–52.

36 Tassies D, Freire C, Pijoan J, et al. Pharmacogenetics of acenocoumarol: cytochrome P450 CYP2C9 polymorphisms influence dose requirements and stability of anticoagulation. *Haematologica* 2002; **87:** 1185–91.

37 Thijssen HH, Verkooijen IW, Frank HL. The possession of the CYP2C9*3 allele is associated with low dose requirement of acenocoumarol. *Pharmacogenetics* 2000; **10:** 757–60.

38 Thijssen HH, Drittij MJ, Vervoort LM, de Vries-Hanje JC. Altered pharmacokinetics of *R*- and *S*-acenocoumarol in a subject heterozygous for CYP2C9*3. *Clin Pharmacol Ther* 2001; **70:** 292–98.

39 Bodin L, Verstuyft C, Tregouet DA, et al. Cytochrome P450 2C9 (CYP2C9) and vitamin K epoxide reductase (VKORC1) genotypes as determinants of acenocoumarol sensitivity. *Blood* 2005; **106:** 135–40.

40 Visser LE, van Vliet M, van Schaik RH, et al. The risk of overanticoagulation in patients with cytochrome P450 CYP2C9*2 or CYP2C9*3 alleles on acenocoumarol or phenprocoumon. *Pharmacogenetics* 2004; **14:** 27–33.

41 Kamali F, Edwards C, Butler TJ, Wynne HA. The influence of (*R*)- and (*S*)-warfarin, vitamin K and vitamin K epoxide upon warfarin anticoagulation. *Thromb Haemost* 2000; **84:** 39–42.

42 Kohnke H, Sorlin K, Granath G, Wadelius M. Warfarin dose related to apolipoprotein E (APOE) genotype. *Eur J Clin Pharmacol* 2005; **61:** 381–88.

43 Wadelius M, Sorlin K, Wallerman O, et al. Warfarin sensitivity related to CYP2C9, CYP3A5, ABCB1 (MDR1) and other factors. *Pharmacogenomics J* 2004; **4:** 40–48.

44 Zanger UM, Raimundo S, Eichelbaum M. Cytochrome P450 2D6: overview and update on pharmacology, genetics, biochemistry. *Naunyn Schmiedebergs Arch Pharmacol* 2004; **369:** 23–37.

45 Ingelman-Sundberg M. Genetic polymorphisms of cytochrome P450 2D6 (CYP2D6): clinical consequences, evolutionary aspects and functional diversity. *Pharmacogenomics J* 2005; **5:** 6–13.

46 Phillips KA, Van Bebber SL. Measuring the value of pharmacogenomics. *Nat Rev Drug Discov* 2005; **4:** 500–09.

47 Heim M, Meyer UA. Genotyping of poor metabolizers of debrisoquine by allele-specific PCR amplification. *Lancet* 1990; **336:** 529–32.

48 Cytochrome P450 (CYP) Allele Nomenclature Committee. Available at: http://www.imm.ki.se/CYPalleles (accessed February 2007).

49 Kirchheiner J, Nickchen K, Bauer M, et al. Pharmacogenetics of antidepressants and antipsychotics: the contribution of allelic variations to the phenotype of drug response. *Mol Psychiatry* 2004; **9:** 442–73.

50 de Leon J, Armstrong SC, Cozza KL. Clinical guidelines for psychiatrists for the use of pharmacogenetic testing for CYP450 2D6 and CYP450 2C19. *Psychosomatics* 2006; **47:** 75–85.

51 Kawanishi C, Lundgren S, Agren H, Bertilsson L. Increased incidence of CYP2D6 gene duplication in patients with persistent mood disorders: ultrarapid metabolism of antidepressants as a cause of nonresponse. A pilot study. *Eur J Clin Pharmacol* 2004; **59:** 803–07.

52 Chou WH, Yan FX, de Leon J, et al. Extension of a pilot study: impact from the cytochrome P450 2D6 polymorphism on outcome and costs associated with severe mental illness. *J Clin Psychopharmacol* 2000; **20:** 246–51.

53 Rau T, Wohlleben G, Wuttke H, et al. CYP2D6 genotype: impact on adverse effects and nonresponse during treatment with antidepressants – a pilot study. *Clin Pharmacol Ther* 2004; **75:** 386–93.

54 Lessard E, Yessine MA, Hamelin BA, et al. Influence of CYP2D6 activity on the disposition and cardiovascular toxicity of the antidepressant agent venlafaxine in humans. *Pharmacogenetics* 1999; **9:** 435–43.

55 Kirchheiner J, Fuhr U, Brockmoller J. Pharmacogenetics-based therapeutic recommendations – ready for clinical practice? *Nat Rev Drug Discov* 2005; **4:** 639–47.

56 Wang JH, Liu ZQ, Wang W, et al. Pharmacokinetics of sertraline in relation to genetic polymorphism of CYP2C19. *Clin Pharmacol Ther* 2001; **70:** 42–47.

57 Yu BN, Chen GL, He N, et al. Pharmacokinetics of citalopram in relation to genetic polymorphism of CYP2C19. *Drug Metab Dispos* 2003; **31:** 1255–59.

58 Sindrup SH, Brosen K. The pharmacogenetics of codeine hypoalgesia. *Pharmacogenetics* 1995; **5:** 335–46.

59 Gasche Y, Daali Y, Fathi M, et al. Codeine intoxication associated with ultrarapid CYP2D6 metabolism. *N Engl J Med* 2004; **351:** 2827–31.

60 Desmeules J, Gascon MP, Dayer P, Magistris M. Impact of environmental and genetic factors on codeine analgesia. *Eur J Clin Pharmacol* 1991; **41:** 23–26.

61 Caraco Y, Sheller J, Wood AJ. Impact of ethnic origin and quinidine coadministration on codeine's disposition and pharmacodynamic effects. *J Pharmacol Exp Ther* 1999; **290:** 413–22.

62 Evans DAP. *Genetic Factors in Drug Therapy. Clinical and Molecular Pharmacogenetics.* Cambridge: Cambridge University Press, 1993.

63 Weber WW. *The Acetylator Genes and Drug Response.* New York: Oxford University Press, 1987.

64 Huang YS, Chern HD, Su WJ, et al. Polymorphism of the *N*-acetyltransferase 2 gene as a susceptibility risk factor for antituberculosis drug-induced hepatitis. *Hepatology* 2002; **35:** 883–89.

65 Huang YS, Chern HD, Su WJ, et al. Cytochrome P450 2E1 genotype and the susceptibility to antituberculosis drug-induced hepatitis. *Hepatology* 2003; **37:** 924–30.

66 Ohno M, Yamaguchi I, Yamamoto I, et al. Slow *N*-acetyltransferase 2 genotype affects the incidence of isoniazid and rifampicin-induced hepatotoxicity. *Int J Tuberc Lung Dis* 2000; **4:** 256–61.

67 Ohno M, Kubota R, Yasunaga M, et al. Population phamacokinetics and pharmacogenetics trial of isonizaid. In: Anderson W, ed. *8th World Conference on Clinical Pharmacology and Therapeutics, 2004.* Brisbane: Blackwell, 2004: A138.

68 Meyer UA, Zanger UM. Molecular mechanisms of genetic polymorphisms of drug metabolism. *Annu Rev Pharmacol Toxicol* 1997; **37:** 269–96.

69 Iyer L, Ratain MJ. Pharmacogenetics and cancer chemotherapy. *Eur J Cancer* 1998; **34:** 1493–99.

70 Evans WE, Relling MV. Pharmacogenomics: translating functional genomics into rational therapeutics. *Science* 1999; **286:** 487–91.

71 Weinshilboum RM, Otterness DM, Szumlanski CL. Methylation pharmacogenetics: catechol *O*-methyltransferase, thiopurine methyltransferase, and histamine *N*-methyltransferase. *Annu Rev Pharmacol Toxicol* 1999; **39:** 19–52.

72 Green MR. Targeting targeted therapy. *N Engl J Med* 2004; **350:** 2191–93.

73 Marsh S, McLeod HL. Cancer pharmacogenetics. *Br J Cancer* 2004; **90:** 8–11.

74 Nebert DW, Jorge-Nebert L, Vesell ES. Pharmacogenomics and 'individualized drug therapy': high expectations and disappointing achievements. *Am J Pharmacogenomics* 2003; **3:** 361–70.

75 Holtzmann NA. Clinical utility of pharmacogenetics and pharmacogenomics. In: Rothstein MA, ed. *Pharmacogenomics. Social, Ethical, and Clinical Dimensions.* Hoboken, NJ: Wiley, 2003: 163–85.

76 Tucker G. Pharmacogenetics – expectations and reality. *BMJ* 2004; **329:** 4–6.

77 Weinshilboum R, Wang L. Pharmacogenomics: bench to bedside. *Nat Rev Drug Discov* 2004; **3:** 739–48.

78 Zineh I, Gerhard T, Aquilante CL, et al. Availability of pharmacogenomics-based prescribing information in drug package inserts for currently approved drugs. *Pharmacogenomics J* 2004; **4:** 354–58.

79 De Leon J, Susce MT, Murray-Carmichael E. The Amplichip CYP450 genotyping test: integrating a new clinical tool. *Mol Diagn Ther* 2006; **10:** 135–51.

80 Bell J. Predicting disease using genomics. *Nature* 2004; **429:** 453–56.

11

Reliable estimation and interpretation of the effects of treatment in subgroups

Peter M. Rothwell

Introduction

> *The combination of some data and an aching desire for an answer does not ensure that a reasonable answer can be extracted from a given body of data.* (John W. Tukey, 1986[1])

Large pragmatic trials with broad eligibility criteria and high inclusion rates provide the most reliable data on the effects of treatments.[2] Trials should also, however, be designed, analysed and reported in a way that leads to the most effective use of treatments in routine practice. As discussed in Chapter 9, subgroup analyses are important if there are potentially large differences between groups in the risk of a poor outcome with or without treatment, if there is potential heterogeneity of treatment effect in relation to pathophysiology, if there are practical questions about when to treat (e.g. stage of disease or timing of treatment), or if there are doubts about benefit in specific groups, such as the elderly, which are leading to undertreatment. However, as detailed in panel 11.1, misinterpreted or inappropriate subgroup analyses can be very harmful, and it is essential therefore that analyses are planned, performed, reported and interpreted as reliably as possible. Yet, there are no guidelines on the analysis and interpretation of subgroup effects, no consensus on the implications for trial design, and the CONSORT statement on reporting of trials includes only a few lines on subgroup analysis.[25]

This chapter will therefore suggest some guidelines for the performance, reporting and interpretation of subgroup analyses, and briefly review their justification and background. The guidelines are outlined in panel 11.2 and can be roughly divided into those relating to trial design, those relating to statistical analysis and reporting, and those relating to interpretation. The overall aim of the guidelines is to avoid the errors illustrated in panel 11.1 whilst allowing researchers to identify clinically important heterogeneity of treatment effects of the sort discussed in Chapter 9.

Trial design

Many of the problems that have stemmed from subgroup analysis could be avoided if any such analyses were considered in detail during the early stages of trial design and if trials were thereby designed with eventual subgroup analyses in mind. Subgroups should be defined in detail at the design stage and should be limited to a small number of clinically important questions. It is essential that there is *expert* clinical input into the design of subgroup analyses, so that all relevant baseline clinical and other data are recorded. The direction and magnitude of anticipated subgroup effects should be stated at the outset, and the exact definitions and categories of the subgroup variables should

Panel 11.1: **Ten examples of subgroup analyses that have shown apparently clinically important heterogeneity of treatment effect but which have subsequently been shown to be false**

Observation	Refutation
• Aspirin is ineffective in secondary prevention of stroke in women[3, 4]	Antiplatelet Trialists Collaboration[5]
• Antihypertensive treatment for primary prevention is ineffective in women[6, 7]	Gueyffier et al.[8]
• Antihypertensive treatment is ineffective or harmful in the elderly[9]	Gueyffier et al.[10]
• Angiotensin-converting enzyme (ACE) inhibitors do not reduce mortality and hospital admission in patients with heart failure who are also taking aspirin[11]	Flather et al.[12]
• Beta-blockers are ineffective after acute myocardial infarction in the elderly[13] and in patients with inferior myocardial infarction[14]	Yusuf et al.[15]
• Thrombolysis is ineffective when given > 6 hours after acute myocardial infarction[16]	ISIS-2 Collaborative Group[17]
• Thrombolysis for acute myocardial infarction is ineffective or harmful in patients with a previous myocardial infarction[16]	Fibrinolytic Therapy Trialists' Collaborative Group[18]
• Tamoxifen is ineffective in women with breast cancer aged < 50 years[19]	Early Breast Cancer Trialists' Collaborative Group[20]
• Benefit from carotid endarterectomy for symptomatic stenosis is reduced in patients taking only low-dose aspirin due to an increased operative risk[21]	Taylor et al.[22]
• Amlodipine reduces mortality in patients with chronic heart failure due to non-ischaemic cardiomyopathy but not in patients with ischaemic cardiomyopathy[23]	Wijeysundera et al.[24]

be defined explicitly in order to avoid post hoc data-dependent variable or category definitions. For continuous or hierarchical variables the cut-off points for analysis should be predefined. Finally, if relative treatment effect is likely to be related to baseline risk, the analysis plan should include a stratification of the results by predicted risk. The risk score or model should be selected in advance so that the relevant baseline data can be recorded. Stratification of randomisation by important subgroup variables should be considered, if appropriate.

Failure to consider subgroup analyses at the outset, coupled with the performance of multiple post hoc analyses, has been at the root of most of the erroneous subgroup observations that have been made in the past. In one trial of beta-blockers after myocardial infarction,[26] for example, 146 subgroup analyses were done,[27] several of which showed apparent differences in the effect of treatment. None were confirmed by subsequent studies.[28] Assmann et al.[28] reviewed 50 trials published in major journals in 1997 and found that 70% reported a median of four subgroup analyses, which was little changed from the number reported in the review by Pocock et al.[29] 10 years previously. The reliability of subgroup observations depends to a great extent on whether they were predefined and how many other analyses were done but not reported. For most of these trials it was uncertain whether the subgroups had been defined in detail in the initial trial protocols. Selective reporting of post hoc subgroup observations, which are generated by the data rather than tested by them, is of course analogous to placing a bet on a horse after watching the race. There is certainly evidence of selective reporting of statistically significant or otherwise interesting analyses,[30–32] but this is difficult to judge when assessing an individual trial. The only solution is for a small number of potentially important subgroups to be predefined in the trial protocol, along with their anticipated directions. Post hoc observations are not automatically invalid (many medical discoveries have been fortuitous), but they should be regarded as unreliable unless they can be replicated.

It is also essential that if clinically important subgroup–treatment effect interactions are anticipated, trials should ideally be powered to detect them reliably. If trials are powered to determine the overall effect of treatment, virtually all subgroup analyses will be underpowered. If a genuine subgroup–treatment effect interaction exists, the chance of a false-negative result with a formal test of interaction will therefore be far greater than the 5% false-positive rate in a trial where no true interaction exists. The ability of formal tests of interaction correctly to identify subgroup effects also depends on the size of the interaction relative to the overall treatment effect. For example, if a trial has 80% power to detect the overall effect of treatment (not uncommon), reliable detection of an interaction of the same magnitude as the overall effect (i.e. potentially clinically important) would require a four-fold greater sample size.[33]

Trial stopping rules should take also into account any potentially important subgroup–treatment effect interactions that are anticipated and not simply the overall effect of treatment. Separate stopping rules for different subgroups is one possibility, and such an approach was used very effectively in the trials of endarterectomy for symptomatic carotid stenosis, in which there was independent stopping and reporting in different subgroups of patients according to the degree of carotid stenosis.[34]

In large trials, randomisation ensures that the prognosis in the different treatment groups is similar at baseline, but this cannot be assumed in subgroups unless randomisation was appropriately stratified.[35] If not, it is important to check that differences in treatment effect between subgroups are not due to baseline imbalances between the treatment arms – although the power of testing for balance between treated and control arms in subgroups will usually be low.

Statistical analysis and reporting

Subgroup analyses can be wrong in two ways. First, they can falsely indicate that treatment is beneficial in a particular subgroup when the trial shows no overall effect – the

Panel 11.2: Rules of subgroup analysis: a proposed guideline for design, analysis, interpretation and reporting

Trial design

- Subgroup analyses should be defined prior to starting the trial and should be limited to a small number of clinically important questions
- It is essential that there is *expert* clinical input into the design of subgroup analyses so that all relevant baseline clinical and other data are recorded
- The direction and magnitude of anticipated subgroup effects should be stated at the outset
- The exact definitions and categories of the subgroup variables should be defined explicitly at the outset in order to avoid post hoc data-dependent variable or category definitions. For continuous or hierarchical variables the cut-off points for analysis should be predefined
- Stratification of randomisation by important subgroup variables should be considered
- If important subgroup–treatment effect interactions are anticipated, trials should ideally be powered to detect them reliably
- Trial stopping rules should take into account anticipated subgroup–treatment effect interactions, and not simply the overall effect of treatment
- If relative treatment effect is likely to be related to baseline risk, the analysis plan should include a stratification of the results by predicted risk. The risk score or model should be selected in advance so that the relevant baseline data can be recorded

Analysis and reporting

- The above design issues should be reported in the methods section along with details of how and why subgroups were selected
- Statistical significance of the effect of treatment in individual subgroups should not be reported; rates of false-negative and false-positive results are extremely high. The only reliable statistical approach is to test for a subgroup–treatment effect interaction
- All subgroup analyses that were done should be reported, i.e. not only the number of subgroup variables but also the number of different outcomes analysed by subgroup, different lengths of follow-up, etc.
- Statistical significance of pre hoc subgroup–treatment effect interactions should be adjusted when multiple subgroup analyses are performed
- Subgroup analyses should be reported as absolute risk reductions as well as relative risk reductions. Where relevant, the statistical significance of differences in absolute risk reductions should be tested
- Ideally, only one outcome should be studied and this should usually be the primary trial outcome, irrespective of whether this is a single outcome or a clinically important composite outcome
- Comparability of treatment groups for prognostic factors should be checked within subgroups
- If multiple subgroup–treatment effect interactions are found, further analysis is required to check whether their effects are independent

Continued

Panel 11.2: Continued

Interpretation

- Reports of the statistical significance of the effect of treatment in individual subgroups should be ignored, particularly reports of lack of benefit in a particular subgroup in a trial in which there is overall benefit, unless there is a significant subgroup treatment effect interaction
- Genuine *unanticipated* subgroup–treatment effect interactions are rare (assuming that *expert* clinical opinion was sought in order to predefine potentially important subgroups) and so apparent interactions that are discovered post hoc should be interpreted with caution. No test of statistical significance is reliable in this situation
- Pre hoc subgroup analyses are not intrinsically valid and should still be interpreted with caution. The false-positive rate for tests of subgroup–treatment effect interaction where no true interaction exists is 5% per subgroup
- The best test of validity of subgroup–treatment effect interactions is their reproducibility in other trials
- Few trials are powered to detect subgroup effects and so the false-negative rate for tests of subgroup–treatment effect interaction where a true interaction exists will usually be high

situation in which subgroup analyses are most commonly performed.[36, 37] Simulations of randomised controlled trials (RCTs) powered to determine the overall effect of treatment suggest that false subgroup effects will be found by chance in 7–21% of analyses depending on other factors.[33] More commonly (41–66% of simulated subgroups) they can falsely indicate that there is no treatment effect in a particular subgroup when the trial shows benefit overall.[33] Benefit is most likely to be absent in small subgroups, which probably explains the recurrent and usually mistaken finding that treatments are ineffective in women,[3, 6, 38] and in the elderly,[6, 9] both of whom tend to be underrepresented in RCTs.[39] The mistake here, of course, it to place any emphasis on the statistical significance of the treatment effect in one subgroup or the other.

The correct analysis is not the statistical significance of the treatment effect in one subgroup or the other, but whether the effect is significantly *different* between the subgroups – the test of subgroup–treatment effect interaction. For example, although endarterectomy for severe stenosis in the European Carotid Surgery Trial (ECST)[40] was only significantly beneficial in patients born on certain days of the week (figure 11.1), this was, of course, due to chance and there was no subgroup–treatment effect interaction ($p = 0.83$). Simulation studies have shown that tests of subgroup–treatment effect interaction are reliable, with a false-positive rate of 5% at $p < 0.05$, which is robust to differences in the size of subgroups, the number of categories and to continuous data.[33] However, although testing of subgroup–treatment effect interactions has long been recommended,[28, 29, 35–37, 41] the review by Assmann et al.[28] showed that 37% of RCTs reported only p values for treatment effect within subgroups and only 43% reported tests of interaction.

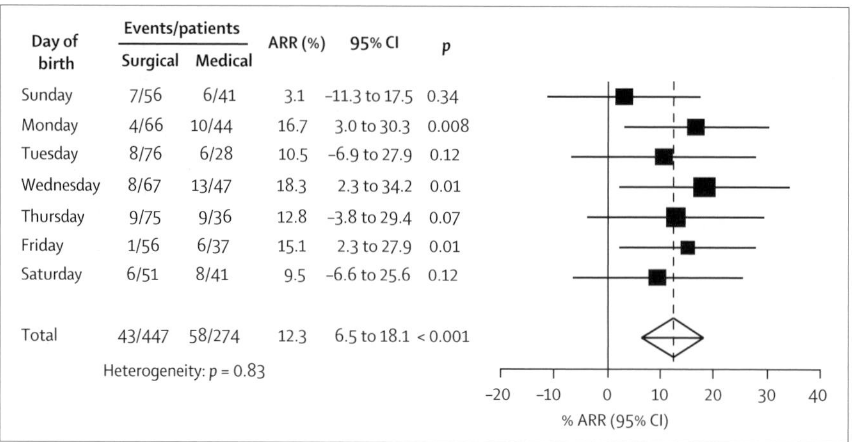

Day of birth	Events/patients Surgical	Events/patients Medical	ARR (%)	95% CI	p
Sunday	7/56	6/41	3.1	-11.3 to 17.5	0.34
Monday	4/66	10/44	16.7	3.0 to 30.3	0.008
Tuesday	8/76	6/28	10.5	-6.9 to 27.9	0.12
Wednesday	8/67	13/47	18.3	2.3 to 34.2	0.01
Thursday	9/75	9/36	12.8	-3.8 to 29.4	0.07
Friday	1/56	6/37	15.1	2.3 to 27.9	0.01
Saturday	6/51	8/41	9.5	-6.6 to 25.6	0.12
Total	43/447	58/274	12.3	6.5 to 18.1	< 0.001

Heterogeneity: $p = 0.83$

***Figure* 11.1: The effect of carotid endarterectomy in patients with ≥ 70% symptomatic stenosis in the ECST[40] according to the day of the week on which patients were born. (Reprinted from Rothwell,[51] copyright 2005, with permission from Elsevier.)**

The choice and number of outcomes studied will also, of course, affect the validity of subgroup analyses. Outcomes that are not directly affected by treatment, as is often the case for all-cause mortality, should be avoided. For example, in the Medical Research Council (MRC) trial of blood pressure lowering in mild hypertension, treatment reduced all-cause mortality in men but increased mortality in women.[7] However, the excess mortality in women on active treatment was due entirely to non-cardiovascular deaths and treatment reduced the risk of stroke in both sexes. Ideally, only one outcome should be studied, and this should usually be the primary outcome for the trial, irrespective of whether it is a single or a composite outcome. For example, sex had no effect on benefit from endarterectomy for 50–69% symptomatic carotid stenosis in the pooled RCTs if the analysis was based on the risk of ipsilateral ischaemic stroke only (i.e. the outcome that surgery prevents), but there was harm in women and benefit in men (interaction: $p = 0.008$) if the clinically relevant composite outcome of ipsilateral ischaemic stroke plus operative stroke or death (the primary outcome in the trials) was considered.[34] The overall effect of surgery depends on the balance of two outcomes which have different mechanisms and risk factors. Women had a lower risk of stroke on medical treatment than men (hazard ratio (HR) = 0.79, 95% confidence interval (CI) 0.64 to 0.97, $p = 0.03$) but a higher operative risk (HR = 1.50, 95% CI 1.14 to 1.97, $p = 0.004$).[34] There is an argument in situations such as this for modelling risk and benefit separately, but patients and clinicians still need to know what the overall effect of treatment on the composite outcome is.

Further in relation to reporting of subgroup analyses, the design issues detailed in the first part of this chapter should be reported in the methods section along with details of how and why subgroups were selected. All subgroup analyses that were done should be reported (i.e. not only the number of subgroup variables but also the number of different outcomes analysed, etc.).

Finally, in order to determine the likelihood of individual benefit, subgroup analyses must be expressed in terms of absolute risk reductions as well as in terms of relative treatment effects. A lack of a statistically significant difference in relative treatment effect between subgroups does not indicate that there is no difference in absolute risk reduction. Figure 11.2 shows the effect of carotid endarterectomy for severe symptomatic stenosis in patients presenting with retinal ischaemic events versus cerebral hemispheric events.[34] There is no significant heterogeneity of relative treatment effect (interaction: $p = 0.55$) but there is a statistically significant ($p = 0.01$) and clinically important three-fold difference in absolute treatment effect. This inconsistency is inevitable if relative risk reductions are similar in two subgroups but the absolute risks without treatment are sufficiently different. The difference in absolute treatment effect between these subgroups is clinically very important and is of an order that will influence the decisions of patients about whether to submit themselves to surgery. Yet most trials report subgroup analyses only in terms of relative treatment effects.

It cannot even be assumed that any difference in absolute risk reduction between subgroups will be in the same direction as that for the relative risk reduction (RRR). For example, in a pooled analysis of data from trials of lipid lowering in prevention of vascular events, the relative treatment effect was significantly lower in patients with hypertension than in those with no hypertension (RRR = 14%, 95% CI 2 to 24 versus 33%, 95% CI 25 to 40; interaction: $p = 0.003$) but absolute benefit was still greater in the patients with hypertension because of their greater absolute risk without treatment.[42] These considerations are crucial in the elderly, in whom relative treatment effects are sometimes less than in younger patients, often because disease is more advanced, but absolute treatment effects are frequently greater because the absolute risk of a poor outcome without treatment is higher.

In summary, the statistical significance of the effect of treatment in individual subgroups should not be reported; rates of false-negative and false-positive results are extremely high. The only reliable statistical approach is to test for a subgroup–treatment effect interaction. However, if multiple subgroup analyses are performed, the statistical significance of pre hoc subgroup–treatment effect interactions should be adjusted accordingly. Only one outcome should be studied and this should usually be the primary

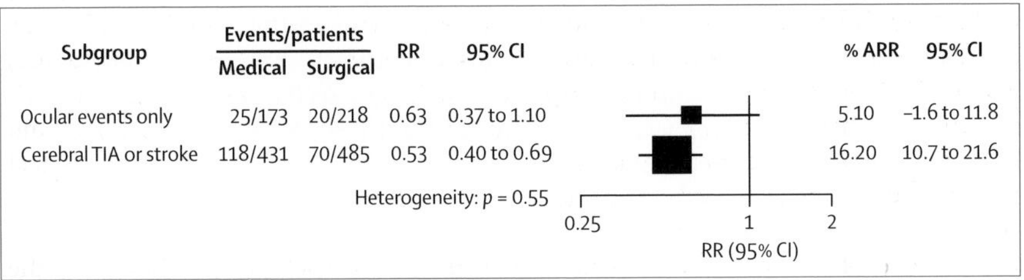

Figure 11.2: **A comparison of the relative (RR) and absolute (ARR) reductions in the risk of stroke with treatment in two subgroups of patients in a randomised comparison of the effect of carotid endarterectomy for ≥ 70% symptomatic stenosis (patients presenting with ocular ischaemic events versus cerebral hemispheric events).[34]**

trial outcome, irrespective of whether this is a single outcome or a clinically important composite outcome. Comparability of treatment groups for prognostic factors should be checked within subgroups and, as discussed later in this chapter, if multiple subgroup–treatment effect interactions are found, further analysis is required to check whether their effects are independent. Finally, subgroup analyses should be expressed in terms of absolute risk reductions as well as in terms of relative treatment effects, with separate subgroup–treatment effect interactions.

Interpretation

Interpretation of subgroup analyses would be made much easier if the guidelines on design, analysis and reporting in panel 11.2 were adhered to. However, this is frequently not the case and clinicians must, therefore, try to make a judgement about likely validity. In this respect, it is essential to understand quite how powerful the effects of chance can be. The effect of chance on subgroup analyses is usually illustrated with the ISIS-2 trial example (aspirin versus placebo in acute myocardial infarction), in which aspirin was ineffective in patients born under the star signs of Libra and Gemini (150 deaths on aspirin versus 147 on placebo, $2p = 0.5$) but was beneficial in the remainder (654 deaths on aspirin versus 869 on placebo, $2p << 0.0001$).[43–45] The statistical significance of this subgroup treatment effect interaction has never been reported, but it appears to be $p = 0.01$ (Breslow Day test). However, Libra and Gemini are not adjacent on the Zodiac and simply splitting a trial of an effective treatment into 12 subgroups and comparing the two subgroups with the least evidence of benefit with the remainder will almost inevitably produce significant heterogeneity. The more appropriate test of the subgroup–treatment effect interaction across the 12 separate birth signs would undoubtedly be non-significant in ISIS-2.

However, highly statistically significant subgroup–treatment effect interactions can occur by chance. Figure 11.3 shows the effect of endarterectomy for severe carotid stenosis by month of birth in the ECST (interaction: $p < 0.001$ across the 12 months).[40] The remarkable trend in benefit ($p < 0.0000001$), maximum in patients born in May (absolute relative risk (ARR) = 37.5%, 95% CI 16.3 to 58.7) or June (ARR = 29.7%, 95% CI 8.1 to 51.1) and falling smoothly to possible harm in March (ARR = −7.2%, 95% CI −22.3 to 7.9) and April (ARR = −10.5%, 95% CI −32.8 to 11.8), would have been very difficult to ignore if it had been in relation to age, blood pressure, or some other plausible variable – illustrating the unreliability of unanticipated post hoc subgroup effects. One of the most damaging unanticipated post hoc subgroup interactions ($p = 0.003$) was the observation in the Canadian Cooperative Study Group trial[3] that aspirin was effective in preventing stroke and death in men (RR = 0.52, $p < 0.005$) but not in women (RR = 1.42, $p = 0.35$). Women were undertreated for at least a decade before subsequent trials and overviews showed benefit.

In fact, the best test of the validity of subgroup analyses is not statistical significance but replication. Predictably, for example, the month of birth interaction was not replicated in ECST patients with < 70% stenosis (figure 11.4) or in other trials, whereas the effect of the timing of surgery on benefit from endarterectomy was present in the two different stenosis groups (see Chapter 9, figure 9.2) and in two independent trials (figure 11.5). For post hoc analyses, replication is absolutely essential, irrespective of plausibility or

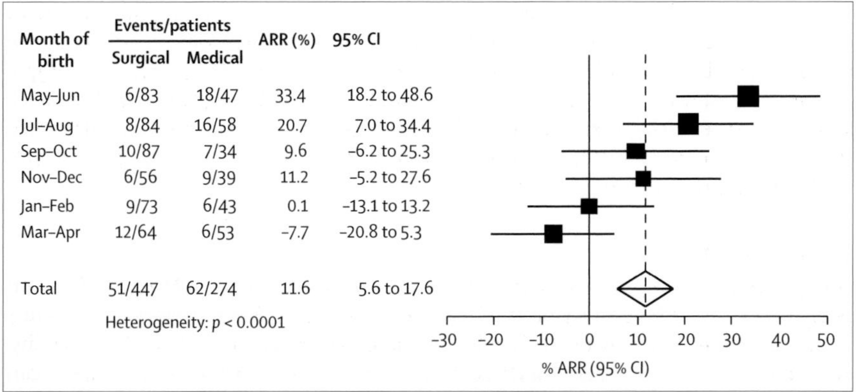

Month of birth	Events/patients Surgical	Events/patients Medical	ARR (%)	95% CI
May–Jun	6/83	18/47	33.4	18.2 to 48.6
Jul–Aug	8/84	16/58	20.7	7.0 to 34.4
Sep–Oct	10/87	7/34	9.6	–6.2 to 25.3
Nov–Dec	6/56	9/39	11.2	–5.2 to 27.6
Jan–Feb	9/73	6/43	0.1	–13.1 to 13.2
Mar–Apr	12/64	6/53	–7.7	–20.8 to 5.3
Total	51/447	62/274	11.6	5.6 to 17.6

Heterogeneity: $p < 0.0001$

–30
–20
–10
0
10
20
30
40
50
% ARR (95% CI)

***Figure** 11.3:* **The effect of carotid endarterectomy in patients with ≥ 70% symptomatic stenosis in the ECST[40] according to month of birth in six 2-month periods. (Reprinted from Rothwell,[51] copyright 2005, with permission from Elsevier.)**

Month of birth	Events/patients Surgical	Events/patients Medical	ARR (%)	95% CI
≥ 70% stenosis				
May–Aug	13/168	32/105	25.6	15.0 to 36.2
Sep–Dec	12/142	14/73	11.0	0.2 to 21.8
Jan–Apr	18/137	12/96	-1.1	-10.5 to 8.2
	Heterogeneity: p = 0.008			
< 70% stenosis				
May–Aug	51/454	13/299	-8.0	-12.3 to 3.6
Sep–Dec	53/409	25/292	-5.1	-10.5- to 0.2
Jan–Apr	55/489	40/343	0.6	-5.8- to 7.1
	Heterogeneity: p = 0.02			
All patients				
May–Aug	64/624	45/404	1.2	-3.3- to 5.6
Sep–Dec	65/556	39/368	-1.3	-6.0 to 3.5
Jan–Apr	73/627	52/439	0.2	-4.2 to 4.7
	Heterogeneity: p = 0.84			
Total	202/1807	136/1211	0.1	-2.5 to 2.7

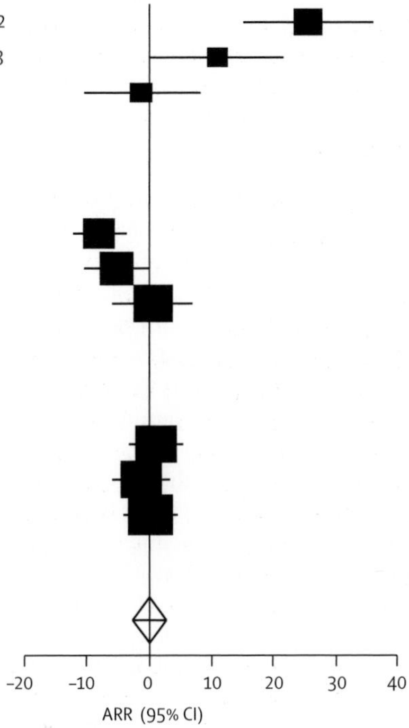

-20
-10
0
10
20
30
40
ARR (95% CI)

***Figure** 11.4:* **The effect of carotid endarterectomy in the ECST[40] according to month of birth in three 4-month periods in patients with ≥ 70%, < 70% and all degrees of symptomatic stenosis. (Reprinted from Rothwell,[51] copyright 2005, with permission from Elsevier.)**

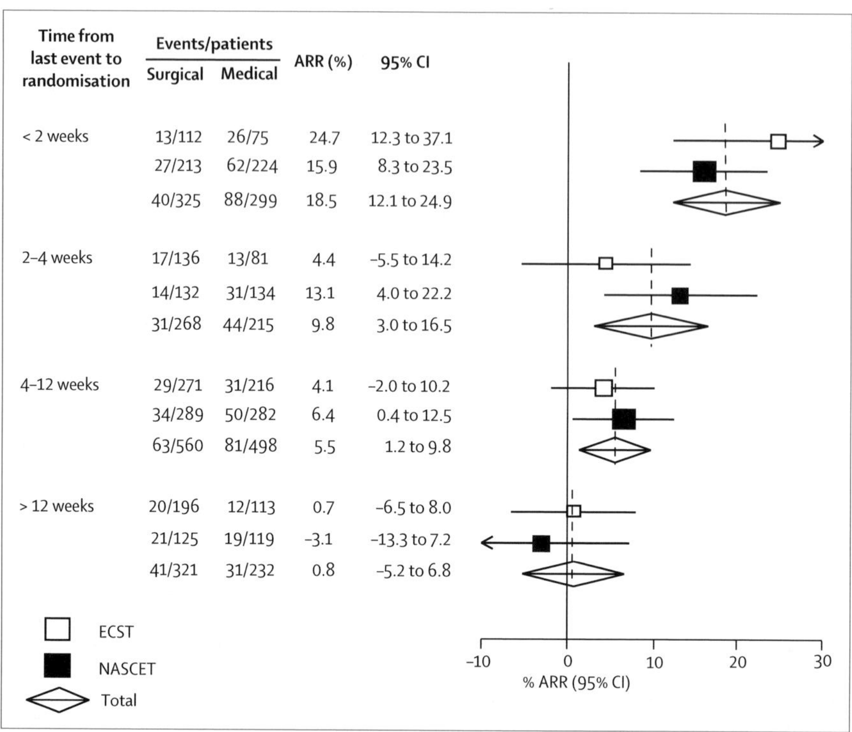

Figure 11.5: The effect of carotid endarterectomy in patients with 50–99% symptomatic stenosis in relation to the time from the last symptomatic ischaemic event to randomisation in the ECST[40] and the North American Symptomatic Carotid Endarterectomy Trial.[34] (Reprinted from Rothwell,[51] copyright 2005, with permission from Elsevier.)

statistical significance. For example, a rigorous pooled analysis of RCTs of tamoxifen in breast cancer showed that treatment was ineffective in women aged < 50 years (mainly premenopausal) but very effective in older women (mainly postmenopausal).[19] The interaction was highly significant ($p < 0.0001$), but was shown to be false in subsequent trials. Similarly, a large RCT of a calcium antagonist in chronic heart failure reported no reduction in mortality in patients with ischaemic cardiomyopathy (relative risk (RR) = 1.04, 95% CI 0.83 to 1.29) but major benefit (RR = 0.64, 95% CI 0.37 to 0.79) in patients with non-ischaemic cardiomyopathy (interaction: $p = 0.004$).[23] This effect was also manifest as a difference between patients with and without angina (RR = 1.09, 95% CI 0.84 to 1.42 versus RR = 0.59, 95% CI 0.44 to 0.81; $p = 0.002$). However, the direction of these interactions was opposite to that expected, and a subsequent trial failed to confirm the benefit in non-ischaemic cardiomyopathy.[24]

Anticipated subgroup–treatment effect interactions that are underpowered but which are reproducible are very probably more reliable than unanticipated interactions, no matter how statistically significant. For example, although an early RCT of coronary artery bypass grafting that showed that survival benefit was mainly confined to patients with left main coronary artery disease or three-vessel disease had only a few hundred patients,[46] the observation was very clinically plausible and was reproduced in a subsequent trial.[47] However, it was not until 20 years later that a pooled analysis of seven RCTs had sufficient power to demonstrate a statistically significant interaction.[48]

Multidimensional subgroup analysis

Subgroup–treatment effect interactions cannot, of course, be interpreted in isolation. Firstly, it is important to understand that apparent subgroup effects can be due to interactions between the subgroup variable and other important patient characteristics. For example, in the pooled analysis of RCTs of carotid endarterectomy, benefit from surgery across all degrees of carotid stenosis was similar in patients with ocular ischaemic events versus hemispheric ischaemic events (i.e. the same for patients presenting with strokes affecting the eye or the brain).[34] However, the mean degree of carotid stenosis was higher in patients with ocular events (54% versus 41%, $p < 0.0001$), which would increase their likelihood of benefiting from surgery. Surgery was more effective in patients with hemispheric than ocular events when subgroup analyses were stratified by degree of stenosis.[34]

Secondly, subgroup analyses are almost always performed only in relation to a single baseline variable at a time, and can sometimes therefore be of limited use to clinicians if there are several clinical characteristics that are likely to have important effects on the risks or benefits of treatment. Absolute risk reductions for patients with multiple specific characteristics cannot be derived indirectly from separate univariate subgroup analyses. Even relative risk reductions cannot be derived indirectly (i.e. if two clinical characteristics were each associated with a doubling of the relative risk reduction with treatment in univariate subgroup analyses, benefit will not necessarily be four times greater in a patient who possesses both characteristics than in a patient who possesses neither). It is possible, however, to perform multivariate subgroup analysis to estimate benefit. For example, it has been shown that carotid endarterectomy for symptomatic carotid stenosis is less effective in women than in men (interaction: $p = 0.007$), and that benefit is also very closely related to the time elapsed since the presenting transient ischaemic attack (TIA) or stroke (interaction: $p = 0.006$).[34] Figure 11.6 shows the effect of surgery in the relevant subgroups in patients with 50–99% stenosis. Interestingly, although the univariate subgroups are independent (i.e. there was no difference in the mean delay in men and women) the subgroup effects are not. The effect of the delay to surgery on benefit is much greater in women (difference in trend: $p < 0.001$), probably as a result of sex differences in the pathology of symptomatic carotid plaque.[50] In practice, of course, statistical power in RCTs is often insufficient for univariate subgroup analyses, and so reliable multifactorial subgroup analysis will seldom be possible in individual trials, but is possible in pooled analyses of individual patient data from multiple trials.

Conclusions

Large pragmatic trials with broad eligibility criteria and high inclusion rates provide the most reliable data on the effects of treatments, but should be designed, analysed and

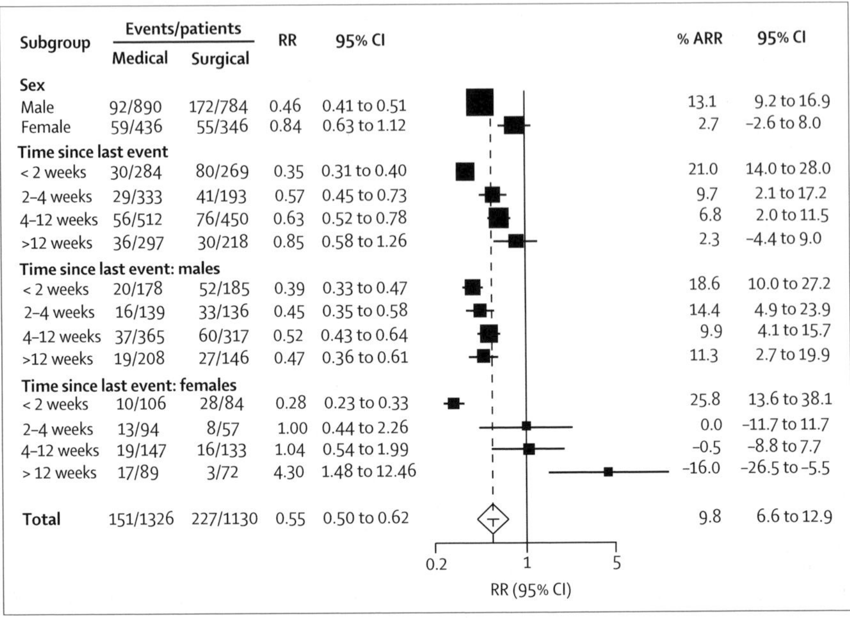

***Figure* 11.6: The interaction between two independent univariate subgroup analyses of the effect of carotid endarterectomy for ≥ 50% symptomatic stenosis in the Carotid Endarterectomy Trialists' Collaboration showing the independent effects of sex and the time from last symptomatic ischaemic event and randomisation on the benefit from surgery (upper portion) and the effect of time from last symptomatic ischaemic event and randomisation on the benefit from surgery in males and females separately.[49] (Reprinted from Rothwell et al.,[52] copyright 2005, with permission from Elsevier.)**

reported in a way that leads to the most effective use of treatments in routine practice. Subgroup analyses are important if there are potentially large differences between groups in the risk of a poor outcome with or without treatment, if there is potential heterogeneity of treatment effect in relation to pathophysiology, if there are practical questions about when to treat, or if there is uncertainty about benefit and consequent undertreatment in specific groups. Analyses must be predefined, carefully justified and limited to a few clinically important questions, and post hoc observations should be treated with scepticism, irrespective of their statistical significance. If important subgroup effects are anticipated, trials should either be powered to detect them reliably or pooled analyses of multiple trials should be undertaken. Adherence to the guidelines for planning, analysis and reporting of subgroup analyses proposed in panel 11.2 would increase reliability. Indeed, none of the flawed subgroup observations listed in panel 11.1 satisfies the guidelines in panel 11.2.

References

1 Tukey JW. Sunset salvo. *Am Stat* 1986; **40:** 72–76.

2 Yusef S, Collins R, Peto R. Why do we need some large, simple randomized trials? *Stat Med* 1984; **3:** 409–20.

3 The Canadian Cooperative Study Group. A randomised trial of aspirin and sulfinpyrazone in threatened stroke. *N Engl J Med* 1978; **299:** 53–59.

4 Fields WS, Lemak NA, Frankowski RF, Hardy RJ. Controlled trial of aspirin in cerebral ischaemia. *Stroke* 1977; **8:** 301–16.

5 Antiplatelet Trialists' Collaboration. Collaborative overview of randomised trials of antiplatelet therapy. I: Prevention of death, myocardial infarction, and stroke by prolonged antiplatelet therapy in various categories of patients. *BMJ* 1994; **308:** 81–106.

6 Anastos K, Charney P, Charon RA, et al. Hypertension in women: what is really known? *Ann Intern Med* 1991; **115:** 287–93.

7 Medical Research Council Working Party. MRC trial of treatment of mild hypertension: principal results. *BMJ* 1985; **291:** 97–104.

8 Gueyffier F, Boutitie F, Boissel J-P, et al. Effect of antihypertensive drug treatment on cardiovascular outcomes in men and women. *Ann Intern Med* 1997; **126:** 761–67.

9 Amery A, Birkenhager W, Brixko P, et al. Influence of antihypertensive drug treatment on morbidity and mortality in patients aged over 60 years: EWPHW results: subgroup analysis based on entry stratification. *J Hypertens* 1986; **4** (suppl 6): S642–47.

10 Gueyffier F, Bulpitt C, Boissel J-P, et al., for the INDANA Group. Antihypertensive drugs in very old people: a subgroup meta-analysis of randomised controlled trials. *Lancet* 1999; **353:** 793–96.

11 Cleland JGF, Bulpitt CJ, Falk RH, et al. Is aspirin safe for patients with heart failure? *Br Heart J* 1995; **74:** 215–19.

12 Flather MD, Yusuf S, Kober L, et al for the ACE-Inhibitor Myocardial Infarction Collaborative Group. Long-term ACE-inhibitor therapy in patients with heart failure or left-ventricular dysfunction: a systematic overview of data from individual patients. *Lancet* 2000; **355:** 1575–81.

13 Anderson MP, Bechsgaard P, Frederiksen J, et al. Effects of alprenolol on mortality among patients with definite or suspected acute myocardial infarction: preliminary results. *Lancet* 1979; **2:** 865–68.

14 Multicenter International Study: Supplemental report: reduction in mortality after myocardial infarction with long-term beta-adrenoreceptor blockade. *BMJ* 1977; **2:** 419–21.

15 Yusuf S, Peto R, Lewis J, et al. Beta blockade during and after acute myocardial infarction: an overview of the randomized trials. *Prog Cardiovasc Dis* 1985; **27:** 335–71.

16 Gruppo Italiano per lo Studio della Streptochinasi nell'Infarcto Myocardico (GISSI). Effectiveness of intravenous thrombolytic treatment in acute myocardial infarction. *Lancet* 1986; **1:** 397–401.

17 ISIS-2 Collaborative Group. Randomised trial of IV streptokinase, oral aspirin, both, or neither among 17,187 cases of suspected acute myocardial infarction. *Lancet* 1988; **2:** 349–60.

18 Fibrinolytic Therapy Trialists' (FTT) Collaborative Group. Indications for fibrinolytic therapy in suspected acute myocardial infarction: collaborative overview of early mortality and major morbidity results from all randomised trials of more than 1000 patients. *Lancet* 1994; **343:** 311–22.

19 Early Breast Cancer Trialists' Collaborative Group. Effects of adjuvant tamoxifen and of cytotoxic therapy on mortality in early breast cancer. *N Engl J Med* 1988; **319:** 1681–92.

20 Early Breast Cancer Trialists' Collaborative Group. Tamoxifen for early breast cancer. *Cochrane Database Systematic Reviews* 2001; (1): CD000486.

21 North American Symptomatic Carotid Endarterectomy Trialists' Collaborative Group. The final results of the NASCET trial. *N Engl J Med* 1998; **339:** 1415–25.

22 Taylor DW, Barnett HJ, Haynes RB, et al. Low-dose and high-dose acetylsalicylic acid for patients undergoing carotid endarterectomy: a randomised controlled trial. ASA and Carotid Endarterectomy (ACE) Trial Collaborators. *Lancet* 1999; **353:** 2179–84.

23 Packer M, O'Connor CM, Ghali JK, et al., for the Prospective Randomised Amlodipine Survival Evaluation Study Group. Effect of amlodipine on morbidity and mortality in severe chronic heart failure. *N Engl J Med* 1996; **335:** 1107–14.

24 Wijeysundera HC, Hansen MS, Stanton E, et al., for the PRAISE II Investigators. Neurohormones and oxidative stress in nonischemic cardiomyopathy: relationship to survival and the effect of treatment with amlodipine. *Am Heart J* 2003; **146:** 291–97.

25 Altman DG, Schulz KF, Moher D, et al., for the CONSORT Group. The revised CONSORT statement for reporting randomised trials: explanation and elaboration. *Ann Intern Med* 2001; **134:** 663–94.

26 Beta-blocker Heart Attack Trial Research Group. A randomised trial of propranolol in patients with acute myocardial infarction. I. Mortality results. *JAMA* 1982; **247:** 1701–14.

27 Furberg CD, Byington RP. What do subgroup analyses reveal about differential response to beta-blocker therapy? *Circulation* 1983; **67:** I98–110.

28 Assmann SF, Pocock SJ, Enos LE, Kasten LE. Subgroup analysis and other (mis)uses of baseline data in clinical trials. *Lancet* 2000; **355:** 1064–69.

29 Pocock SJ, Hughes MD, Lee RJ. Statistical problems in the reporting of clinical trials. *N Engl J Med* 1987; **317:** 426–32.

30 Tannock IF. False positive results in clinical trials: multiple significance tests and the problem of unreported comparisons. *J Natl Cancer Inst* 1996; **88:** 206–07.

31 Gelber RD, Goldhirsch A. Interpretation of results from subset analyses within overviews of randomised clinical trials. *Stat Med* 1987; **6:** 371–78.

32 Hahn S, Williamson PR, Hutton L, et al. Assessing the potential for bias in meta-analysis due to selective reporting of subgroup analysis within studies. *Stat Med* 2000; **19:** 3325–36.

33 Brookes ST, Whitley E, Peters TJ, et al. Subgroup analyses in randomised controlled trials: quantifying the risks of false-positives and false-negatives. *Health Technol Assess* 2001; **5**(33). Available at: http://www.ncchta.org (accessed February 2007).

34 Rothwell PM, Eliasziw M, Gutnikov SA, et al., for the Carotid Endarterectomy Trialists' Collaboration. Effect of endarterectomy for recently symptomatic carotid stenosis in relation to clinical subgroups and the timing of surgery. *Lancet* 2004; **363:** 915–24.

35 Cui L, Hung HNJ, Wang SJ, Tsong Y. Issues related to subgroup analysis in clinical trials. *J Biopharm Stat* 2002; **12:** 347–58.

36 Stallones RA. The use and abuse of subgroup analysis in epidemiological research. *Prev Med* 1987; **16:** 183–94.

37 Pocock SJ, Hughes MD. Estimation issues in clinical trials and overviews. *Stat Med* 1990; **9:** 657–71.

38 Frasure-Smith N, Lesperance F, Prince RH, et al. Randomised trial of home-based psychological nursing intervention for patients recovering from myocardial infarction. *Lancet* 1997; **350:** 473–79.

39 Rothwell PM. External validity of randomised controlled trials: To whom do the results of this trial apply? *Lancet* 2005; **365:** 82–93.

40 European Carotid Surgery Trialists' Collaborative Group. Randomised trial of endarterectomy for recently symptomatic carotid stenosis: final results of the MRC European Carotid Surgery Trial (ECST). *Lancet* 1998; **351:** 1379–87.

41 Yusuf S, Wittes J, Probstfield J, Tyroler HA. Analysis and interpretation of treatment effects in subgroups of patients in randomised clinical trials. *JAMA* 1991; **266:** 93–98.

42 Sacks FM, Tonkin AM, Shepherd J, et al., for the Prospective Pravastatin Pooling Project Investigators Group. Effect of pravastatin on coronary disease events in subgroups defined by coronary risk factors. *Circulation* 2000; **102:** 1893–900.

43 Peto R. Statistics of cancer trials. In: Halan KE, ed. *Treatment of Cancer.* London: Chapman & Hall, 1981.

44 Collins R, Peto R, Gray R, Parish S. Large-scale randomised evidence: trials and overviews. In: Weatherall DJ, Ledingham JGG, Warrell DA, eds. *Oxford Textbook of Medicine.* Oxford: Oxford University Press, 1996.

45 Collins R, MacMahon S. Reliable assessment of the effects of treatment on mortality and major morbidity, I: clinical trials. *Lancet* 2001; **357:** 373–80.

46 Takaro T, Hultgren HN, Lipton MJ, Detre KM. The VA cooperative randomised study of surgery for coronary arterial occlusive disease. II. Subgroup with significant left main lesions. *Circulation* 1976; **54** (suppl 3): 107–17.

47 European Coronary Surgery Study Group. Long-term results of a prospective randomised study of coronary artery bypass surgery in stable angina patients. *Lancet* 1982; **II:** 1173.

48 Yusuf S, Zucker D, Peduzzi P, et al. Effect of coronary artery bypass graft surgery on survival: overview of 10-year results from randomised trials by the Coronary Artery Bypass Graft Surgery Trialists' Collaboration. *Lancet* 1994; **344:** 563–70.

49 Rothwell PM, Gutnikov SA, Eliasziw M, et al. Sex difference in effect of time from symptoms to surgery on benefit from endarterectomy for transient ischaemic attack and non-disabling stroke. *Stroke* 2004; **35:** 2855–61.

50 Schulz UGR, Rothwell PM. Sex differences in the angiographic and gross pathological appearance of carotid atherosclerotic plaques. *J Neurol Sci* 2001; **187** (suppl 1): S127.

51 Rothwell PM. Treating individuals 2. Subgroup analysis in randomised controlled trials: importance, indications, and interpretation. *Lancet* 2005; **365:** 176–86.

52 Rothwell PM, Mehta Z, Howard SC, et al. Treating individuals 3: from subgroups to individuals: general principles and the example of carotid endarterectomy. *Lancet* 2005; **365:** 256–65.

12

Can meta-analysis help target interventions at individuals most likely to benefit?

Simon G. Thompson and Julian P. T. Higgins

Introduction

Systematic reviews of healthcare interventions are an attempt to collate information from all relevant studies and, if deemed appropriate, combine their results using meta-analysis.[1] This process inevitably brings together studies that are diverse in their designs (e.g. in terms of outcomes assessed and length of follow-up), in the specific interventions used (method, intensity and duration) and in the types of patients studied (demographic and clinical characteristics). Thus the results, based on such a broad range of evidence, can seem remote from the issue of how to treat individual patients, and even somewhat irrelevant to clinical practice.[2] Nevertheless, it is incontrovertible that treatment decisions should be based on evidence when it exists, and that good-quality systematic reviews provide an essential mechanism in reviewing available evidence.[3] The issue is how best to bridge the gap between evidence based on many patients and making decisions about treating individuals.

The larger randomised trials are, the less their results will be subject to chance. Many patients are needed to distinguish true treatment benefits that are clinically important, but moderate in size, from chance effects.[4] Increasing numbers of patients by combining results across trials provides a principal rationale for meta-analysis.[3] At the other extreme, *n*-of-1 trials attempt to isolate effective treatments for a particular individual;[5] however, such trials can only be undertaken in specific clinical situations (e.g. to relieve symptoms in chronic disorders), and do not provide evidence about medical policy that can be generalised to new patients. In between these extremes lies the aim of targeting interventions by identifying subgroups of patients most likely to benefit. Subgroup analyses within a clinical trial investigate the effects of an intervention for specific groups of patients, for example defined by their clinical characteristics, in an attempt to refine how the treatment might best be used in practice.[6] Such analyses are, however, inevitably plagued by chance effects – both wider confidence intervals due to the fewer patients involved, leading to more uncertain inferences, and false-positive results arising from the multiplicity of subgroups typically investigated.[7]

Comparing patient subgroups within a meta-analysis might help to ameliorate the tension between decision-making in clinical medicine and overall statements of evidence in systematic reviews. Researchers have suggested that meta-analysis might go beyond estimating one overall effect:[8–10] an aim should be to estimate how treatment effectiveness varies according to patients' characteristics.[11] In this chapter, we discuss the extent to which this aim is achievable, and investigate whether we can progress beyond the general statement that meta-analytic conclusions should be 'borne in mind' in clinical decision-making. In doing so, we need to distinguish the relative risk reductions usually summarised in meta-analyses from their implications for absolute risks, which describe how much patients benefit.

Conventional meta-analysis

To focus the discussion, we introduce a specific example. The effectiveness of platelet glycoprotein IIb/IIIa inhibitors (PGIs) in acute coronary syndromes (non-Q-wave infarction and unstable angina) has received much attention, being the subject of a *Health Technology Assessment* review,[12] National Institute for Health and Clinical Excellence guidance[13] and a Cochrane Systematic Review.[14] Although PGIs reduce the risk of death and myocardial infarction in patients undergoing percutaneous coronary intervention,[14] their role in acute coronary syndromes in which coronary revascularisation is not planned is more uncertain. We focus on this issue by undertaking a meta-analysis of six large randomised trials (each > 1000 patients) as reviewed by Boersma et al.[15]

The six trials (PRISM, PRISM-PLUS, PARAGON, PURSUIT, GUSTO IV-ACS and PARAGON-B)[16–21] included 31 402 patients with unstable angina or myocardial infarction without persistent ST-segment elevation, who were not routinely scheduled for early revascularisation. PGIs were given intravenously (bolus plus infusion) and compared with placebo or control (aspirin or heparin). The PGI drugs used varied between trials (abciximab, eptifibatide, lamifiban and tirofiban), as did the doses and durations (24–120 hours) of infusion. Myocardial infarction was defined objectively in every study, with slightly varying criteria for cardiac enzyme concentrations. We consider the risk of death and myocardial infarction up to 30 days after randomisation, as all trials reported results at this time point. A total of 3530 events occurred, an average risk of 11%.

The meta-analysis yields an overall odds ratio of 0.91 (95% confidence interval (CI) 0.85 to 0.98, $p = 0.02$; figure 12.1). Since relative risks and odds ratios are similar for risks up

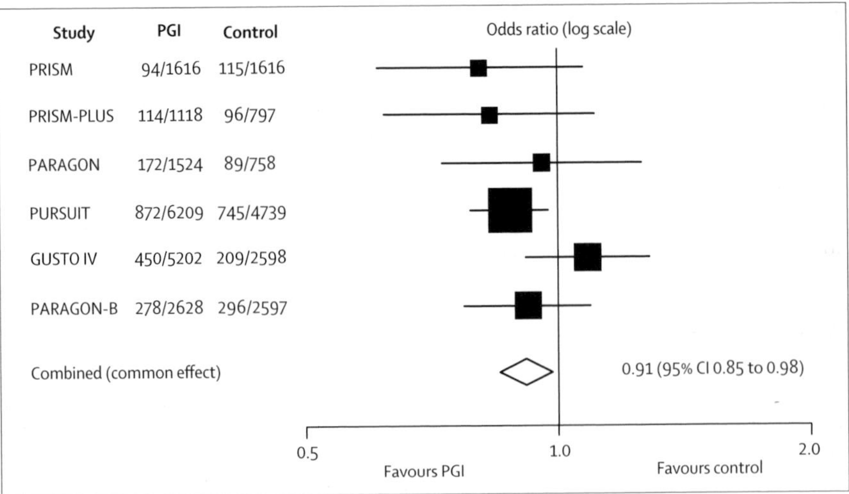

Figure 12.1: Meta-analysis of six trials of platelet glycoprotein IIb/IIIa inhibitors (odds ratios and 95% CI). Numbers are the number of deaths and myocardial infarctions up to 30 days/the total number of patients randomised. (Reprinted from Thompson and Higgins,[54] copyright 2005, with permission from Elsevier.)

to about 20%, this result corresponds to a 9% reduction in risk from the use of PGIs. The analysis is based on an assumption of a common effect across all trials. The failure to show direct statistical evidence against this assumption (the test for heterogeneity is not significant, $p = 0.33$) does not, however, mean that the underlying odds ratio in every trial is in fact the same. The test for heterogeneity lacks statistical power[22] and cannot distinguish true differences between the results in the different trials from chance effects. Indeed, in view of the clinical diversity of the trials, an assumption of a common effect is highly implausible. From a clinical standpoint, it would be convenient to assume that the 9% reduction in risk applies to all patients with acute coronary syndromes. Unfortunately, this assumption would be unjustified, not only because the test for heterogeneity lacks power but also because the test only addresses differences between trials (e.g. because of varying treatment protocols) rather than potential differences between patients with varying characteristics.

Absolute risks are more informative for clinical decision-making than are relative measures such as the relative risk or odds ratio.[23] The absolute risk difference estimates the risk reduction that is expected on average for every patient. For the six PGI trials, a meta-analysis of the differences in the proportions of patients dying or having a myocardial infarction within 30 days yields an overall absolute risk difference of 0.89% (95% CI 0.17 to 1.60) in favour of PGIs. This finding corresponds to an expected number needed to treat to prevent one event of 112 (95% CI 63 to 590). In this case, we might argue that the absolute risk differences are as likely to be consistent between the trials as are the odds ratios, as the period of follow-up for the outcome considered is identical. In general, and especially for trials with different follow-up periods, the relative risks or odds ratios are more likely to be consistent between trials and patients.[24] Extrapolation to a specific patient group then involves applying the relative risk reduction from the meta-analysis to the group's baseline level of risk.[25–27]

Conventional meta-analysis thus does not effectively identify groups of patients who might benefit most from an intervention. To do this, the extent of treatment benefit should be related to the patients' characteristics. On the basis of published data, one way to link benefit to characteristics is to relate the treatment effect in every trial to some average characteristic of the patients in that trial (e.g. mean age or proportion of women). Such an analysis is called meta-regression,[28] which, although straightforward to do, is subject to substantial difficulties in interpretation.

Meta-regression

Meta-regression aims to relate the treatment effects recorded in different trials to the overall characteristics of those trials. We consider here the example of whether the effectiveness of PGIs is different between men and women. The basic characteristics of patients recruited into trials are usually reported fully in publications. For example, we can relate the odds ratio noted in every trial to the proportion of women in that study (figure 12.2). Meta-regression assesses the strength of the relationship between the two. In this case, the log(odds ratio) for the effect of PGIs is estimated to increase by 0.044 (standard error (SE) 0.024, $p = 0.06$) for every 1% rise in the proportion of women. This result could be taken to imply that the odds ratio for women is 81 times that in men, corresponding to studies of 100% women and 0% women, respectively (exponential of $100 \times 0.044 = 81$). This conclusion is clearly totally implausible, even though the relationship is of borderline significance.

First, we note some technical issues about undertaking meta-regression, as they are sometimes incorrectly done.[29] Odds ratios or relative risks are usually log-transformed because they can more justifiably be regarded as normally distributed. The regression also has to be weighted, taking into account not only the precision of every trial's result (as shown by the size of the circles in figure 12.2) but also the extent of residual differences between their results not attributable to the characteristic being considered.[30] Statistical software to do such analyses is now widely available.[31] To investigate directly whether the treatment effect (e.g. odds ratio or absolute risk difference) varies with the baseline risk of the patients in the different trials is tempting. However, the baseline risk can usually only be measured by the reported risk in the control groups, which directly enters the calculation of the treatment effect. Therefore, simple meta-regression can give biased results.[32] Although more appropriate statistical methods can be used for such analyses,[33] results are not necessarily robust.

Even if meta-regression is undertaken correctly from a technical point of view, relationships with averages of patients' characteristics are potentially misleading. First, meta-

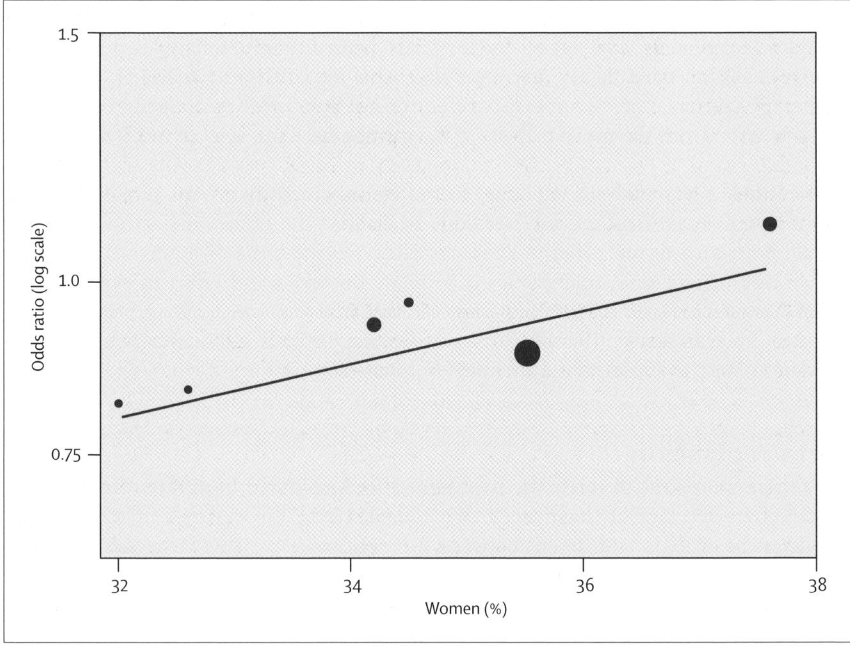

Figure 12.2: **Meta-regression relationship of the log(odds ratio) values across trials. The size of each circle is proportional to the precision of each log(odds ratio) estimate. (Reprinted from Thompson and Higgins,[54] copyright 2005, with permission from Elsevier.)**

regression describes observational relationships across studies, which are subject to confounding by other characteristics that vary between the trials. Even though every trial is randomised, meta-regression is only the study of the epidemiology of trials[34] and relationships may well not be causal. For example, many (and probably more important) characteristics vary across the PGI trials than merely the proportion of women, but which might be correlated with it. Thus, the relationship of the odds ratio with the proportion of women could be attributable to other factors. A second difficulty is the limited range of characteristics when they are averaged over all the patients in a trial. For example, across the six PGI trials the proportions of women vary only from 32% to 38%, whereas individual patients are either 0% or 100% female. Similarly, mean ages vary from 62 to 66 years, whereas the individual patients' ages have a much wider spread (typically 45–85 years), suggesting that little statistical power exists to detect relationships by meta-regression.[35] In the extreme case, in which the proportions of women are identical in every trial, there is no possibility of detecting a relationship. One final difficulty is that, in any systematic review, many characteristics (of trials or their patients) could be investigated by meta-regression, but there are usually only a few trials.[36] This fact leads to the likelihood of data dredging and the reporting in publications of only significant findings. These are therefore likely to be false-positive results, which are misleading for both clinical practice and future research.[30]

Thus, there are many reasons why meta-regression should be avoided. Its use should be restricted to the investigation of differences between trials that relate to trial features (e.g. treatment regimen) and patients' characteristics that vary substantially across trials and not within trials, when these features have been prespecified and many trials are available.[36] Although data for average patients' characteristics are usually available, and meta-regression is easily undertaken, this does not mean that findings can be reliably interpreted. To provide a way of investigating patients' characteristics we have to move away from looking at relationships across trials, to inspection of relationships within trials. So we need to compare subgroups of patients within every trial (e.g. men versus women) and then combine these results over trials.

Meta-analysis of subgroup differences

Most large trials report whether certain baseline patients' characteristics are effect modifiers, that is whether the treatment effect varies according to these characteristics. For example, treatment effects in men and women, or by age group, are calculated and presented separately. Evidence for differential effects should be assessed by a statistical test of interaction.[37] In principle, we should be able to extract this information from every trial: for example, calculate the difference in log(odds ratio) values between subgroups in every trial, and undertake a meta-analysis of these differences across all trials to assess the evidence for, and extent of, any overall treatment interaction. However, to undertake this analysis, sufficient numerical information must be present in the publication, enabling calculation of both the log(odds ratio) values within subgroups and their SEs, which is uncommon in practice.

For example, in the six PGI trials,[16–21] to what extent is such within-trial information on the sex difference in treatment effect available? Only one trial gave the basic numerical information from which the relevant quantities could be calculated for men and women. Another did not present any subgroup findings, but the remaining four provided some information for men and women separately. However, these data were presented as diagrams rather than tables, with commentary in the text restricted to the issue of the significance of the interactions. For characteristics other than sex, greater problems arose. For continuous characteristics, such as age, or more complex categorical variables, such as electrocardiography (ECG) findings, different groupings were used in the trial reports. Moreover, the variables chosen for presentation were not consistent between trials. For example, of the five trials presenting any subgroup findings, only two presented subgroup results by weight, another two by smoking category and one by previous use of beta-blockers. A concern here is that the selection of variables for presentation might have been determined by the results obtained, leading to false-positive interactions. A final difficulty was that the outcome chosen for detailed subgroup analysis varied substantially between the trials: different combinations of death, myocardial infarction, refractory ischaemia and unstable angina were used, at time points ranging from 2 days to 6 months.

The example of the PGI trials is no doubt typical. Even if one extracted as much information as possible out of the subsidiary publications from every trial, we would be unlikely to resolve the difficulties. Without sufficient and consistent information from every trial, a meta-analysis of within-trial subgroup findings, which would overcome some of the worst drawbacks of meta-regression, cannot be undertaken. Two solutions can be considered. The first is that tabulated information in a consistent format is requested from every group of trialists. Such a request might be successful, but sharing of individual patient data from different trials is usually more fruitful. This has many additional advantages,[38] including the possibility to check basic data and analyses, to improve consistency between trials (e.g. in terms of definition of outcomes), to undertake extra analyses and to consider confounding of subgroup effects by other individual characteristics.

Individual patient data meta-analysis

The trialists from the six large PGI trials undertook a collaborative project in which data for every patient were collated centrally and analysed.[15] Again we focus on the 30-day outcome of death or myocardial infarction. A simple meta-analysis based on these data gave the overall odds ratio noted before (i.e. 0.91, 95% CI 0.85 to 0.98). Now, however, the results by subgroup could be extracted in a consistent manner. For example, by logistic regression,[15] the estimated odds ratio was 0.81 for men (a beneficial effect of PGIs) and 1.15 for women (an apparent adverse effect) as shown in figure 12.3. This differential treatment effect was highly significant ($p < 0.0001$, a test of interaction based on a meta-analysis of within-trial differences). The investigators also reported whether 12 other baseline characteristics modified the overall odds ratio. None was as convincing as the sex difference, but there was some evidence that the benefit of PGIs was greater in younger people ($p = 0.10$) and in those without ST-segment depression ($p = 0.06$).

How should such interactions, based on individual patient data, be judged? One consideration is the extent to which the results are compatible with chance, which depends not only on the p value for the interaction test but also on how many characteristics have been investigated (which might be more than the number reported). With a simple adjustment for multiple testing,[39] one might reasonably regard the sex difference in the PGI trials as most unlikely to have arisen by chance, but judge that the differential effects by age and ST-segment depression are unconvincing because at least 13 characteristics have been investigated. The magnitude of the sex difference might be exaggerated merely because it was the most extreme among many interactions investigated. A second issue is the extent to which the findings are biologically plausible, although such arguments are prone to post hoc speculation. Some researchers argue that qualitative interactions (treatment effects in opposite directions) are intrinsically implausible. A third point is whether the relationship revealed might be attributable to other characteristics. In the case of the sex difference for the effect of PGIs, one relevant consideration is the concentration of troponin, a marker of the extent of myocardial damage. Boersma et al.[15] argue that, as men generally had higher concentrations of troponin than did women, a sex difference might be caused by differential effects of PGIs in those with different levels of myocardial damage. However, men also had other characteristics that differed from women, such as age and prevalence of a history of myocardial infarction and diabetes.

With individual patient data we can, in principle, investigate this type of confounding. By adjustment simultaneously for the potential confounding variables, one can see whether the sex difference becomes compatible with chance. In the case of the PGI trials, this possibility was not the case, with one exception. When adjusting for baseline troponin concentration, the sex difference was no longer evident.[15] Although such findings are observational in nature, and can be subject to residual confounding and measurement error,[40] it suggests that troponin might be the more important moderator of the effect of PGIs than sex per se. However, troponin data were only available for 35% of the entire population, and when restricting the analysis to this subgroup the unadjusted sex difference was no longer evident. Had complete data for troponin been available from the trials, the confounding of sex and troponin concentration could have been addressed fully. With incomplete data available, the answer remains uncertain. This difficulty is typical of other individual patient data meta-analyses, when different baseline data have been obtained in the included trials.

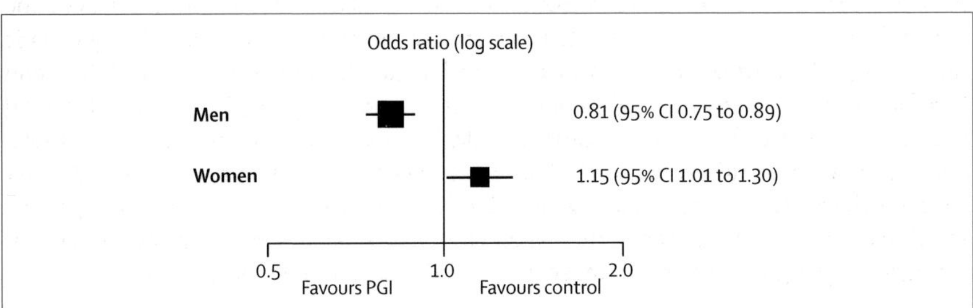

***Figure* 12.3: Odds ratios (95% CI) of death or myocardial infarction in men and women based on individual patient data. (Reprinted from Thompson and Higgins,[54] copyright 2005, with permission from Elsevier.)**

The technical demands of individual patient data meta-analyses are substantially greater than are those of meta-analysis or meta-regression.[41] Indeed, statistical methods need to be developed in this area. In general, we would suggest that the estimated relationships between the extent of treatment benefit and patients' characteristics are derived only from within-trial information, so that confounding because of differences between trials is avoided. As discussed above, such confounding is one issue that affects meta-regression. To avoid this problem, interaction effects (e.g. the differences between men and women) are calculated in every trial separately and then combined over trials. When some studies contain only women or only men, they contribute no within-trial information to the evidence about a sex difference in treatment effect and so would be omitted from the analysis. Such a method is designed to reduce bias, at the expense of losing some precision. Some multilevel model methods of analysis do not clearly separate within and between trial information, and can consequently result in misleading conclusions.[42]

The conclusions from the PGI trials' individual patient data meta-analysis might reasonably be that the proportionate risk reduction for men of 19% seems to apply reasonably uniformly across patient subgroups. For women, the results do not seem encouraging, with a reported 15% increase in risk. Whether this finding is attributable to an intrinsic difference between the sexes, or to the generally less severe myocardial damage in women, remains uncertain.

Discussion

Identification of patient groups who benefit most from an intervention is never going to be easy, since it is a task for which enormous quantities of randomised evidence are necessary. Even in large trials, apparent subgroup differences can result merely from chance. Meta-analyses of large trials based on individual patient data allow subgroups to be contrasted within trials, and for these results to be combined across trials, producing more reliable evidence. Individual patient data also allow investigation of whether treatment interactions associated with one clinical characteristic are potentially confounded by another. Attempts to target treatments by meta-regression of overall trial results and averages of patients' characteristics are generally misleading. For example, in the PGI trials, a completely unrealistic estimate of the sex difference in treatment effect was obtained from a meta-regression across trials.

Although we have considered only the role of meta-analyses of clinical trials, meta-analyses of other types of study can help inform which patients are more likely to benefit from an intervention. Prognostic factors are inherently taken into account when deciding among treatment options. Thus, meta-analyses of associations between patient characteristics and risk or progression of disease provide essential contributions to evidence-based practice. The emerging area of pharmacogenetics (the use of genetic data to individualise treatment choice, dose and monitoring) raises further possibilities. Although pharmacogenetic strategies will need to be evaluated in randomised trials, insight often comes from genetic association studies and meta-analyses of them. For example, carriers of the Pl^{A2} variant of the gene encoding glycoprotein IIIa has been demonstrated through meta-analysis to have a higher risk of coronary artery disease.[43] Furthermore, since an in vitro study found that platelets carrying this variant are more sensitive to abciximab,[44] there has been interest in whether individuals Pl^{A2} carriers will respond differently to PGIs.[43, 45] However, initial findings have not been supported by subsequent studies,[46, 47] and a meta-analysis of these studies may be warranted.

Clinical decisions for the individual patient, and medical policy decisions, have always to be made, at least to some degree, on the basis of incomplete or insufficient evidence. When we do not have evidence about treatment effects in specific subgroups of patients, these decisions have to be based on evidence about overall effectiveness. We should only make different decisions for specific patient groups when strong evidence supporting this becomes available. For policy decisions at a national level, cost-effectiveness has to be considered in addition to clinical effectiveness.[48] A treatment should be targeted at those for whom it is most cost-effective, ideally individuals who get the greatest clinical benefit with the least use of medical resources. In general, we are far from having sufficient information to make reliable policy decisions on this basis.

Evidence of generally consistent relative risk reductions has been a striking finding in some meta-analyses. For example, antiplatelet treatment produced a relative reduction in risk of serious vascular events of about 25% across a wide range of patient groups,[49] and fibrinolytic treatment after myocardial infarction showed about a 20% reduction in mortality.[50] In such situations, the benefit for specific patient groups depends crucially on their baseline risk; those with low baseline risk have little to gain, but those with high baseline risk have much to gain. There are, however, some exceptions to consistent relative effects: the PGI trials apparently showed beneficial effects in men and adverse effects in women; for antiplatelet treatment, there was a lesser proportionate reduction in the risk of serious vascular events in patients with acute stroke than in other high risk groups;[49] for endarterectomy in patients with carotid stenosis, benefit was restricted to those with at least 70% stenosis.[51]

Even when relative risk reductions are used as the summary of effects in meta-analysis of individual patient data, absolute risk reductions should be estimated explicitly for specific patient groups.[49] Estimation of the baseline risks for different patient groups is conventionally not part of meta-analyses. Nevertheless, it can be done, with either data from the trials themselves[51] or from external observational studies.[52] Such analyses would add to the clinical usefulness of the usual meta-analytic summaries of relative risk reductions.[53] Individual patient data meta-analysis should be seen as more than merely a gold standard method for doing simple meta-analysis. For example, patient subgroups can be consistently defined and systematically contrasted for evidence of possible differential treatment effects. Prespecification of a limited number of such patient subgroups can help guard against the risk of false-positive results. Individual patient data meta-analyses would then be explicitly designed to address directly the best targeting of interventions.

Acknowledgments

We thank Eric Boersma, Colin Baigent, John Danesh and Shah Ebrahim for their helpful comments on an earlier version of this chapter. Both authors are funded by the UK Medical Research Council. The chapter is a slightly revised version of a previous article (*Lancet* 2005; **365**: 341–346), reprinted with permission.

12 Using meta-analysis to target interventions at individuals

References

1 Egger M, Davey Smith G, Altman DG. *Systematic Reviews in Health Care: Meta-Analysis in Context.* London: BMJ Books, 2001.

2 Wittes RE. Problems in the medical interpretation of overviews. *Stat Med* 1987; **6:** 269–80.

3 Mulrow CD. Rationale for systematic reviews. *BMJ* 1994; **309:** 597–99.

4 Peto R. Why do we need systematic overviews of randomised trials? *Stat Med* 1987; **6:** 233–40.

5 Guyatt G, Sackett D, Taylor DW, et al. Determining optimal therapy: randomized trials in individual patients. *N Engl J Med* 1986; **314:** 889–92.

6 Rothwell PM. Can overall results of clinical trials be applied to all patients? *Lancet* 1995; **345:** 1616–19.

7 Oxman AD, Guyatt GH. A consumers guide to subgroup analyses. *Ann Intern Med* 1992; **116:** 78–84.

8 Thompson SG. Why sources of heterogeneity in meta-analysis should be investigated. *BMJ* 1994; **309:** 1351–55.

9 Berlin JA. Benefits of heterogeneity in meta-analysis of data from epidemiologic studies. *Am J Epidemiol* 1995; **142:** 383–87.

10 Davey Smith G, Egger M, Phillips AN. Meta-analysis: beyond the grand mean? *BMJ* 1997; **315:** 1610–14.

11 Lau J, Ioannidis JPA, Schmid CH. Summing up evidence: one answer is not always enough. *Lancet* 1998; **351:** 123–27.

12 McDonagh MS, Bachmann LM, Golder S, et al. A rapid and systematic review of the clinical effectiveness and cost-effectiveness of glycoprotein IIb/IIIa antagonists in the medical management of unstable angina. *Health Technol Assess* 2000; **4:** 1–95.

13 National Institute for Health and Clinical Excellence. *Guidance on the Use of Glycoprotein IIb/IIIa Inhibitors in the Treatment of Acute Coronary Syndromes.* Technology Appraisal Guidance No. 12. London: NICE, 2000.

14 Bosch X, Marrugat J. Platelet glycoprotein IIb/IIIa blockers for percutaneous coronary revascularization, and unstable angina and non-ST-segment elevation myocardial infarction (Cochrane Review). *Cochrane Database Systematic Review* 2001; **4:** CD002130.

15 Boersma E, Harrington RA, Moliterno DJ, et al. Platelet glycoprotein IIb/IIIa inhibitors in acute coronary syndromes: a meta-analysis of all major randomised clinical trials. *Lancet* 2002; **359:** 189–98.

16 The Platelet Receptor Inhibition in Ischemic Syndrome Management (PRISM) Study Investigators. A comparison of aspirin plus tirofiban with aspirin plus heparin for unstable angina. *N Engl J Med* 1998; **338:** 1498–505.

17 The Platelet Receptor Inhibition in Ischemic Syndrome Management in Patients Limited by Unstable Signs and Symptoms (PRISM-PLUS) Study Investigators. Inhibition of the platelet glycoprotein IIb/IIIa receptor with tirofiban in unstable angina and non-Q-wave myocardial infarction. *N Engl J Med* 1998; **338:** 1488–97.

18 The PARAGON Investigators. International, randomized, controlled trial of lamifiban (a platelet glycoprotein IIb/IIIa inhibitor), heparin, or both in unstable angina. *Circulation* 1998; **97:** 2386–95.

19 The PURSUIT Trial Investigators. Inhibition of platelet glycoprotein IIb/IIIa with eptifibatide in patients with acute coronary syndromes. *N Engl J Med* 1998; **339:** 436–43.

20 The GUSTO IV-ACS Investigators. Effect of glycoprotein IIb/IIIa receptor blocker abciximab on outcome in patients with acute coronary syndromes without early coronary revascularisation: the GUSTO IV-ACS randomised trial. *Lancet* 2001; **357:** 1915–24.

21 The Platelet IIb/IIIa Antagonist for the Reduction of Acute Coronary Syndrome Events in a Global Organization Network (PARAGON-B) Investigators. Randomized, placebo-controlled trials of titrated intravenous lamifiban and acute coronary syndromes. *Circulation* 2002; **105:** 316–21.

22 Hardy RJ, Thompson SG. Detecting and describing heterogeneity in meta-analysis. *Stat Med* 1998; **17:** 841–56.

23 Sackett DL, Deeks JJ, Altman DG. Down with odds ratios! *Evidence Based Med* 1996; **1:** 164–66.

24 Deeks JJ. Issues in the selection of a summary statistic for meta-analysis of clinical trials with binary outcomes. *Stat Med* 2002; **21:** 1575–600.

25 Bailey KR. Generalizing the results of randomized clinical trials. *Control Clin Trials* 1994; **15:** 15–23.

26 Smeeth L, Haines A, Ebrahim S. Numbers needed to treat derived from meta-analyses: sometimes informative, usually misleading. *BMJ* 1999; **318:** 1548–51.

27 Glasziou PP, Irwig LM. An evidence based approach to individualizing treatment. *BMJ* 1995; **311:** 1356–59.

28 Berkey CS, Hoaglin DC, Mosteller F, Colditz GA. A random-effects regression model for meta-analysis. *Stat Med* 1995; **14:** 395–411.

29 Thompson SG, Sharp SJ. Explaining heterogeneity in meta-analysis: a comparison of methods. *Stat Med* 1999; **18:** 2693–708.

30 Thompson SG, Higgins JPT. How should meta-regression analyses be undertaken and interpreted? *Stat Med* 2002; **21:** 1559–74.

31 Sharp S. Meta-analysis regression. *Stat Tech Bull* 1998; **42:** 16–22.

32 Sharp SJ, Thompson SG, Altman DG. The relation between treatment benefit and underlying risk in meta-analysis. *BMJ* 1996; **313:** 735–38.

33 Sharp SJ, Thompson SG. Analysing the relationship between treatment benefit and underlying risk in meta-analysis: comparison and development of approaches. *Stat Med* 2000; **19:** 3251–74.

34 Sterne JAC, Jüni P, Schulz KF, et al. Statistical methods for assessing the influence of study characteristics on treatment effects in 'meta-epidemiological' research. *Stat Med* 2002; **21:** 1513–24.

35 Lambert PC, Sutton AJ, Abrams KR, Jones DR. A comparison of summary patient-level covariates in meta-regression with individual patient data meta-analysis. *J Clin Epidemiol* 2001; **55:** 86–94.

36 Higgins J, Thompson S, Deeks J, Altman D. Statistical heterogeneity in systematic reviews of clinical trials: a critical appraisal of guidelines and practice. *J Health Serv Res Policy* 2002; **7:** 51–61.

37 Assmann SF, Pocock SJ, Enos LE, Kasten LE. Subgroup analysis and other (mis)uses of baseline data in clinical trials. *Lancet* 2000; **355:** 1064–69.

38 Stewart LA, Clarke MJ. Practical methodology of meta-analyses (overviews) using updated individual patient data. *Stat Med* 1995; **14:** 2057–79.

39 Altman DG. *Practical Statistics for Medical Research.* London: Chapman and Hall, 1991.

40 Phillips AN, Davey Smith G. The design of prospective epidemiological studies: more subjects or better measurements? *J Clin Epidemiol* 1993; **46:** 1203–11.

41 Higgins JPT, Whitehead A, Turner RM, et al. Meta-analysis of continuous outcome data from individual patients. *Stat Med* 2001; **20:** 2219–41.

42 Thompson SG, Turner RM, Warn DE. Multilevel models for meta-analysis, and their application to absolute risk differences. *Stat Meth Med Res* 2001; **10:** 375–92.

43 Di Castelnuovo A, de Gaetano G, Donati MB, Iacoviello L. Platelet glycoprotein IIb/IIIa polymorphism and coronary artery disease: implications for practice. *Am J Pharmacogenet* 2005; **5:** 93–99.

44 Michelson AD, Furman MI, Goldschmidt-Clermont P, et al. Platelet GP IIIa Pl(A) polymorphisms display different sensitivities to agonists. *Circulation* 2000; **101:** 1013–18.

45 Meisel C, Lopez JA, Stangl K. Role of platelet glycoprotein polymorphisms in cardiovascular diseases. *Naunyn Schmiedebergs Arch Pharmacol* 2004; **369:** 38–54.

46 Wheeler GL, Braden GA, Bray PF, et al. Reduced inhibition by abciximab in platelets with the PlA2 polymorphism. *Am Heart J* 2002; **143:** 76–82.

47 Weber AA, Jacobs C, Meila D, et al. No evidence for an influence of the human platelet antigen-1 polymorphism on the antiplatelet effects of glycoprotein IIb/IIIa inhibitors. *Pharmacogenetics* 2002; **12:** 581–83.

48 National Institute for Health and Clinical Excellence. *Guide to the Methods of Technology Appraisal.* London: NICE, 2004.

49 Antiplatelet Trialists' Collaboration. Collaborative meta-analysis of randomised trials of antiplatelet therapy for prevention of death, myocardial infarction, and stroke in high risk patients. *BMJ* 2002; **324:** 71–86.

50 Fibrinolytic Therapy Trialists' Collaborative Group. Indications for fibrinolytic therapy in suspected acute myocardial infarction: collaborative overview of early mortality and major morbidity results from all randomised trials of more than 1000 patients. *Lancet* 1994; **343:** 311–22.

51 Rothwell PM, Warlow CP. Prediction of benefit from carotid endarterectomy in individual patients: a risk-modelling study. *Lancet* 1999; **353:** 2105–10.

52 Yusuf S, Zucker D, Peduzzi P, et al. Effect of coronary artery bypass graft surgery on survival: overview of 10-year results from randomised trials by the Coronary Artery Bypass Graft Surgery Trialists Collaboration. *Lancet* 1994; **344:** 563–70.

53 Bobbio M, Demichelis B, Giustetto G. Completeness of reporting trial results: effect on physicians' willingness to prescribe. *Lancet* 1994; **343:** 1209–11.

54 Thompson SG, Higgins JPT. Can meta-analysis help target interventions at individuals most likely to benefit? *Lancet* 2005; **365:** 341–46.

13

Use of risk models to predict the likely effects of treatment in individuals

Peter M. Rothwell

Introduction

Clinicians have a responsibility both to try to provide the most appropriate treatment for each individual patient and to use limited healthcare resources efficiently. Both these aims require that treatments be targeted at those individuals who are likely to benefit, and avoided in those with little chance of benefit or in whom the risks of treatment are too great. Many treatments, such as blood pressure lowering in uncontrolled hypertension, are indicated in the vast majority of patients. However, a targeted approach based on risk is useful for treatments with modest benefits (e.g. lipid lowering in primary prevention of vascular disease),[1] for costly treatments with moderate overall benefits (e.g. β-interferon in multiple sclerosis),[2] if the availability of treatment is limited (e.g. organ transplantation),[3] in developing countries with very limited healthcare budgets and, most importantly, for treatments which, although of overall benefit in large trials, are associated with a significant risk of harm.[4, 5] The crux of the problem is how to use data from large pragmatic randomised controlled trials (RCTs), which, as discussed in Chapter 1 provide the most reliable estimates of the overall average effects of treatment, to determine the likely effect of treatment in an individual. This chapter illustrates the use of risk models and scores to predict the likely effects of treatment in individuals, and the next chapter considers some of the technical and practical issues related to their derivation and validation.

Individual variation in absolute risk

As discussed in previous chapters, when considering the potential benefit of an intervention in an individual patient it is essential to consider the absolute risk reduction (ARR) with treatment in the relevant RCT or the number needed to treat (NNT) to prevent an adverse event. An ARR tells us what chance an individual has of benefiting from treatment (i.e. an ARR of 25% indicates that there is a one in four chance of benefit; NNT = 4). Differences in the likelihood of benefit from an intervention between individuals are also therefore best expressed in terms of their likely absolute benefits. For treatments that do not have a clinically significant complication rate themselves, the likely absolute benefit for an individual will often be directly proportional to their absolute risk of a poor outcome without treatment, which is often termed the 'baseline risk'. Even when treatments do have a risk of harm as well as benefit, individual baseline risk without treatment is usually still correlated fairly closely with the absolute benefit from treatment, even if it does also correlate to some extent with the risk of complications of treatment. For most interventions, therefore, the ability reliably to predict the likelihood of benefit in an individual will depend on the extent to which outcome without treatment varies between individuals and the extent to which that outcome can be predicted in an individual. Differences in baseline risk will not, of course, be helpful in conditions in which outcome without treatment is uniformly poor, such as, for example, in a highly aggressive form of cancer. In this situation, there may well be biological reasons why a particular treatment might be more beneficial in some patients than others, but consideration of baseline risk will not usually be helpful.

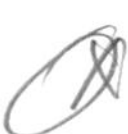

In many conditions, however, there are marked differences in outcome between individuals, and hence the potential to identify predictors of baseline risk. For example, patients with transient ischaemic attacks (TIAs) are at relatively high risk of stroke over the next few days and weeks, but 95% of patients referred to hospital with a diagnosis of possible TIA will not have an early recurrent stroke.[6] Thus, any aggressive inpatient investigation and treatment to prevent stroke could be highly beneficial in a high-risk minority, but would be unlikely to be cost-effective in patients with a stroke risk of less than 1%, for example. The potential for targeting treatment in this way depends, therefore, on the extent to which it is possible to predict the risk of stroke in individuals.

In the TIA example, we do in fact have some simple but powerful risk scores.[7,8] Table 13.1 shows a multivariate model for the risk of stroke during the 7 days after a TIA, which contains some very powerfully predictive risk factors. Table 13.2 shows the observed 7-day risk of stroke in a cohort of patients referred with possible TIA, stratified according to a simple risk score derived from the variables in table 13.1.[8] In individuals with an ABCD score of less than 4, absolute benefit from acute intervention would be very small (accepting that the observed stroke risk of 0% was an underestimate of the likely true risk). In patients with higher scores, however, the absolute benefit of an effective intervention could be substantial. About one in three patients with an ABCD score of six will have a stroke during the 7 days after the TIA. A treatment that reduced this risk by 50% in relative terms would, therefore, have an NNT of about 6 in this

Risk factor	HR (95% CI)	*p*
Age ≥ 60 years	2.57 (0.75 to 8.81)	0.133
Systolic BP > 140 mmHg or diastolic BP ≥ 90 mmHg	9.67 (2.23 to 41.94)	0.002
Clinical features		
Unilateral weakness	6.61 (1.53 to 28.50)	
Speech disturbance without weakness	2.59 (0.50 to 13.56)	
Other	1	0.016
Duration of symptoms		
≥ 60 minutes	6.17 (1.43–26.62)	
10–59 minutes	3.08 (0.64–14.77)	
< 10 minutes	1	0.019
Diabetes	4.39 (1.36–14.22)	0.014

BP, blood pressure; HR, hazard ratio. *Data from the Oxford Community Stroke Project and the Oxford Vascular Study.[8]

Table** **13.1: Multivariate regression analysis of predictors of the 7-day risk of stroke in patients with probable or definite TIA derived from the pooled data (stratified by study)*

group, compared with an NNT of around 200 in patients with an ABCD score of less than 4 (if we assume that the stroke risk in this group might be as high as 1% in reality). These figures do not, of course, represent a reliable prediction of benefit or otherwise for every *individual* – we are still talking in terms of *groups* – but they represent a substantial step in that direction when compared with the average NNT of around 40 in the population in table 13.2 as a whole.

The example of carotid endarterectomy

Consideration of individual outcomes is more complicated for treatments that have associated risks as well as benefits, such as surgical interventions like carotid endarterectomy. For an individual there are only two possible outcomes (stroke or no stroke), but surgery can have four possible effects:

- harm (i.e. an operative stroke in a patient who would not otherwise have had a stroke)
- benefit (i.e. prevention of a stroke that would have occurred if the patient had not had surgery)
- no stroke but no benefit (i.e. the patient did not have a stroke but would not have had a stroke without surgery anyway)
- stroke but no harm (i.e. the patient had a stroke but would also have had a stroke without surgery).

Figure 13.1 shows the relative risks of stroke with endarterectomy for patients with 50–69% stenosis and 70–99% stenosis, as well as the distribution of individuals across these four different outcomes. The difficulty for clinicians is that only a relatively small proportion of individuals benefit from surgery because the majority of patients are destined to remain stroke-free without surgery. Most patients face the anxiety and discomfort of surgery without any potential for benefit, and a significant proportion are harmed

ABCD score	No. (%) of patients	All strokes		Excludes strokes prior to seeking medical attention	
		Events (%)	% Risk (95% CI)	Events (%)	% Risk (95% CI)
≤1	28 (7)	0 (0)	0	0 (0)	0
2	74 (20)	0 (0)	0	0 (0)	0
3	82 (22)	0 (0)	0	0 (0)	0
4	90 (24)	1 (5)	1.1 (0 to 3.3)	0 (0)	0
5	66 (18)	8 (40)	12.1 (4.2 to 20.0)	5 (33)	7.6 (1.2 to 14.0)
6	35 (9)	11 (55)	31.4 (16.0 to 46.8)	10 (67)	28.6 (13.6 to 43.5)
Total	375 (100)	20 (100)	5.3 (3.0 to 7.5)	15 (100)	4.0 (2.0 to 6.0)

***Table** 13.2:* **The 7-day risk of stroke stratified according to the ABCD score at first assessment in all referrals with suspected transient ischaemic attack in the Oxford Vascular Study[8]**

13 Use of risk models to predict the likely effects of treatment

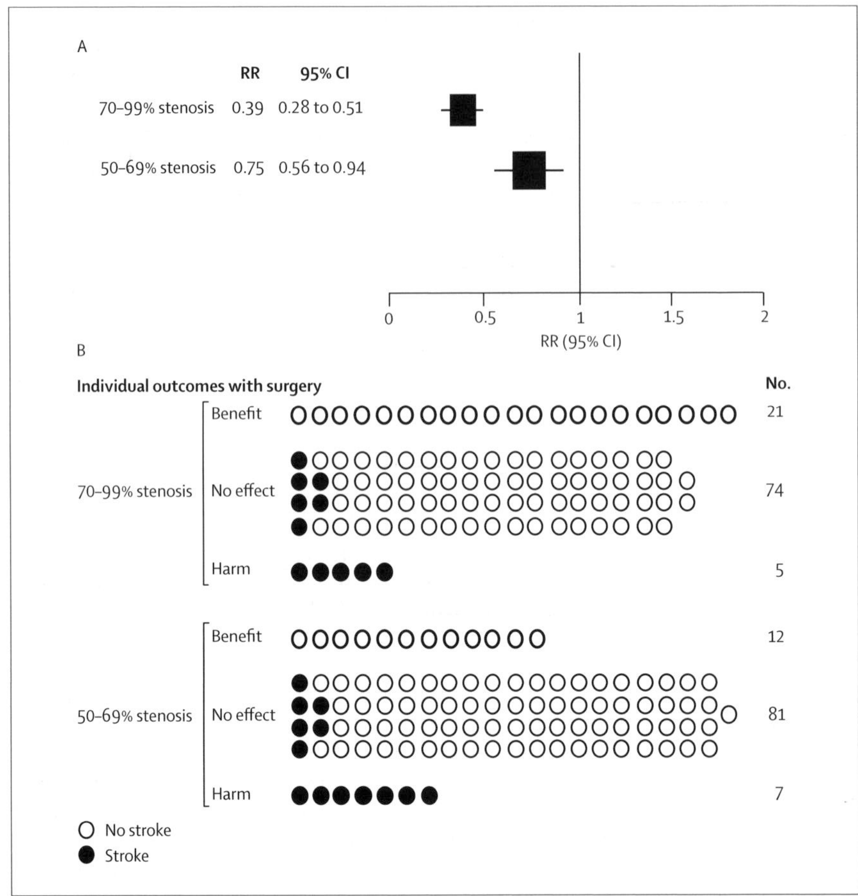

Figure 13.1: The effect of carotid endarterectomy for ≥ 70% and 50–69% symptomatic stenosis on the 5-year risk of stroke and operative death in RCTs of endarterectomy versus medical treatment alone.[7] (A) The relative risk reductions shown in standard format. (B) The effect of endarterectomy on individual patients: the actual outcomes after endarterectomy in 100 individuals with 70–99% stenosis and 100 individuals with 50–69% stenosis. There are four possible outcomes. Some patients are harmed by surgery (i.e. they had an operative stroke but would not have had a stroke if they had not been operated on). Only a relatively small proportion of patients actually benefit from surgery (i.e. they would have had a stroke but it was prevented by surgery). The vast majority of patients do not benefit, but are not harmed. Either they had a stroke but would have had one without surgery anyway, or they did not have a stroke but would not have had a stroke without surgery. The calculation of outcomes is based on the first stroke during follow-up, and assumes that the risk of stroke on medical treatment and the operative risk with surgical treatment are independent, and that strokes which occur after the postoperative period would have occurred had the patient not had surgery.

Absolute risk reduction = $N_{benefit} - N_{harm}$

Relative risk = $(N_{no\text{-}effect\ strokes} + N_{harm})/(N_{no\text{-}effect\ strokes} + N_{benefit})$

(Reprinted from Rothwell et al.,[43] copyright 2005, with permission from Elsevier.)

as a consequence of the 5–7% operative risk of stroke. Evidence-based guidelines recommend operating on all patients similar to those in the trials, but clinicians understandably want to operate on only the small subset of patients who will benefit.

Absolute risk reductions in subgroups can be useful in predicting the likely effect of treatment on individuals, but analyses are usually performed only in relation to a single baseline variable and are of limited use if there are several clinical characteristics that are likely to have important effects on the risks or benefits of treatment. Absolute risk reductions for patients with multiple specific characteristics cannot be derived from separate univariate subgroup analyses, and, although multidimensional subgroup analyses are possible (see Chapter 11), as statistical power in RCTs is usually insufficient even for univariate subgroup analyses, reliable multifactorial subgroup analysis will rarely be possible in practice. Yet, benefit from endarterectomy for symptomatic carotid stenosis has been shown in univariate subgroup analyses to depend on age, sex, the type of presenting event, plaque surface morphology and the time since the last symptomatic event.[9] What then would be the likely benefit from surgery, for example, in a 78-year-old (increased benefit) woman (reduced benefit) with 80% stenosis who presented within 2 weeks (increased benefit) of an ocular ischaemic event (reduced benefit) and was found to have an ulcerated carotid plaque (increased benefit)? On the basis of the clinical characteristics of the patients in the RCTs of endarterectomy, in order to have an adequate sample of patients (say, 2000) with the same characteristics as this patient, a total trial population of about 200 000 would be required.

A more realistic approach is to abandon any attempt to consider the effect of treatment in subgroups based on particular characteristics, and to base decisions on the predicted absolute risks of a poor outcome with each treatment option in individual patients. It is usually suggested that the best way to determine the likely effect of treatment in an individual is simply to multiply the overall relative risk reduction from a relevant trial or systematic review by whatever absolute risk of a poor outcome it is estimated that the current patient faces without treatment[10–12] – as in the example of the hypothetical treatment to prevent stroke after TIA that was discussed above. However, problems arise when there is clinically important heterogeneity of relative treatment effect (see Chapter 9), particularly when the relative treatment effect itself depends on the absolute risk of a poor outcome in the control group,[4, 13–23] such that the two variables cannot simply be multiplied as if they were independent. Moreover, without formal risk models, clinicians are often inaccurate in assessing risk in their patients,[24] and there is frequently a lack of high-quality and up-to-date natural history data on which to base estimates.[25]

A better approach is to use risk models to predict the absolute risks of a poor outcome with each treatment option in individual patients.[4, 26] Validated prognostic models are available for many medical conditions (although not nearly enough),[27, 28] and there are several for prediction of individual risk of coronary heart disease and stroke,[1, 4, 19, 23, 28–37] especially in primary prevention (see Chapter 16).[35–37] Although trial populations do, on average, have a lower absolute risk of a poor outcome than patients in routine clinical practice, they do usually contain some high-risk patients,[38] and do therefore allow determination of the effect of treatment in individuals with a reasonable range of baseline risk. The usefulness of this approach in exploring the relationship between the effects of treatment in RCTs and the baseline absolute risk of a poor outcome in trials in vascular medicine is illustrated by the demonstration of qualitative heterogeneity of relative treatment effect in relation to baseline risk for carotid endarterectomy for symptomatic stenosis,[4] anticoagulation in primary prevention of stroke in patients with non-valvular atrial fibrillation,[13] coronary artery bypass grafting[14] and antiarrhythmic drugs following myocardial infarction.[23] Clinically important heterogeneity of relative treatment effect by baseline risk has also been demonstrated for blood pressure lowering,[15] aspirin,[16] and lipid lowering[17] in primary prevention, for benefit from treatment with clopidogrel[18] and with enoxaparin[19, 20] in patients with acute coronary syndromes, and in many other areas of medicine and surgery.[21, 22] Weightings based on patient preferences for different outcomes can be built in,[39–41] and modelling also allows the interactions between the effects of different characteristics to be determined and incorporated.

Predicting benefit from carotid endarterectomy

The potential usefulness of a risk modelling approach is illustrated below with the example of carotid endarterectomy for recently symptomatic carotid stenosis. There are several validated models to predict stroke risk in different situations,[29, 31, 32, 42] but these models were derived in populations with a low prevalence of carotid disease and did not include the degree of carotid stenosis. Given the importance of the latter in determining the risk of stroke on medical treatment in patients with recently symptomatic carotid disease,[5] models are required for use in this specific clinical situation. One such model was derived from the patients randomised in the European Carotid Surgery Trial (ECST).[4]

The ECST risk model could not at first be validated on data from another similar trial because of differences in the method of measurement of the degree of carotid stenosis

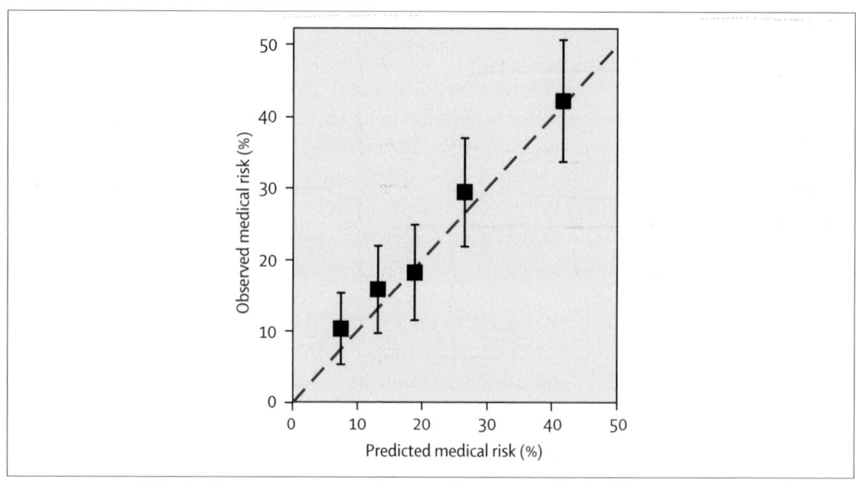

***Figure* 13.2: Reliability of the ECST prognostic model (see table 13.3) for the 5-year risk of stroke on medical treatment in patients with 50–99% stenosis in the NASCET.[43] Observed medical risk is plotted against predicted medical risk by quintile groups of predicted risk. Error bars represent 95% CIs.**

and in the definition of outcome events.[7] However, after re-measurement of the degree of stenosis on the pre-randomisation angiograms and revision of the definition of outcome events, the ECST data were made consistent with data from the North American Symptomatic Carotid Endarterectomy Trial (NASCET),[5] and the ECST model was re-derived (table 13.3).[43] The potential usefulness of the model is illustrated in figure 13.2, which shows the risk of stroke on medical treatment in patients with 50–99% symptomatic carotid stenosis who were randomised to medical treatment in NASCET stratified into quintiles of predicted risk according to the ECST model.[43] There was close agreement between predicted and observed medical risk ($\chi^2_{Heterogeneity} = 43.1$, df = 4, $p < 0.0001$). The model was not able to identify patients with 0% risk or 100% risk as would be required in order to be certain of the effect of treatment, but it did reliably distinguish between quintiles with 10% and nearly 50% risks of ipsilateral ischaemic stroke after 5 years of follow-up. The likelihood of benefit from endarterectomy, which has a 7% operative risk of stroke and death followed by a residual stroke risk of about 1% per year,[5] is clearly very different in these two groups of individuals.

To assess the usefulness of risk models in targeting treatment it is necessary to use the model to stratify the effect of treatment in RCTs by the predicted risk of a poor outcome in individuals. Clinically important heterogeneity of both relative and absolute treatment effect has been demonstrated for many interventions in vascular medicine in this way.[4, 13–23] Figure 13.3 shows the effect of endarterectomy in NASCET in patients with 50–69% and ≥70% stenosis stratified into quintiles of predicted risk of stroke on medical treatment with the ECST model. Benefit from surgery was restricted to the highest quintile of medical risk in patients with 50–69% stenosis and to the three highest quintiles in patients with 70–99% stenosis. Heterogeneity in absolute risk reduction

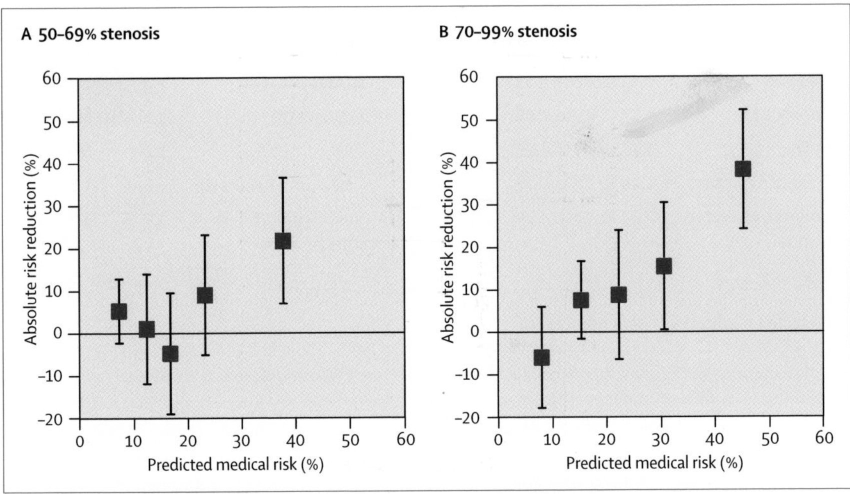

Figure 13.3: **The effect of surgery measured by absolute risk reduction in patients with (A) 50–69% stenosis and (B) 70–99% stenosis in the NASCET by quintile groups of predicted risk based on the ECST prognostic model (see table 13.3).[43] Error bars represent 95% CIs.**

Model			**Scoring system**		
Risk factor	HR (95% CI)	*p*	Risk factor	Score	Example
Stenosis (per 10%)	1.18 (1.10 to 1.25)	< 0.0001	Stenosis (%)		
			50–59	2.4	2.4
			60–69	2.8	
			70–79	3.3	
			80–89	3.9	
			90–99	4.6	
Near occlusion	0.49 (0.19 to 1.24)	0.1309	Near occlusion	0.5	No
Male sex	1.19 (0.81 to 1.75)	0.3687	Male sex	1.2	No
Age (per 10 years)	1.12 (0.89 to 1.39)	0.3343	Age (years)		
			31–40	1.1	
			41–50	1.2	
			51–60	1.3	
			61–70	1.5	1.5
			71–80	1.6	
			81–90	1.8	
Time since last event (per 7 days)			Time since last event (days)		
	0.96 (0.93 to 0.99)	0.0039	0–13	8.7	8.7
			14–28	8.0	
			29–89	6.3	
			90–365	2.3	
Presenting event		0.0067	**Presenting event**		
Ocular	1.000		Ocular	1.0	
Single TIA	1.41 (0.75 to 2.66)		Single TIA	1.4	
Multiple TIAs	2.05 (1.16 to 3.60)		Multiple TIAs	2.0	
Minor stroke	1.82 (0.99 to 3.34)		Minor stroke	1.8	
Major stroke	2.54 (1.48 to 4.35)		Major stroke	2.5	2.5
Diabetes	1.35 (0.86 to 2.11)	0.1881	Diabetes	1.4	1.4
Previous MI	1.57 (1.01 to 2.45)	0.0471	Previous MI	1.6	No
PVD	1.18 (0.78 to 1.77)	0.4368	PVD	1.2	No
Treated hypertension	1.24 (0.88 to 1.75)	0.2137	Treated hypertension	1.2	1.2
Irregular/ulcerated plaque	2.03 (1.31 to 3.14)	0.0015	Irregular/ulcerated plaque	2.0	2.0
Total risk score				263	
Predicted medical risk using nomogram					37

CI, confidence interval; HR, hazard ratio; MI, myocardial infarction; PVD, peripheral vascular disease; TIA, transient ischaemic attack. *The model differs slightly from one previously published[4] in that the degree of stenosis and the definition of the outcome event are based on those used in the NASCET trial.[5] Hazard ratios derived from the model are used for the scoring system. The score for the 5-year risk of stroke is the product of the individual scores for each of the risk factors present. The score is converted into a risk, as shown by the example in figure 13.4.

Table* 13.3: A Cox model for the 5-year risk of ipsilateral ischaemic stroke on medical treatment in patients with recently symptomatic carotid stenosis derived from the ECST

across the quintile groups was highly significant ($p = 0.001$). This stratification of trial data using an independently derived model is essential, even if the model has been validated previously in non-trial cohorts, because although trials tend to recruit relatively low-risk individuals, the distribution of risks in patients who are considered for treatment in clinical practice may well also be different from that in the non-trial observational cohorts used for derivation and validation of the model. Clinicians will also need to be convinced that use of a risk modelling approach does produce clinically useful heterogeneity of treatment effect.

For most treatments, in which the risk of harm from the treatment itself is very much lower than the risk of a poor outcome without treatment, it is only necessary to model the risk of a poor outcome without treatment. However, for treatments that have a significant risk of harm, the risk of a poor outcome with treatment should be considered separately because its determinants may be different.[4, 9] For carotid endarterectomy, for example, female sex is associated with a low risk of stroke on medical treatment but a higher operative risk of stroke and death,[9, 44] whereas increasing age and a very recent symptomatic ischaemic event are associated with a high risk of stroke on medical treatment but not with an increased operative risk.[9, 30, 44, 45] A modelling process that provides estimates of the likely individual risks with both treatment options is therefore required.[4] Figures 13.2 and 13.3 show that risk modelling is a useful approach to targeting carotid endarterectomy, but a more sophisticated model that includes interactions (e.g. between sex and the effect of the timing of surgery) and also takes into account predicted individual operative risk might be more effective.

Making the results of risk models accessible to busy clinicians

Prediction of risk using models requires a computer, a pocket calculator with an exponential function, or internet access to use the model online.[46] As an alternative when access to computing facilities or the internet is not possible, a simplified risk score based on the hazard ratios derived from the relevant risk model can be helpful.[47, 48] For example, table 13.3 also shows a score for the 5-year risk of stroke on medical treatment in patients with recently symptomatic carotid stenosis derived from the ECST model. Clinicians calculate the total risk score as the product of scores for each risk factor. Figure 13.4 shows a plot of the total risk score against the 5-year predicted risk of ipsilateral carotid territory ischaemic stroke derived from the full model, and is used as a nomogram for the conversion of the score into a prediction of the percentage risk. An example of the use of the risk score is also shown in table 13.3.

An alternative approach to provide clinicians with a tool to target treatment that has been used widely in the primary prevention of vascular disease is the derivation of risk tables, which are often colour coded.[1, 49–51] This approach is best suited to situations in which there are a relatively small number of important variables to consider and has the major advantage that it does not require the calculation of any score by the clinician or patient. Figure 13.5 shows a risk table indicating the 5-year risk of ipsilateral ischaemic stroke in patients with recently symptomatic carotid stenosis on medical treatment. To limit the number of separate tables necessary, only the five variables that were both significant predictors of risk in the ECST model (see table 13.3) and yielded

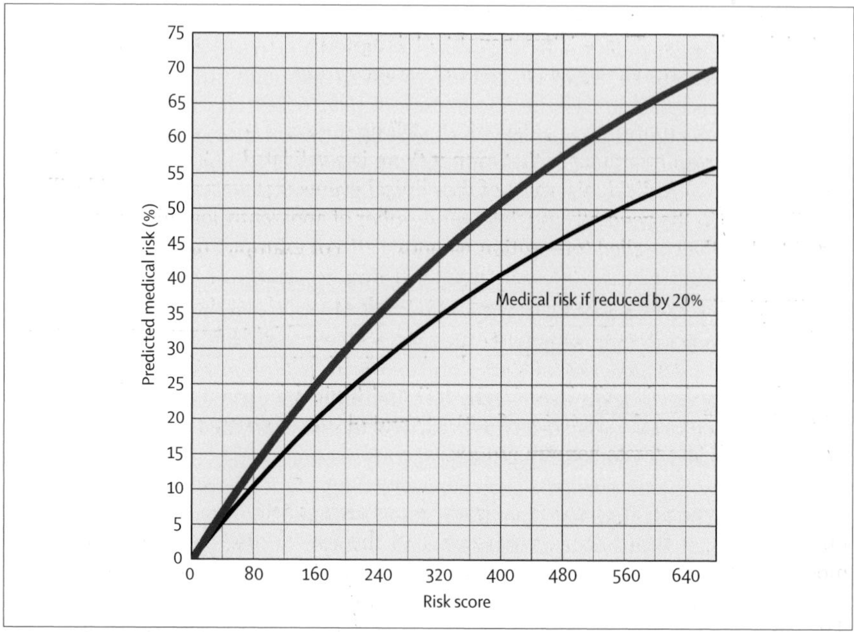

Figure 13.4: A plot of the total risk score derived from table 13.3 against the 5-year predicted risk of ipsilateral carotid territory ischaemic stroke derived from the full model in the table in patients in the ECST (green line).[43] This should be used as a nomogram for the conversion of the score into a prediction of the percentage risk. The black line represents a 20% reduction in risk as might be seen with more intensive medical treatment than was available in the ECST in the late 1980s and 1990s. (Reprinted from Rothwell et al.,[43] copyright 2005, with permission from Elsevier.)

clinically important univariate subgroup treatment effect interactions in the analysis of pooled data from the relevant trials[9] are included: sex, age, time since last symptomatic event, type of presenting event(s) and carotid plaque surface morphology (each categorised as in the previous subgroup analysis).[9]

Problems with using individual risk to target treatment

The use of risk models to target treatment is not without problems. Models tend to overpredict (i.e. to label high-risk patients as higher risk, and low-risk patients as lower risk, than they really are), and it is therefore essential that they are externally validated and adjusted if there is overprediction (see Chapter 14). Models rarely perform as well on independent populations as in the derivation population, and are usually less effective when validated by groups other than those who derived the model.[52, 53] Nevertheless, as shown in figures 13.2 and 13.3, they can still be clinically useful. There are also problems with rigid risk cut-off points below which treatment should not be given, which are usually based on relatively short follow-up periods. In primary prevention of vascular disease, for example, it does not necessarily make long-term sense to withhold treatment from young low-risk patients and only commence treatment when they have reached an age and an absolute risk that mean that they have already developed serious underlying disease. The relative benefit of long-term early treatment may well be greater than in short-term trials done in older age groups.

One of the main arguments against risk modelling to select individual patients with the most to gain from treatment is that even if there is a validated risk score that is able to identify high-risk individuals, most of the clinical events that we want to avoid will still usually occur in the generally much larger number of apparently low and moderate risk individuals – the so-called 'prevention paradox'.[54, 55] For example, figure 13.6 shows the results of RCTs of three antithrombotic treatments for acute coronary syndromes[18–20] stratified by the independently derived TIMI risk score.[19] In all three trials, the intervention was of no benefit in low-risk patients but was highly beneficial in high-risk cases. However, the figure also shows that in each trial the proportion of patients with low risk scores (no benefit from treatment) and high risk scores (major benefit) was relatively small, and the majority of patients and of events prevented were in the large moderate risk (moderate benefit) groups.

However, the prevention paradox is by no means an inevitable result of the risk modelling approach; it is simply a consequence of the use of relatively poorly predictive models. Admittedly, risk models are sometimes poorly predictive, either because the outcome has few known risk factors or, more commonly, because there are insufficient data from high-quality cohort studies with which to derive and validate models. The more powerfully predictive risk scores for patients with TIA (see tables 13.1 and 13.2) and patients with symptomatic carotid stenosis (see table 13.3 and figures 13.2 and 13.3) illustrate the potential of the risk-based approach to allow clinicians to target interventions such that as many adverse outcomes are prevented by treating a subset of patients as by treating all patients. The prevention paradox is unlikely to be a problem for the ABCD score, for example, given that 55% of stroke outcomes occurred in the 9% of patients with the highest risk score, or that 95% of outcomes occurred in the 27% of patients with a score of 5 or more (see table 13.2).

Finally, if effective new treatments are introduced, models derived in the past may overestimate current risks. For example, the ECST medical risk model was derived from data that were collected before the use of statins was widespread. However, such improvements in treatment pose more problems for interpretation of the overall trial results than for the risk modelling approach. For example, it would take only a relatively modest improvement in the effectiveness of medical treatment to erode the overall benefit of endarterectomy in patients with 50–69% stenosis in figure 13.1. In contrast, very major improvements in medical treatment would be required in order significantly to reduce the benefit from surgery in patients in the high predicted risk quintile in figure 13.2. Thus, the likelihood that ancillary treatments have improved, and are likely to continue to improve, is an argument in favour of a risk-based approach to targeting treatment. It would be reasonable in a patient on treatment with a statin, for example, to reduce the risks derived from the risk models in table 13.1 by 20% in relative terms in order to account for the likely benefit of that treatment. The same approach can be used to account for any reductions in the risks of treatment in models such as that shown in figure 13.5. The operative risk of stroke and death due to endarter-

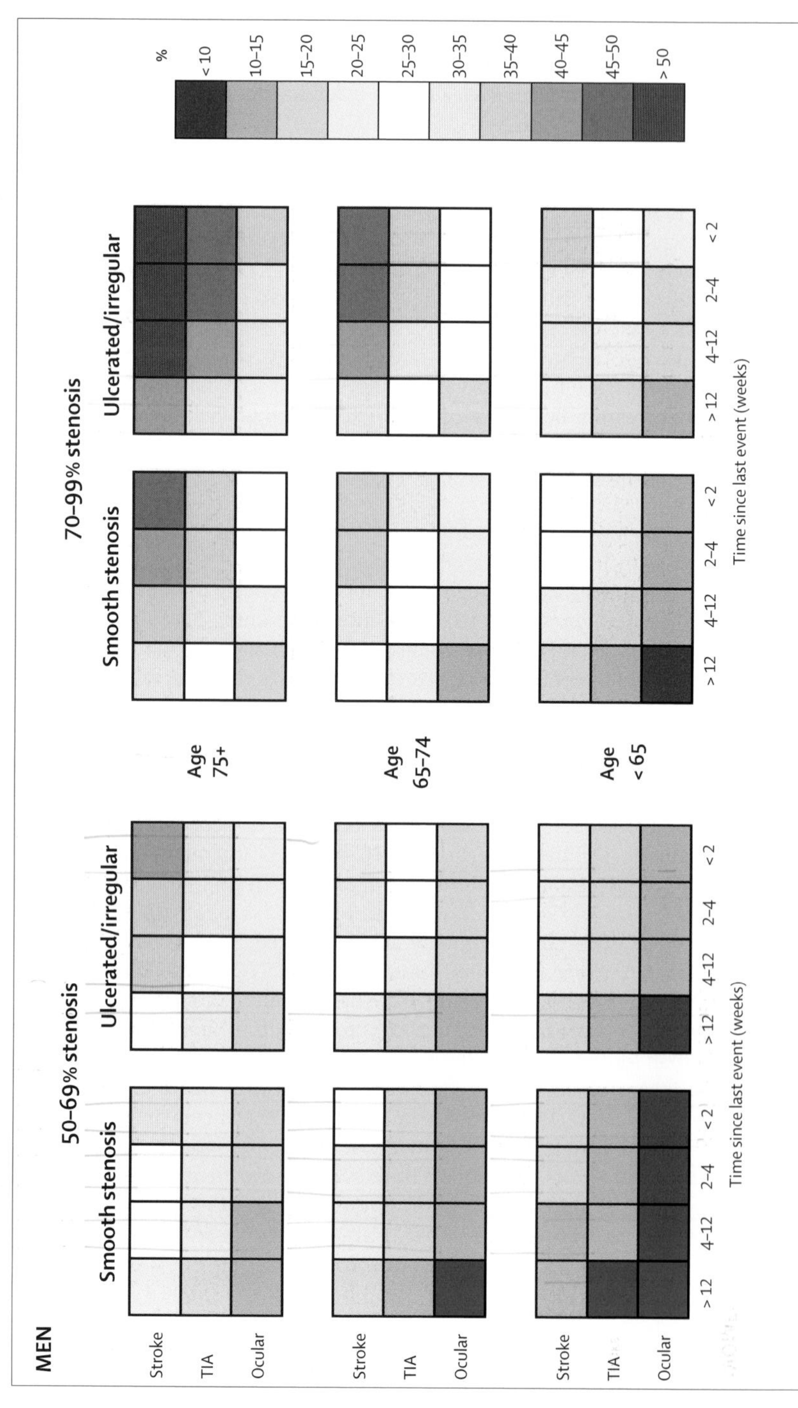

MEN
50–69% stenosis
70–99% stenosis
Smooth stenosis
Ulcerated/irregular
Smooth stenosis
Ulcerated/irregular
Stroke
TIA
Ocular
Age
75+
Age
65–74
Age
< 65
> 12
4–12
2–4
< 2
Time since last event (weeks)
%
< 10
10–15
15–20
20–25
25–30
30–35
35–40
40–45
45–50
> 50

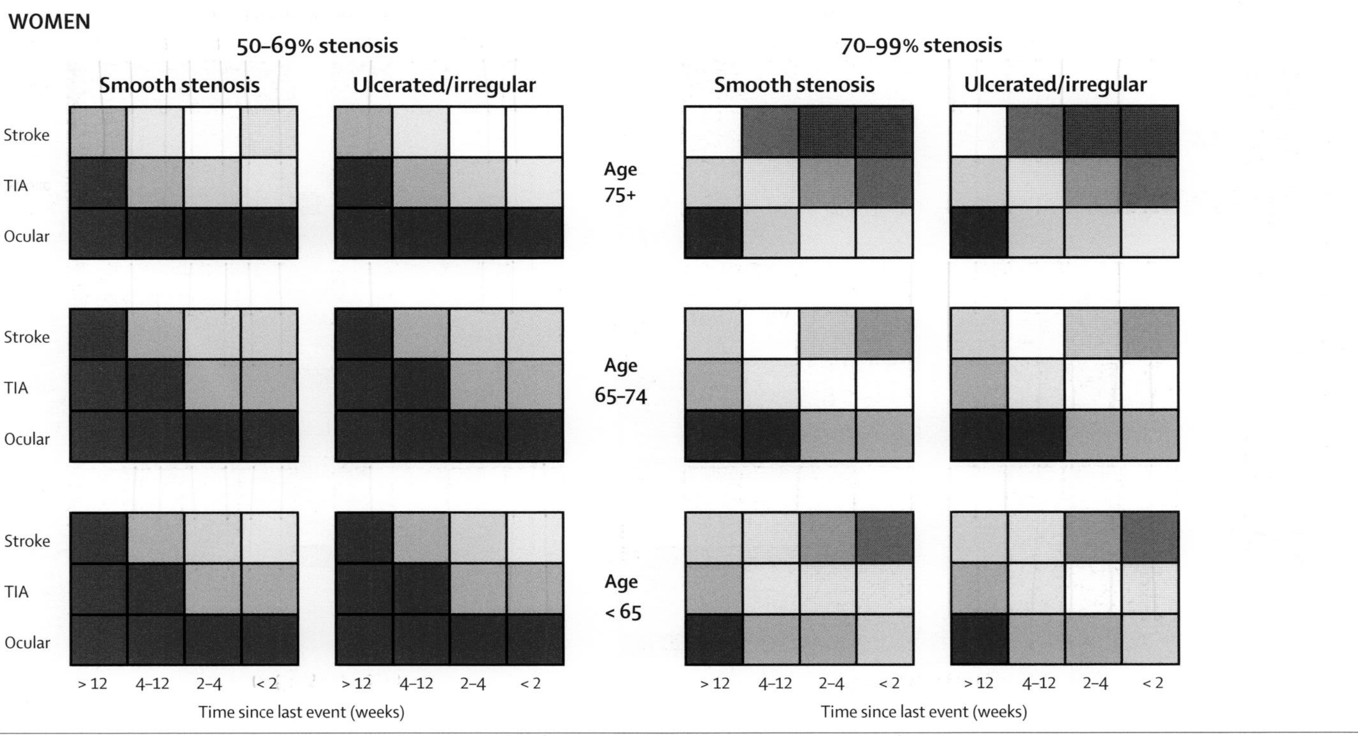

Figure 13.5: **A table of the predicted absolute risk of ipsilateral ischaemic stroke on medical treatment in ECST patients with recently symptomatic carotid stenosis derived from a Cox model and based on six clinically important patient characteristics.[43] (Reprinted from Rothwell et al.,[43] copyright 2005, with permission from Elsevier.)**

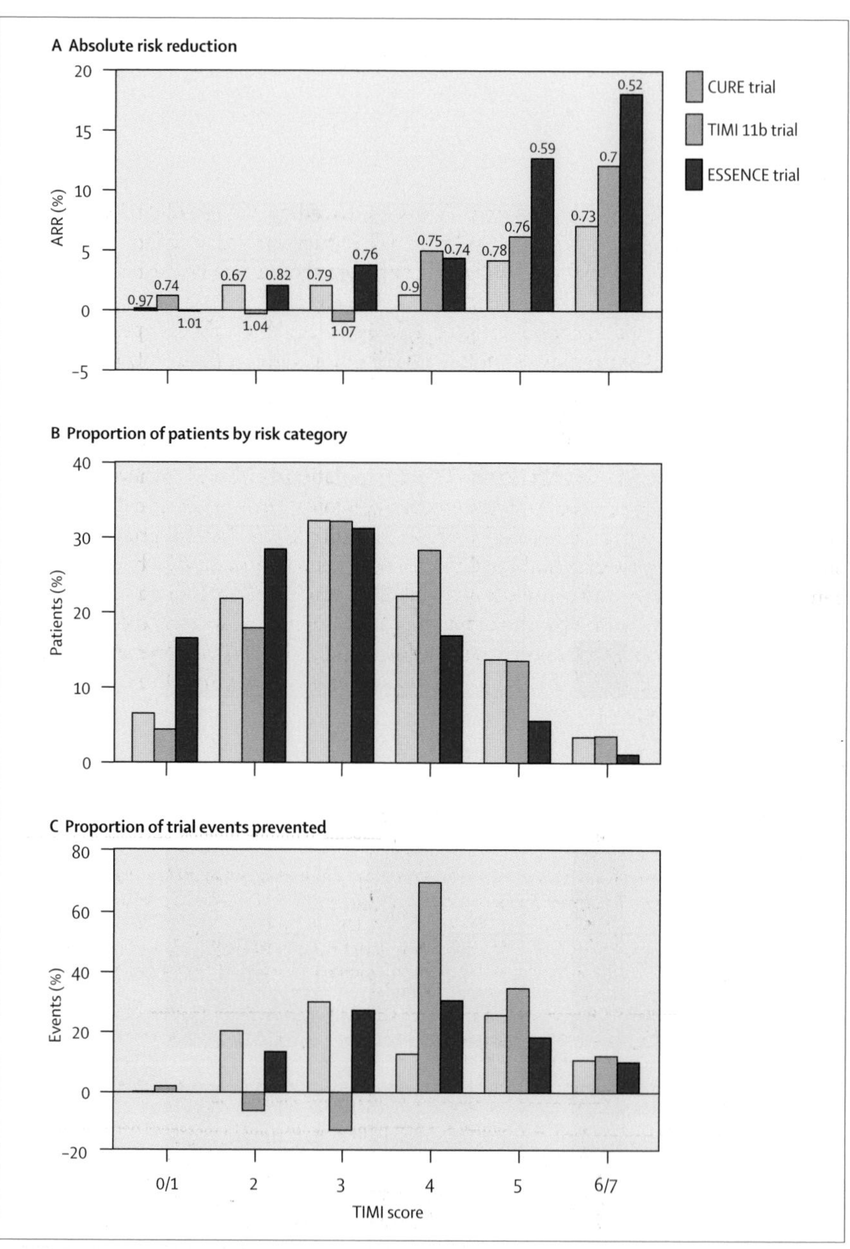

Figure 13.6: **The results of three RCTs of treatments for acute coronary syndromes[18-20] stratified by the independently derived TIMI risk score.[19] For each trial, the absolute risk reduction with treatment (A), the proportion of patients (B) and the proportion of events prevented (C) are shown in each risk category.[43] (A) The numbers given above the bars are the relative risks. (Reprinted from Rothwell et al.,[43] copyright 2005, with permission from Elsevier.)**

ectomy was 7% in the large trials,[9] and does not appear to have fallen since, at least in published series,[56] but may also be reduced in future or be less for carotid angioplasty with cerebral protection.[57]

Conclusions

Clinicians must often make treatment decisions based on the absolute likelihood of benefit for individual patients. Since relative risk reductions are uninformative in this regard, overall results of trials and subgroup analyses should also be expressed as absolute risk reductions. Where there are multiple clinically important subgroup–treatment effect interactions, multifactorial subgroup analysis could, in theory, provide useful information, but very large trials or meta-analyses of individual patient data from several trials are required. Alternatively, and particularly for clinical conditions or interventions where benefit is likely to be highly dependent on the absolute risk of adverse outcomes with and/or without treatment, the effect of baseline risk on benefit from treatment should be determined by stratification of trial populations with independently derived and validated prognostic models. Risk modelling avoids some of the problems of subgroup analysis, including chance findings due to multiple post hoc subgroup comparisons, and is a more powerful tool for differentiating between patients who are likely to benefit from treatment and those who are not. Risk models allow clinicians to take into account the multiple particular characteristics of an individual patient and their interactions in a logical and systematic manner, to consider the risks and benefits of interventions separately if required, and to provide patients with personalised estimates of their likelihood of benefit.

References

1 Haq IU, Jackson PR, Yeo WW, Ramsay LE. Sheffield risk and treatment table for cholesterol lowering for primary prevention of coronary heart disease. *Lancet* 1995; **346:** 1467–71.

2 Filippini G, Munari L, Incorvaia B, et al. Interferons in relapsing remitting multiple sclerosis: a systematic review. *Lancet* 2003; **361:** 545–52.

3 Morris PJ, Johnson RJ, Fuggle SV, et al., on behalf of the HLA Task Force of the Kidney Advisory Group of the United Kingdom Transplant Support Service Authority (UKTSSA). Analysis of factors that affect outcome of primary cadaveric renal transplantation in the UK. *Lancet* 1999; **354:** 1147–52.

4 Rothwell PM, Warlow CP, on behalf of the European Carotid Surgery Trialists' Collaborative Group. Prediction of benefit from carotid endarterectomy in individual patients: a risk modeling study. *Lancet* 1999; **353:** 2105–10.

5 Rothwell PM, Gutnikov SA, Eliasziw M, et al., for the Carotid Endarterectomy Trialists' Collaboration. Pooled analysis of individual patient data from randomised controlled trials of endarterectomy for symptomatic carotid stenosis. *Lancet* 2003; **361:** 107–16.

6 Coull A, Lovett JK, Rothwell PM, on behalf of the Oxford Vascular Study. Early risk of stroke after a TIA or minor stroke in a population-based incidence study. *BMJ* 2004; **328:** 326–28.

7 Johnston SC, Gress DR, Browner WS, Sidney S. Short-term prognosis after emergency department diagnosis of TIA. *JAMA* 2000; **284:** 2901–06.

8 Rothwell PM, Giles MF, Flossmann E, et al. A simple score (ABCD) to identify individuals at high early risk of stroke after a transient ischaemic attack. *Lancet* 2005; **366:** 29–36.

9 Rothwell PM, Eliasziw M, Gutnikov SA, et al., for the Carotid Endarterectomy Trialists' Collaboration. Effect of endarterectomy for recently symptomatic carotid stenosis in relation to clinical subgroups and the timing of surgery. *Lancet* 2004; **363:** 915–24.

10 Sackett DL, Straus SE. Finding and applying evidence during clinical rounds: the 'evidence cart'. *JAMA* 1998; **280:** 1336–38.

11 Sackett DL. Applying overviews and meta-analyses at the bedside. *J Clin Epidemiol* 1995; **48:** 61–70.

12 Ellis J, Mulligan I, Rowe J, Sackett DL. Inpatient general medicine is evidence based. *Lancet* 1995; **346:** 407–10.

13 Laupacis A, Boysen G, Connolly S, et al. Risk factors for stroke and efficacy of antithrombotic therapy in atrial fibrillation. Analysis of pooled data from five randomised controlled trials. *Arch Intern Med* 1994; **154:** 1449–57.

14 Yusuf S, Zucker D, Peduzzi P, et al. Effect of coronary artery bypass graft surgery on survival: overview of 10-year results from randomised trials by the Coronary Artery Bypass Graft Surgery Trialists' Collaboration. *Lancet* 1994; **344:** 563–70.

15 Li W, Boissel JP, Girard P, et al. Identification and prediction of responders to a therapy: a model and its preliminary application to actual data. *J Epidemiol Biostat* 1998; **3:** 189–97.

16 Sanmuganathan PS, Ghahramani P, Jackson PR, et al. Aspirin for primary prevention of coronary heart disease: safety and absolute benefit related to coronary risk derived from meta-analysis of randomised trials. *Heart* 2001; **85:** 265–71.

17 West of Scotland Coronary Prevention Group. West of Scotland Coronary Prevention Study: identification of high-risk groups and comparison with other cardiovascular intervention trials. *Lancet* 1996; **348:** 1339–42.

18 Bundaj A, Yusuf S, Mehta SR, et al., for the Clopidogrel in Unstable Angina to Prevent Recurrent Events (CURE) Trial Investigators. Benefit of clopidogrel in patients with acute coronary syndromes without ST-segment elevation in various risk groups. *Circulation* 2002; **106:** 1622–26.

19 Antman EM, Cohen M, Bernink PJLM, et al. The TIMI risk score for unstable angina/non-ST elevation MI. A method for prognostication and therapeutic decision making. *JAMA* 2000; **284:** 835–42.

20 Cohen M, Demers C, Garfinkel EP, et al. A comparison of low molecular weight heparin with unfractionated heparin for unstable coronary artery disease. *N Engl J Med* 1997; **337:** 447–52.

21 Pagliaro L, D'Amico G, Soronson TIA, et al. Prevention of bleeding in cirrhosis. *Ann Intern Med* 1992; **117:** 59–70.

22 International Study of Unruptured Intracranial Aneurysms Investigators. Unruptured intracranial aneurysms – risks of rupture and risks of surgical intervention. *N Engl J Med* 1998; **339:** 1725–33.

23 Boissel JP, Collet JP, Lievre M, Girard P. An effect model for the assessment of drug benefit: example of antiarrhythmic drugs in postmyocardial infarction patients. *J Cardiovasc Pharmacol* 1993; **22:** 356–63.

24 Grover SA, Lowensteyn I, Esrey KL, et al. Do doctors accurately assess coronary risk in their patients? Preliminary results of the coronary health assessment study. *BMJ* 1995; **310:** 975–78.

25 Rothwell PM. Incidence, risk factors and prognosis of stroke and transient ischaemic attack: the need for high-quality large-scale epidemiological studies. *Cerebrovasc Dis* 2003; **16** (suppl 3): 2–10.

26 Rothwell PM. Can overall results of clinical trials be applied to all patients? *Lancet* 1995; **345:** 1616–19.

27 Braitman LE, Davidoff F. Predicting clinical states in individual patients. *Ann Intern Med* 1996; **125:** 406–12.

28 Nanchahal K, Duncan JR, Durrington PN, Jackson RT. Analysis of predicted coronary heart disease risk in England based on Framingham study risk appraisal models published in 1991 and 2000. *BMJ* 2002; **325:** 194–95.

29 Hankey GJ, Slattery JM, Warlow CP. Transient ischaemic attacks: which patients are at high (and low) risks of serious vascular events? *J Neurol Neurosurg Psychiatry* 1992; **55:** 640–52.

30 Rothwell PM, Slattery J, Warlow CP. A systematic review of clinical and angiographic predictors of stroke and death due to carotid endarterectomy. *BMJ* 1997; **315:** 1571–77.

31 Pearce LA, Hart RG, Halpern JL. Assessment of three schemes for stratifying stroke risk in patients with non-valvular atrial fibrillation. *Am J Med* 2000; **109:** 45–51.

32 Kernan WN, Viscoli CM, Brass LM, et al. The Stroke Prognosis Instrument II (SPI II): a clinical prediction instrument for patients with transient ischaemia and non-disabling ischaemic stroke. *Stroke* 2000; **31:** 456–62.

33 Lauer MS. Aspirin for primary prevention of coronary events. *N Engl J Med* 2002; **346:** 1468–74.

34 Baker S, Priest P, Jackson R. Using thresholds based on risk of cardiovascular disease to target treatment for hypertension: modelling events averted and number treated. *BMJ* 2000; **320:** 680–85.

35 Isles CG, Ritchie LD, Murchie P, Norrie J. Risk assessment in primary prevention of coronary heart disease: randomised comparison of three scoring methods. *BMJ* 2000; **320:** 690–91.

36 Montgomery AA, Fahey T, Peters TJ, et al. Evaluation of computer based clinical decision support system and risk chart for management of hypertension in primary care: randomised controlled trial. *BMJ* 2000; **320:** 686–90.

37 Robson J, Boomla K, Hart B, Feder G. Estimating cardiovascular risk for primary prevention: outstanding questions for primary care. *BMJ* 2000; **320:** 702–04.

38 Ionnidis JPA, Lau J. The impact of high-risk patients on the results of clinical trials. *J Clin Epidemiol* 1997; **50:** 1089–98.

39 Nadeau SE. The use of expected value as an aid to decisions regarding anticoagulation in patients with atrial fibrillation. *Stroke* 1993; **24:** 2128–34.

40 Elwyn G, Edwards A, Eccles M, Rovner D. Decision analysis in patient care. *Lancet* 2001; **358:** 571–74.

41 Thomson R, Parkin D, Eccles M, et al. Decision analysis and guidelines for anticoagulant therapy to prevent stroke in patients with atrial fibrillation. *Lancet* 2000; **355:** 956–62.

42 Laupacis A, Boysen G, Connolly S, et al. Risk factors for stroke and efficacy of antithrombotic therapy in atrial fibrillation. Analysis of pooled data from five randomised controlled trials. *Arch Intern Med* 1994; **154:** 1449–57.

43 Rothwell PM, Mehta Z, Howard SC, et al. From subgroups to individuals: general principles and the example of carotid endartectomy. *Lancet* 2005; **365:** 256–65.

44 Bond R, Rerkasem K, Cuffe R, Rothwell PM. A systematic review of the associations between age and sex and the operative risks of carotid endarterectomy. *Cerebrovasc Dis* 2005; **20:** 69–77.

45 Bond R, Rerkasem K, Rothwell PM. A systematic review of the risks of carotid endarterectomy in relation to the clinical indication and the timing of surgery. *Stroke* 2003; **34:** 2290–301.

46 ECST model available at: http://www.stroke.ox.ac.uk (accessed February 2007).

47 Pocock SJ, McCormack V, Gueyffier F, et al., on behalf of the INDANA Project Steering Committee. A score for predicting risk of death from cardiovascular disease in adults with raised blood pressure, based on individual patient data from randomised controlled trials. *BMJ* 2001; **323:** 75–81.

48 Leteurtre S, Martinot A, Duhamel A, et al. Validation of the paediatric logistic organ dysfunction (PELOD) score: prospective, observational, multicentre study. *Lancet* 2003; **362:** 192–97.

49 Jackson R. Updated New Zealand cardiovascular disease risk–benefit prediction guide. *BMJ* 2000; **320:** 709–10.

50 Ramsay LE, Haq IU, Jackson PR, et al. Targeting lipid-lowering drug therapy for primary prevention of coronary disease: an updated Sheffield table. *Lancet* 1996; **348:** 387–88.

51 Kanis JA. Diagnosis of osteoporosis and assessment of fracture risk. *Lancet* 2002; **359:** 1929–36.

52 Altman DG, Royston P. What do we mean by validating a prognostic model? *Stat Med* 2000; **19:** 453–73.

53 Rathore SS, Weinfurt KP, Gross CP, Krumholz HM. Validity of a simple ST-elevation acute myocardial infarction risk index: are randomised trial prognostic estimates generalizable to elderly patients? *Circulation* 2003; **107:** 811–16.

54 Rose G. Strategy of prevention: lessons from cardiovascular disease. *BMJ* 1981; **282:** 1847–51.

55 Rose G. Sick individuals and sick populations. *Int J Epidemiol* 1985; **14:** 32–38.

56 Bond R, Rerkasem K, Shearman CP, Rothwell PM. Time trends in the published risks of stroke and death due to endarterectomy for symptomatic carotid stenosis. *Cerebrovasc Dis* 2004; **18:** 37–46.

57 Kastrup A, Groschel K, Krapf H, et al. Early outcome of carotid angioplasty and stenting with and without cerebral protection devices: a systematic review of the literature. *Stroke* 2003; **34:** 813–19.

Evaluating the performance of prognostic models

Douglas G. Altman and Patrick Royston

Background

Even when a randomised trial shows a clear benefit of a new treatment, not all future patients meeting the trial's eligibility criteria will benefit. It is increasingly recognised that treatments need to be targeted at individuals. As reviewed in Chapter 13, a common approach is to base treatment decisions on each patient's predicted risk of the relevant clinical outcome, but this practice relies on good-quality information about that patient's prognosis. In general, there are several risk factors that are not independent. Prognostic models are widely used in medicine for predicting patient outcome in relation to multiple patient and disease characteristics. They are used in many medical fields, but their use is especially common in cancer and cardiovascular disease. In this chapter we consider how models are derived and issues in obtaining evidence that they are reliable, in the sense that they perform well in new patients.

The key characteristic of a prognostic model is the statistical combination of at least two separate variables to predict patient outcome. Models yielding prognostic indices or risk scores are also known as probability models,[1] risk stratification schemes or clinical prediction rules (as illustrated in Chapters 16–18).[2] An example is the model to predict survival among patients with end-stage liver disease (MELD),[3] from which the prognostic score is calculated as:

0.957 log(creatinine)
+ 0.378 log(bilirubin)
+ 1.120 log(international normalised ratio for prothrombin time)
+ 0.643 (if cause of cirrhosis was not alcohol-related liver disease or cholestatic liver disease)

The numerical weights for each variable are coefficients from a fitted regression model.[4] Simplified scoring systems require categorisation of continuous variables, and thus some loss of information.

Models help to stratify patients according to their risk of adverse outcomes. Such models may allow the (reasonably) reliable classification of patients into two or more risk groups with different prognoses. Such classification schemes can be used to inform patients, influence choice of therapy and perhaps save patients from unnecessary referrals or procedures. Models can also be used to compare performance of different institutions via case-mix adjustment.

Prognostic studies may be pragmatic or explanatory.[1] Pragmatic studies aim to produce a clinically useful measure of risk (e.g. for decision support). Explanatory studies are mainly concerned with scientific understanding, to answer such questions as: 'Which factors influence the course of disease *X*?' Here we focus our attention on pragmatic studies.

14 Evaluating the performance of prognostic models

A multiple regression model can be derived from any set of data, but it is clear that a prognostic model will have no clinical value unless it has been shown to predict outcome with some success.[5,6] A crucial idea, therefore, considered in some detail below, is that to be credible a model must be shown to perform adequately, not just on the data from which it was derived, but also on data from further patients. The concept is sometimes referred to as 'generalisability' or 'validity', and a model that is found to pass such a test is said to have been 'validated'. While there are many sources of advice on the technical aspects of developing statistical models, there is rather little guidance on the issues associated with the assessment of whether a model works well in practice, or 'validation'.[7]

Developing a useful prognostic model

Although prognostic models are sometimes developed to predict a continuous outcome, for most the aim is to quantify the risk of a specific event, possibly in relation to length of follow-up; examples are the risk of operative mortality or risk of recurrence of breast cancer, respectively. A basic issue relating to predicting events is that binary outcome data have considerable irreducible variability. The data are all zeros and ones, but the predictions are probabilities lying between these extremes.

We need to distinguish between how well a model may predict for groups of patients, and how well for individual patients. If a prognostic model predicts that, say, 85% of a defined set of patients will survive for 5 years after a myocardial infarction, then we would expect that among a large group of similar patients, close to 85% will indeed still be alive after 5 years. If the sample size is large, and thus there is little uncertainty in the prediction, there remains uncertainty about whether or not a particular patient will survive that long. So, although with an excellent model we may successfully distinguish between high- and low-risk patients, and can estimate group survival probabilities with precision, the ability to provide informative prognoses for individuals is almost always limited.[8]

Wyatt and Altman[5] suggested five prerequisites for clinical credibility:

1. 'All clinically relevant patient data should have been tested for inclusion in the model'. Many models are developed in retrospective studies using those variables that happen to have been collected already for other reasons. Thus potentially valuable variables may be omitted if data for them are unavailable.
2. 'It should be simple for doctors to obtain all the patient data required, reliably and without expending undue resources, in time to generate the prediction and guide decisions. Data should be obtainable with high reliability, particularly in those patients for which the model's predictions are most likely to be needed.'
3. 'Model builders should try to avoid arbitrary thresholds for continuous variables.' Categorisation discards potentially useful information. As discussed below, many models include dichotomised variables.
4. 'The model's structure should be apparent and its predictions should make sense to the doctors who will rely on them.' The statistical modelling method must be correctly applied. 'Black box' models, such as artificial neural networks and complex spline models, are less suitable for clinical applications.

5. 'It should be simple for doctors to calculate the model's prediction for a patient.' While not strictly necessary, it is clear that simplicity will increase the likelihood of uptake of a model.

A further aspect, only implicit in the above quote, is that the patients whose data are used to develop a model are precisely those for whom such a model would be used in clinical practice. It follows that it is essential for patient characteristics and the sampling method to be described in reports.

In the context of clinical practice, Reilly and Evans[2] defined five levels of evidence relating to clinical prediction rules (table 14.1). Even verifying that a model does indeed make useful predictions does not end the process, as it should ideally be shown that use of the rule has a beneficial impact (i.e. helps patients). Of 41 rules published in 2000–2003, the numbers of studies at each level of evidence were 10, 10, 16, 1 and 4.[2] Clearly, rather few published models have been evaluated for impact and many have not been evaluated in external contexts. We will not address impact further here, noting only that the best evidence of impact comes from randomised trials, and that such trials should ideally be performed before the model is brought into clinical use.[9] We focus now on aspects of validation studies, and present some case studies.

Why do we need to validate a prognostic model?

To demonstrate that a prognostic model is valuable, we need evidence that it does what it is intended to; that is, its predictions are adequate for the intended use. There are several interrelated reasons why prognostic models may not perform well.

Level	Definition	Standards of evaluation
1	Derivation of the prediction rule	
2	Narrow validation of the prediction rule	Prospective evaluation in one setting
3	Broad validation of the prediction rule	Prospective evaluation in varied settings with wide spectrum of patients and physicians
4	Narrow impact analysis of the prediction rule used as a decision rule	Prospective demonstration in one setting that use of prediction rule improves physicians' decisions
5	Broad impact analysis of the prediction rule used as a decision rule	Prospective demonstration in varied settings that use of prediction rule improves physicians' decisions for wide spectrum of patients

*Based on Reilly and Evans.[2]

Table** 14.1:* **Levels of evidence relating to the development and evaluation of a clinical prediction rule (prognostic model)

Deficiencies in the design of prognostic studies

A reliable prognostic study requires a well-defined cohort of patients all at the same defined point of their disease, often at diagnosis. Protocol-driven prospective studies are the ideal, but most prognostic studies are retrospective investigations of existing data. In cancer, for example, the large majority of prognostic studies are retrospective and, it seems, not protocol driven. The big advantage of retrospective studies for longer term outcomes is the availability of a cohort with a long enough follow-up for assessment of a substantial number of outcome events (e.g. deaths or recurrences). Retrospective studies have several serious disadvantages, however. Foremost among these are problems associated with the lack of a premeditated design for the study: unclear inclusion criteria, unknown completeness of the cohort, lack of standardisation of diagnostic and therapeutic procedures, incomplete baseline data, and unclear completeness of follow-up.[10] The same deficiencies may also affect some prospective studies. The definition of the characteristics of the sample is of clear importance to the clinician who wishes to know whether a model is relevant to a particular patient.

For studies with the aim of developing a prognostic model, the sample size needs to be large enough to outweigh the problems of multiple testing in the selection of variables and the comparison of models. Several authors have addressed the issue of sample size for prognostic studies.[11, 12] It is important to recognise that the power of a study depends on the number of observed events not the number of patients. A small sample with long follow-up may thus yield better information than a large study with short follow-up. Studies with few events per variable (EPV), especially if also small in size, are likely to have unreliable findings. Various authors have suggested that the EPV should be at least 10, and maybe 20–25, times the number of potential prognostic variables investigated.[13–15] Many published models are based on data sets with EPV < 10. The importance of EPV diminishes as the sample size increases; it is unlikely to be important in very large studies with several thousands of individuals. Another important consideration is the information content in a data set as expressed, for example, by the prognostic strength of individual predictors. Without some good predictors no model will be especially helpful. We return to this idea later.

Data quality

Incomplete data is a common and often serious problem for those developing prognostic models. Missing patient data for at least one variable are generally excluded from a modelling exercise. Even when each variable is reasonably complete, there may be many patients who do not have complete data. For example, in one study to develop a prognostic model for patients with ovarian cancer, only 44% of the patients had complete data.[16]

Excluding cases reduces statistical power, but there is also the serious risk of introducing bias. Such selection bias cannot be discerned by readers unless published articles report on the selection of individuals for inclusion in a study. For example, in cancer it may be helpful to present a comparison of the characteristics of those with and without available tumour material.[17] Such information is rarely provided.

The alternative to excluding patients with missing data is to impute the missing values.[18, 19] Imputation requires some quite strong and unverifiable assumptions about the mechanisms that generated the missingness, but so does complete case analysis (although the assumptions are not the same). Imputation, especially 'multiple imputation',[19] may well be preferable to using only complete cases, but at present it is rarely seen in published prognostic studies.[20] Statistical analysis using imputed data is in its infancy. It is not good practice to have data completeness as a criterion for including patients in the study, as it is then impossible to know how complete (and representative) the sample was.

For data that are available there are still quality issues. It is important that measurements are made using reliable and appropriate methods. Ideally, measurements should be recorded without categorisation, to enhance generalisability and improve modelling opportunities. In data sets obtained from multiple centres, it is important to have standardisation of both the methods of measurement and definitions of categorical variables.

Deficiencies of standard modelling methods

For clinical application it is usually necessary for a predictive model to be based on a small number of variables, and it is arguable that parsimony is a desirable feature of a good model.[21] Furthermore, most of the prognostic information is often concentrated in a few variables with 'strong' effects, with the remaining 'weak' variables contributing little to the model's predictive ability.[21] A model comprising only weak variables is likely to be unreliable. For clinical use a rule that can be memorised is appealing – an example is a score based on the number of risk factors present out of four to predict the risk of postoperative nausea and vomiting in children undergoing surgery.[22] Such simplicity will come at a cost, however, and judgement may be required regarding the trade-off between simplicity and predictive ability.

In most studies a large number of 'candidate' variables are available for consideration, and thus there is a need to select the 'important' ones. A balance is needed between fitting the current data as well as possible and developing a model that will work well in other situations. Models that are influenced by the specific features of the derivation data set may perform poorly when evaluated elsewhere; such models are called 'overfitted'.[14, 23]

Standard statistical methods to derive prognostic models do not explicitly address the issue of generalisability. Also, as they have data-dependent aspects, especially relating to variable selection, we would expect them to give an optimistic assessment of predictive performance. There is no simple way to judge the extent of such deficiencies.

Prognostic models are mostly derived using logistic regression for predicting a binary outcome (event) or Cox regression for time-to-event data. The initial set of variables is commonly reduced using a stepwise selection algorithm (often backward elimination or forward selection). The set of variables retained in the final model is based on multiple sequential hypothesis testing of individual variables, usually with $p < 0.05$ as the inclusion criterion (although this value has no specific justification). As often applied, the procedure is fully automated and requires no intellectual input. Although stepwise procedures are undoubtedly convenient, there is no reason why they should yield the model that is best in a predictive sense. It is possible, and also desirable, to use clinical knowledge to override the statistically chosen model – for example, to ensure that a known important variable is included regardless of whether it turns out to be statistically significant in the data set to hand. It may also be sensible to reduce the number of candidate variables using clinical knowledge, especially when there are many of them, before applying the statistical algorithm, thus reducing the risk of an overoptimistic model.[14] Problems arising from data-dependent selection are exacerbated by a small sample size. With a small sample there will be an increased risk of selecting unimportant variables and failing to include important ones.

Before going to multivariable analysis, many authors first reduce the number of candidate variables by means of univariate tests of association with outcome, discarding those that are not significant (perhaps with a high *p* value such as 0.2). There is no need to include this step, and it may introduce bias.[23, 24] By contrast, it makes sense to try to reduce the number of candidate variables using clinical criteria, for example to remove one of a pair of closely related variables, or variables that do not discriminate (e.g. indicators of risk factors that are very rare).

A further issue is that statistical models may not use the full information in the prognostic variables.[25, 26] If continuous predictors are dichotomised, as is common, the effective sample size is reduced by 30% or more and power is reduced.[25] Also, data-derived cutpoints introduce bias, and these are likely to compromise the generalisability of a model.

Models may not be transportable

Clearly a prognostic model that includes all important prognostic variables, appropriately modelled, should be transportable to centres with a different case mix. If, however, one or more important variables is absent, then variation in case mix could lead to quite different performance when a model is used elsewhere. Centres may also differ in other ways, including some factors reflecting differences in healthcare systems; examples include referral patterns, treatment protocols and methods of measurement. The difficulty, of course, is that one can never know whether a model does indeed include all important variables.

Possible weaknesses in the design and analysis plus the risk of omitted variables mean that it is not possible to use the original data to determine reliably the transportability of a model. These and other considerations argue strongly for the need to evaluate the performance of a model on a new series of patients, ideally in a different location. In addition, for a model to be adopted by others requires a degree of confidence in its reliability, which can probably only be gained by empirical demonstration of transportability.[5]

Validation of a prognostic model

Validating a model means establishing that it performs satisfactorily for patients other than those on whose data the model was derived (the 'derivation sample'). It is valuable to compare observed and predicted event rates for groups of patients (calibration), and calculate measures that show how well a model distinguishes between patients who do or do not experience the event of interest (discrimination).[27, 28] The new data may be from the same source as the derivation sample, to assess reproducibility, or from else-

Term	Definition or criteria
Accuracy	The degree to which predicted outcomes match observed outcomes
Calibration	Observed outcome is similar to predicted probability (commonly shown with calibration curves)
Discrimination	Relative ranking of individual risk is in substantially the correct order (observed event rates in those with higher scores are higher); commonly measured with the area under the receiver-operating characteristic curve
Generalisability	Ability of a prognostic system to provide accurate predictions in a new sample of patients
Reproducibility	The system is accurate in patients who were not included in development but who are from an identical population
.Transportability	The system is accurate in patients drawn from a different but related population, or in data collected using methods that differ from those used in development

*Based on Justice et al.[6]

Table** 14.2:* **Criteria for assessing the performance of a prognostic model

where, to assess generalisability (table 14.2). In a validation study the question addressed is whether the performance on the new data matches, or comes close to, the performance in the data on which the model was developed. Even if the performance is less good, it remains possible that the model is adequate for clinical use.[7]

The development of a successful model depends on:

- the potential for accurate prognosis, which is presumably unknown
- the intrinsic prognostic information in the available factors, which depends on many things, including the physiology of the disease in question
- the measurement process, which converts the intrinsic information into numbers, with some measurements being more reliable than others
- the accuracy with which the model converts the measurements into predictions.

We may ask whether, with the available factors, the model is the best that can be found, and also whether the model predicts accurately enough for its purpose.

Below, we consider in turn four main considerations in validating a model.

Study design

A hierarchy of three increasingly stringent validation strategies is:

- internal – procedures restricted to a single data set
- temporal – evaluation on a second data set from the same centre(s)
- external – evaluation on data from one or more other centres, perhaps by different investigators.

Internal validation

One approach is to split the data set into two parts before the modelling begins. The model is derived on the first portion of the data (often called the 'training' set), and its ability to predict outcome is evaluated on the second or 'test' data set. The usual approach of splitting at random must, however, lead to data sets that are essentially the same other than for chance variation (and perhaps smaller sample size), and it is thus a weak procedure.[13, 29] Better internal validation approaches are to use bootstrapping or 'leave one out' cross-validation. A tougher test is to split the data in a non-random way (e.g. by time period or geographical area). From these analyses, shrinkage factors can be estimated and applied to the regression coefficients to attempt to counter over-optimism.[23, 30, 31]

Temporal validation

An alternative is to evaluate the performance of a model on subsequent patients within the same centre(s).[32] Unfortunately, it is no different, in principle, from splitting a single data set by time period, as just mentioned. A better prognostic model would be obtained simply by analysing all the available data because the sample size would be larger. However, temporal validation is at least a prospective evaluation that is (supposedly) independent of the original data and model-fitting process. When the outcome is survival time, a disadvantage can be the need to wait several years to accrue enough events in a further cohort.

External validation

Neither internal nor temporal evaluation addresses the wider issue of the generalisability of the model. It is clearly desirable to evaluate a model on new data collected from an appropriate patient population in one or more different centres. External evaluation can be based on retrospective data, and so is viable for validating survival models needing long follow-up. Further design issues for external validation, such as inclusion criteria and sample size, have as yet not been considered in the literature.

Measuring intrinsic prognostic information

We assume that prognoses are to be framed as predicted probabilities of a particular event, implicitly or explicitly linked to a specific time point (e.g. the chance of surviving for 5 years following initial diagnosis or treatment). The predicted probabilities are obtained as outputs from a prognostic model. Such predicted probabilities can be obtained from models for survival time (Cox regression) and binary regression models (logistic regression).

Intuitively, the idea of prognostic information is straightforward and relates to the spread of event probabilities. For example, in an analysis unadjusted for other factors, the estimated chance of surviving for 3 years following initial treatment for node-positive breast cancer may be about 90% for patients with 1–3 affected lymph nodes, compared with about 60% for those with 10 or more affected nodes. By contrast, predicted 3-year survival probabilities for pre- and postmenopausal patients may be about 84% and 82%, respectively. The prognostic information contained in lymph-node status is clearly much greater than that in menopausal status, since the spread of probabilities is 0.3, as against only 0.02. Solely for the purpose of illustration later, we use this simple approach, referring to the separation between extreme groups as PSEP. This measure is not intended to be definitive. The spread of probabilities from which PSEP is obtained depends on how finely the prognostic factor or index is graded, the distribution of individuals across the groups and the prevalence of the event. We recommend other methods for formal assessment, in particular the index *D*.[33] With just two groups, PSEP is closely related to the positive (PPV) and negative (NPV) predictive values:[7]

$$\text{PSEP} = \text{PPV} + \text{NPV} - 1$$

Comparing predictions with observations

There are several possible approaches to comparing predicted and observed event probabilities. It is helpful to consider both calibration and discrimination, for neither of which is there a standard approach.

Calibration is quite simply assessed by comparing the observed and predicted proportions of events in groups defined by the risk score, possibly accompanied by a test such as the Hosmer–Lemeshow test for binary data. For time-to-event data, observed and expected survival rates can be compared at a chosen time point. Similar analyses may be performed using groups defined by key patient variables, such as diagnostic or demographic subgroups.

Discrimination may be summarised by various single statistics, such as the area under the receiver–operating characteristic (ROC) curve (or the equivalent *c* statistic), R^2 measures or the *D* statistic.[4, 33] The Brier score[34] is a measure of average lack of fit for an individual patient, but it lacks familiarity or an easy interpretation (other than the bigger the score, the worse the predictions). The statistic PSEP, discussed above, is crude but interpretable. Of course more than one measure may be used.

One other aspect of such comparisons deserves mention. When assessing the performance of a model on new data, it is common to treat the predictions from the model as fixed (known, and without error). In reality there is uncertainty in performance measures (hazard ratios, area under the curve (AUC) values, R^2, etc.) in both data sets. Ignoring uncertainty in the derivation data set could lead to false inferences.

Prespecifying adequate performance

In pragmatic studies the idea is to prejudge the quality of predictions from a prognostic model that may or may not be acceptable. In a validation study we seek evidence that the model meets the prestated criterion in new data; if it does, the model may be suitable for clinical use.

Although it is helpful to predefine 'adequate' performance of a model, one feature of a validation study is simply to provide an external estimate of the prediction error of the model.[32] In other words, we should quantify the performance of a model and accept that the final assessment requires clinical judgement and is context dependent. Statistics alone cannot determine clinical validity.

Case studies

We describe here some examples of the development of prognostic models and validation studies. The last example is one of several considered by Altman and Royston.[7]

Predicting 4-year mortality in older adults

Lee et al.[35] described the derivation and validation of a prognostic model that 'could be used for community-dwelling individuals older than 50 for clinical, health policy and epidemiological purposes.' Their data came from a large, prospective, cohort study carried out in the USA. The model was developed using 11 701 individuals (1361 deaths) living in the eastern, western or central regions of the USA, and the evaluation study was done using 8009 individuals (1072 deaths) from the southern region.

Data on 41 variables were considered for inclusion in the model. These included demographic, (co)morbidity, behavioural and functional variables. The investigators excluded a few variables that might be associated with mortality because they might compromise generalisability (e.g. socio-economic status was not considered as it is associated with quality of care). All variables were binary, except for age, which was split into six categories. Only body mass index was a dichotomised continuous variable.

Logistic regression with backward elimination (with $p < 0.05$) gave a model including 16 variables, which was reduced further to 12 variables using the Bayesian Information Criterion. The investigators showed that the same model was obtained using various alternative methods. The resulting model, which included variables from all four categories described above, was turned into a simple scoring scheme by converting the regression coefficients into points: 1–7 points for age, and 1 or 2 points for each of the 11 binary covariates.

The risk of dying within 4 years varied markedly across risk scores, from < 1% for a score of zero to over 50% for scores greater than 12 (about 5% of the sample). The AUC (*c* statistic) was 0.84 in the development cohort and 0.82 in the validation cohort. Figure 14.1 shows that the model was very well calibrated, as the performance of the scoring system was almost identical in both cohorts. In general, given a sensible approach to modelling, we would expect good performance in a very large cohort in which chance plays little role, especially when the data are from the same data collection system, even if from a different geographical area.

This model has thus reached level 2 of evidence (see table 14.1) and, in the terms of Justice et al.,[6] has been shown to be reproducible. The derivation and validation samples were derived from a single cohort with an identical study protocol, however, so generalisability remains to be demonstrated.

Predicting operative mortality of patients undergoing cardiac surgery

The European System for Cardiac Operative Risk Evaluation (EuroSCORE) was developed using data from eight European countries to predict the operative mortality of patients undergoing cardiac surgery. It has been successfully validated in other European cohorts. Yap et al.[36] examined the performance of these models in an Australian cohort.

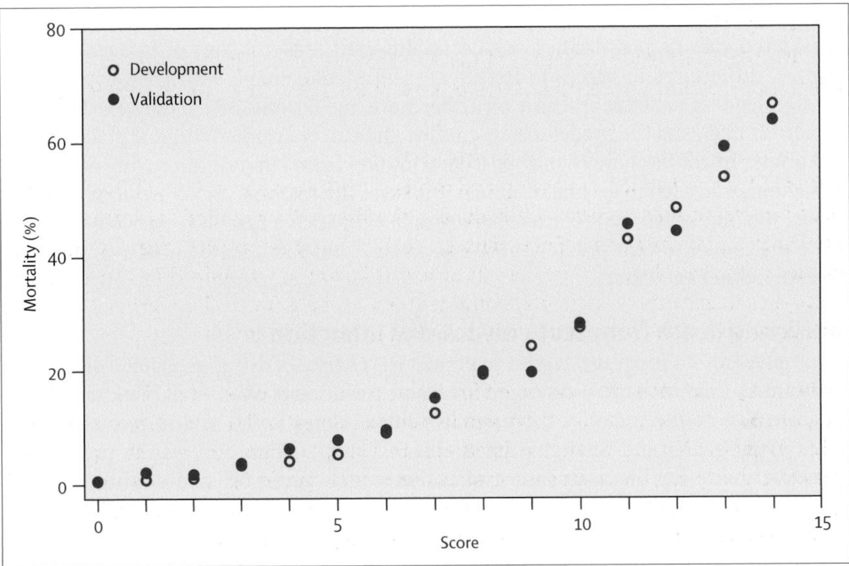

***Figure 14.1:* Risk of dying within 4 years by risk scores among community-dwelling individuals older than 50 years, in the development and validation cohorts. (Based on Lee et al.[35])**

The Australian patients were rather different from the derivation cohort, with a generally higher risk of death. For example, 41% of the Australian patients were aged over 70 years, compared to 27% of the derivation cohort, and there were 15% versus 10%, respectively, with recent myocardial infarction.

Yet the observed mortality in the Australian cohort was consistently much lower than that predicted by both the EuroSCORE models. The predicted and observed survival for three risk groups obtained with the additive EuroSCORE model are shown in table 14.3. Mortality overall was only half the predicted mortality (and a third of that using the alternative logistic EuroSCORE model). The model discriminates in this cohort, but the calibration is very poor.

EuroSCORE additive model	Patients (deaths)	Observed mortality (95% CI)	Predicted mortality (95% CI)
0–2 (low risk)	1955 (8)	0.41% (0.18 to 0.80)	1.03% (0.99 to 1.06)
3–5 (medium risk)	1996 (17)	0.85% (0.50 to 1.36)	3.90% (3.87 to 3.94)
≥ 6 (high risk)	1641 (87)	5.30% (4.27 to 6.50)	8.52% (8.39 to 8.65)
Total	5592 (112)	2.00% (1.65 to 2.40)	4.25% (4.16 to 4.34)

***Table 14.3:* Predicted and observed mortality by EuroSCORE risk level for Australian patients undergoing coronary artery bypass grafting[36]**

Why might the model not have predicted well for the Australian patients? The authors considered various possibilities, including different epidemiology of ischaemic heart disease, differences in access to healthcare and management, with greater resources possibly leading to better outcomes. Furthermore, the EuroSCORE model was based on data from 1995, and the model may not reflect the current cardiac surgical practice even in Europe. In addition, there may be a contribution from survival improving over time, a phenomenon seen in several diseases. Whatever the reasons, they concluded that this model was not appropriate for use in Australia.[36] In such a case, it is possible to recalibrate the model so that predictions are accurate,[37] but the updated model might then require further validation.

Predicting death from acute myocardial infarction

Woo[38] presented a prognostic index to predict the chance of dying in hospital after acute myocardial infarction (MI) among a Chinese population. Woo et al.[39] evaluated the performance of the index in the original centre (Hong Kong) and in two additional cities (Guangzhou and Shanghai in mainland China). Their aim was to provide 'an objective guide for the assessment of patients with acute MI and stratify different grades of clinical severity.'[39] The authors did not suggest what specific clinical actions should be taken as a result of identifying a patient's disease severity grade, so we view the study as explanatory rather than pragmatic.

The index was derived from four continuous and seven binary variables using a non-standard approach based on univariate χ^2 tests of association and linear discriminant analysis of the resulting significant predictors in a multivariable model. Seven factors were rejected as not being univariately associated with mortality. All the continuous factors (age, systolic blood pressure, heart size and blood urea concentration) were initially converted to categoric form by applying cut-points (three categories for age and two for the other predictors).

Woo et al.[39] concluded that 'on the whole, the trend in mortality of the subsets correlated well with that predicted by the prognostic index ... $p > 0.2$, although a possible lower mortality was detected in the groups with prognostic scores between 6 and 7.' Table 14.4 shows a simplified summary of their results.

PSEP is 0.67 in the original (Hong Kong) sample and 0.55 in the validation sample from the same location, showing a reduction in separation typical of overfitting in the original analysis. Nevertheless, the prognostic information seems strong and fairly reproducible. The value of PSEP for the two Chinese mainland cities is 0.76, actually greater than for the original Hong Kong sample. This seems to be mainly due to the relatively high death rate among severely ill patients (index 8 or more) in those cities. Woo et al.[39] interpreted the reduction in death rates in the 1977–1986 Hong Kong cohort compared with 1971–1980 as indicating that the prognostic index could detect secular changes in death rates stratified by disease severity. However, the difference may be caused simply by the overoptimism in the predictive ability of the model; the overall death rates have hardly changed.

We doubt whether the model is the best that can be found with the available factors, because categorising continuous predictors always results in some loss of information.

Index	Original sample		Validation samples			
	Hong Kong 1971–1980		Hong Kong 1977–1986		Guangzhou 1977–1982 and Shanghai 1978–1986	
	Proportion	No. deaths/ No. patients	Proportion	No. deaths/ No. patients	Proportion	No. deaths/ No. patients
≥ 8	0.72	63/87	0.61	49/80	0.79	38/48
6–7	0.54	55/102	0.39	38/97	0.40	27/68
4–5	0.21	39/182	0.16	20/126	0.20	35/172
≤ 3	0.05	14/273	0.06	8/132	0.03	5/163
Total	0.27	171/644	0.26	115/435	0.23	105/451
PSEP (95% CI)	0.67 (0.57 to 0.77)		0.55 (0.44 to 0.61)		0.76 (0.64 to 0.88)	

***Table** 14.4:* **Validation of prognostic index in acute MI[39]**

However, as the model seems capable of predicting probabilities of death reliably over a very wide range, we conclude that it seems potentially clinically valid (and valuable).

Discussion

Lessons from the case studies

The few case studies presented here are not representative of the medical literature, but certain lessons may be drawn from them, those we described before,[7] and other studies we have examined.

Research groups tend to confirm the validity of their own models, but others are less successful in doing so. We can only speculate about the reasons for this. The test (validation) set of patients is often drawn from the same centre as the original set, but at a later time. Clearly, there will be many similarities between the two sets of patients and between the clinical and laboratory techniques used in evaluating them. This will pose a lesser challenge to a prognostic model than will a new setting with different investigators and techniques, and perhaps a more sceptical approach. Also, if the original model and its evaluation with new data are published by the same investigators in a single article, there may be a temptation, if the model does not give a good fit to the new data, to modify it in the light of the new data and publish it as though it was the original model. We have no evidence of such a practice, but it does not seem totally improbable. Our general attitude supports the view of Laupacis et al.:[40] 'It is essential to prospectively validate the rule in a group of patients different from the group in which it was derived, preferably with different clinicians.' Such studies are not commonly reported.[2]

Many authors seem unclear about (or at least do not state clearly) the reason for developing their model. It seems widely believed that demonstration of usefulness may be based on the statistical significance of predictors in a multivariable model. Similarly, and perhaps consequently, when evaluating a model with new data authors seem instinctively to want to calculate *p* values and conclude that the validation is satisfactory if there is no significant difference between, say, observed and predicted event rates.

General points

An important question that arises in an attempt to validate a model with new data is 'What is the final model?'. Van Houwelingen and Thorogood[37] felt that the original model should be updated in light of the new data, and proposed a way of doing that in a survival analysis setting. Their updating method involved a minor calibration of the prognostic index from the original model, rather than a complete reconstruction. Such an approach might also be contemplated in any situation where a model from elsewhere has very good discrimination but poor calibration.

A model is 'a snapshot in place and time, not fundamental truth'.[9] If the case mix in the validation sample differs in a major way from that of the construction sample, the model may fail. However, it may be possible to improve it by including new variable(s) that relate to the different case mix and are found to be prognostic in the new sample. For example, the range of patients' ages in the construction and validation samples might differ markedly, resulting in age not being recognised initially as an important prognostic factor. Such a new model then needs further validation.[41]

Simplicity of models and reliability of measurements are important criteria in developing clinically useful prognostic models.[5] Experience shows that larger models tend to give optimistic predictions, especially when extensive variable selection has been performed.[21] That view may not help when considering a particular data set, however, as so many other factors are relevant. For example, with a very large sample, as in some of the cited examples, the risk of optimism is very much reduced. Shrinkage-based approaches can be applied to reduce optimism[23] and have some appeal; as yet they are not much used.

As the aim of prognostic studies is to create clinically valuable indices, the definition of risk groups should be driven mainly by clinical rather than statistical criteria, particularly in the case of pragmatic studies. If a clinician were to leave untreated a patient with at least a 90% chance of surviving 5 years, apply aggressive therapy if the prognosis was 30% survival or less, and use standard therapy in intermediate cases, then three prognostic groups would appear to be sensible, and validation of the model would address whether the discrimination across those groups was maintained by other investigators in other settings. In explanatory studies the question of how best to define prognostic groups (or even whether to produce groups) remains an open question.

Quantifying performance

The two main aspects of model performance are the amount of prognostic information, which relates to potential clinical usefulness, and the performance of the model with new (external) data. These ideas are largely captured by the notions of discrimination and calibration.

There are many possible ways to define the amount of prognostic information, including R^2, the area under the ROC curve (c statistic), D,[33] and the Brier score.[34] As noted, we do not propose PSEP, the simple measure described above, as a formal method of quantifying prognostic performance. For one thing, its magnitude is strongly influenced by the number of risk groups. However, we have found it useful when describing the results of the analysis of prognostic data in case studies. Analysis of an independent data set will show if that estimate was reasonable. When there are more than two groups, the extreme groups, from which PSEP is calculated, should be large enough and have sufficient events to allow adequate estimation.

PSEP is of course the difference between two proportions, also known as the risk difference, in the context of randomised trials. The reciprocal of PSEP represents the number of extra patients in the high-risk group needed to generate one additional adverse event.[7] In survival studies, PSEP is a function of follow-up time.

Concluding comments

Although they have considerable potential clinical value, prognostic models are not widely used in clinical practice. It is likely that a major contributory factor is that most of these models have not been demonstrated to be effective by other investigators in other centres.[2, 5] To be useful, a prognostic index should be clinically credible, accurate (well calibrated), have generality (i.e. be validated elsewhere) and, ideally, be demonstrated to be clinically effective, in the sense that it provides useful additional information to clinicians.[2, 5]

Studies developing models should be reported in adequate detail. Concato et al.[42] reviewed 44 publications that presented prognostic models. They found frequent methodological shortcomings, including unspecified method for selecting variables in the model, unspecified coding of variables, and risk of overfitting through too few events per variable. Other authors have also found deficiencies in both reporting and methodology used.[40, 43–47] Quality appraisal of studies presenting prognostic models should focus on internal validity, external validity, statistical validity, evaluation of the model and practicality of the model.[43, 45]

In a pragmatic study, the aim of developing a prognostic model is the prediction of outcome for future patients; that objective should be kept in mind when producing a model. Thus study design and model building should anticipate and deal with overoptimism. Further methodological research is needed to investigate which design features and analysis procedures are likely to lead to a good model.

References

1 Braitman LE, Davidoff F. Predicting clinical states in individual patients. *Ann Intern Med* 1996; **125:** 406–12.

2 Reilly BM, Evans AT. Translating clinical research into clinical practice: impact of using prediction rules to make decisions. *Ann Intern Med* 2006; **144:** 201–09.

3 Malinchoc M, Kamath PS, Gordon FD, et al. A model to predict poor survival in patients undergoing transjugular intrahepatic portosystemic shunts. *Hepatology* 2000; **31:** 864–71.

4 Katz MH. Multivariable analysis: a primer for readers of medical research. *Ann Intern Med* 2003; **138:** 644–50.

5 Wyatt JC, Altman DG. Commentary. Prognostic models: clinically useful or quickly forgotten? *BMJ* 1995; **311:** 1539–41.

6 Justice AC, Covinsky KE, Berlin JA. Assessing the generalizability of prognostic information. *Ann Intern Med* 1999; **130:** 515–24.

7 Altman DG, Royston P. What do we mean by validating a prognostic model? *Stat Med* 2000; **19:** 453–73.

8 Henderson R, Keiding N. Individual survival time prediction using statistical models. *J Med Ethics* 2005; **31:** 703–06.

9 Iezzoni LI. Statistically derived predictive models. Caveat emptor. *J Gen Intern Med* 1999; **14:** 388–89.

10 Altman DG, Riley RD. Primer: an evidence-based approach to prognostic markers. *Nature Clin Pract Oncol* 2005; **2:** 466–72.

11 Schmoor C, Sauerbrei W, Schumacher M. Sample size considerations for the evaluation of prognostic factors in survival analysis. *Stat Med* 2000; **19:** 441–52.

12 McShane LM, Simon R. Statistical methods for the analysis of prognostic factor studies. In: Gospodarowicz MK, Henson DE, Hutter RVP, et al., eds. *Prognostic Factors in Cancer.* New York: Wiley-Liss, 2001: 37–48.

13 Feinstein AR. *Multivariable Analysis: An Introduction.* New Haven, CT: Yale University Press, 1996.

14 Harrell FE Jr, Lee KL, Califf RM, et al. Regression modelling strategies for improved prognostic prediction. *Stat Med* 1984; **3:** 143–52.

15 Schumacher M, Holländer N, Schwarzer G, Sauerbrei W. Prognostic factor studies. In: Crowley J, Ankerst DP, eds. *Handbook of Statistics in Clinical Oncology.* Boca Raton, FL: Chapman & Hall/CRC Press, 2006: 289–333.

16 Clark TG, Altman DG. Developing a prognostic model in the presence of missing data: an ovarian cancer case study. *J Clin Epidemiol* 2003; **56:** 28–37.

17 Hoppin JA, Tolbert PE, Taylor JA, et al. Potential for selection bias with tumor tissue retrieval in molecular epidemiology studies. *Ann Epidemiol* 2002; **12:** 1–6.

18 Vach W. Some issues in estimating the effect of prognostic factors from incomplete covariate data. *Stat Med* 1997; **16:** 57–72.

19 Schafer JL, Graham JW. Missing data: our view of the state of the art. *Psychol Methods* 2002; **7:** 147–77.

20 Burton A, Altman DG. Missing covariate data within cancer prognostic studies: a review of current reporting and proposed guidelines. *Br J Cancer* 2004; **91:** 4–8.

21 Sauerbrei W. The use of resampling methods to simplify regression models in medical statistics. *Appl Stat* 1999; **48:** 313–29.

22 Eberhart LH, Morin AM, Guber D, et al. Applicability of risk scores for postoperative nausea and vomiting in adults to paediatric patients. *Br J Anaesth* 2004; **93:** 386–92.

23 Babyak MA. What you see may not be what you get: a brief, nontechnical introduction to overfitting in regression-type models. *Psychosom Med* 2004; **66:** 411–21.

24 Sun GW, Shook TL, Kay GL. Inappropriate use of bivariable analysis to screen risk factors for use in multivariable analysis. *J Clin Epidemiol* 1996; **49:** 907–16.

25 Royston P, Altman DG, Sauerbrei W. Dichotomizing continuous predictors in multiple regression: a bad idea. *Stat Med* 2006; **25:** 127–41.

26 Christensen E. Multivariate survival analysis using Cox's regression model. *Hepatology* 1987; **7:** 1346–58.

27 Harrell FE Jr, Lee KL, Mark DB. Multivariable prognostic models: issues in developing models, evaluating assumptions and adequacy, and measuring and reducing errors. *Stat Med* 1996; **15:** 361–87.

28 Mackillop WJ, Quirt CF. Measuring the accuracy of prognostic judgments in oncology. *J Clin Epidemiol* 1997; **50:** 21–29.

29 Hirsch RP. Validation samples. *Biometrics* 1991; **47:** 1193–94.

30 Schumacher M, Hollander N, Sauerbrei W. Resampling and cross-validation techniques: a tool to reduce bias caused by model building? *Stat Med* 1997; **16:** 2813–27.

31 Verweij PJ, Van Houwelingen HC. Cross-validation in survival analysis. *Stat Med* 1993; **12:** 2305–14.

32 Miller ME, Hui SL, Tierney WM. Validation techniques for logistic regression models. *Stat Med* 1991; **10:** 1213–26.

33 Royston P, Sauerbrei W. A new measure of prognostic separation in survival data. *Stat Med* 2004; **23:** 723–48.

34 Graf E, Schmoor C, Sauerbrei W, Schumacher M. Assessment and comparison of prognostic classification schemes for survival data. *Stat Med* 1999; **18:** 2529–45.

35 Lee SJ, Lindquist K, Segal MR, Covinsky KE. Development and validation of a prognostic index for 4-year mortality in older adults. *JAMA* 2006; **295:** 801–08.

36 Yap CH, Reid C, Yii M, et al. Validation of the EuroSCORE model in Australia. *Eur J Cardiothorac Surg* 2006; **29:** 441–46.

37 Van Houwelingen HC, Thorogood J. Construction, validation and updating of a prognostic model for kidney graft survival. *Stat Med* 1995; **14:** 1999–2008.

38 Woo KS. Coronary prognostic index for the Chinese. *Aust NZ J Med* 1987; **17:** 562–67.

39 Woo KS, Pun CO, Wang RY, et al. Validation of a coronary prognostic index for the Chinese – a tale of three cities. *Int J Cardiol* 1989; **23:** 173–78.

40 Laupacis A, Sekar N, Stiell IG. Clinical prediction rules. A review and suggested modifications of methodological standards. *JAMA* 1997; **277:** 488–94.

41 Hubacek J, Galbraith PD, Gao M, et al. External validation of a percutaneous coronary intervention mortality prediction model in patients with acute coronary syndromes. *Am Heart J* 2006; **151:** 308–15.

42 Concato J, Feinstein AR, Holford TR. The risk of determining risk with multivariable models. *Ann Intern Med* 1993; **118:** 201–10.

43 Counsell C, Dennis M. Systematic review of prognostic models in patients with acute stroke. *Cerebrovasc Dis* 2001; **12:** 159–70.

44 Coste J, Fermanian J, Venot A. Methodological and statistical problems in the construction of composite measurement scales: a survey of six medical and epidemiological journals. *Stat Med* 1995; **14:** 331–45.

45 Jacob M, Lewsey JD, Sharpin C, et al. Systematic review and validation of prognostic models in liver transplantation. *Liver Transpl* 2005; **11:** 814–25.

46 Hackett ML, Anderson CS. Predictors of depression after stroke: a systematic review of observational studies. *Stroke* 2005; **36:** 2296–301.

47 Williams C, Brunskill S, Altman D, et al. Cost effectiveness of using prognostic information to select women with breast cancer for adjuvant systemic therapy of breast cancer. *Health Technol Assess* 2006; **10:** 1–222.

15

Are *n*-of-1 trials of any practical value to clinicians and researchers?

Graeme J. Hankey

Introduction

The optimum estimate of the effectiveness and safety of a treatment in trial populations is derived from a meta-analysis of a systematic review of all published and unpublished randomised controlled trials (RCTs). In many aspects of clinical practice, however, there is a dearth of such high-quality evidence. When it is available, it is commonly not possible to generalise the results beyond the trial populations to individual patients because the populations are inadequately described or highly selected (e.g. exclude the elderly). In addition, when the evidence is widely generalisable, the estimate of the effectiveness and safety of the treatment is only an average treatment effect for the population (e.g. a reduction in the odds of an unfavourable outcome), and not a specific treatment effect for an individual patient. Indeed, most effective treatments are not beneficial for all patients but only a modest proportion.[1] Furthermore, in trials reporting no effect of a treatment, there may be a subgroup of individuals who actually benefited but the sample size was too small for an important treatment effect to be detected reliably.

These concerns about the generalisability (external validity) of the estimates of treatment effects derived from RCTs of *populations* of patients to *individual* patients are one of the many barriers impeding the translation of reliable evidence into clinical practice.[2–4] One strategy to overcome this limitation is to undertake subgroup analyses of data from large RCTs. However, unless predefined (i.e. a priori), subgroup analyses are fraught with random errors and tend to be interpreted incorrectly as a *test* of hypotheses about indicators of outcome among subgroups of individuals rather than as a *generator* of them.[5] Another strategy is to identify patients by genomic profile so that drugs can be tailored to individuals who are likely to have minimal risk of adverse drugs reactions and maximal potential benefits.[6,7] However, the utility of pharmacogenomics in clinical practice remains to be established.

Sometimes the only vehicle for resolving clinical uncertainty about the effect of a treatment in an individual is for clinicians and patients to undertake their own experiments to assess the effectiveness of a treatment. The traditional experiment is a 'trial of therapy'. A patient is assessed at baseline, started on a treatment and followed up by means of regular reassessments. If the patient improves, the treatment is usually judged effective. If the patient does not improve, the treatment is usually judged ineffective. However, other factors, apart from treatment, may influence the outcome for the patient, and bias the study results. These factors include how and by whom outcome is measured, the natural history of the condition and the outcome measurements, and random error (chance). For example, the natural history of the condition may be self-limiting (i.e. the patient was going to improve anyway), the act of taking a treatment may provoke a subjective improvement of symptoms irrespective of any inherent efficacy (the placebo effect),[8, 9] symptoms frequently become less severe when they are reassessed (in the same way that extreme measurements, such as high and low blood pressure, frequently regress to the mean and return toward the individual's normal range when reassessed), and the patient may report favourable benefits simply as a result of optimistic expectations or gratitude (willingness to please bias).

These pitfalls of traditional uncontrolled and unblinded observational case studies, and the limited generalisability of RCTs of trial populations to individual patients, have prompted the development of RCTs in individual patients (*n*-of-1 RCTs) to increase the scientific rigour of individual patient assessments.[10–15]

What are *n*-of-1 trials and how are they done?

Definition

An *n*-of-1 trial is a randomised, controlled, multiple crossover study of an individual patient's responses to treatments.[12–15]

Methods

Setting

The setting is clinical practice, usually primary care and hospital outpatient clinics.

Subject

The subject is an individual patient.

Informed consent

The clinician and patient agree to test a treatment (experimental) for its ability to control or improve the patient's symptoms, signs or other manifestations of the illness (the treatment target).

Readiness of the patient to change their behaviour according to the results of an *n*-of-1 trial

Where the aim of the trial is to identify the efficacy of an existing treatment, screening for readiness to change (according to the stage-of-change model[16]) might provide useful information as to whether the results of the trial will influence whether the patient continues or ceases the treatment after the trial. Finding that the patient is prepared to change, and maintain, their treatment according to the results of an *n*-of-1 trial, rather than simply precontemplating or contemplating changing their treatment, might be the difference between the patient ultimately complying or not complying with the trial results.[17, 18]

Interventions

Usually one treatment and placebo, or two alternative treatments, are compared.[12] More than two treatments can be compared, but this introduces analytical complexity.

Preliminary, unblinded, run-in period of active treatment

A preliminary, unblinded, run-in period of active treatment(s), during which both the clinician and patient know that active treatment is being taken, is commonly undertaken to determine whether the occurrence of intolerable adverse effects or a complete lack of response would obviate the need for further evaluation by means of an *n*-of-1 trial.[19] Furthermore, an open run-in period may facilitate the identification and use of the optimal dose of active medication.

Design

The design is a randomised, controlled, multiple, crossover trial, in which the patient serves as their own control (figure 15.1). It can take several forms, depending on the nature of the clinical question, the characteristics of the disease and the patient, the properties of the treatment being evaluated, the views of the patient, and local circumstances, including availability of trial support services.[11, 15]

Patients may be randomly assigned a set of the treatments (e.g. treatments A and B) individually or within paired treatment periods/cycles (see figure 15.1). For example, treatments A and B may be randomised (r) within sequential pairs (e.g. rAB, rBA, rBA ...) or en bloc (e.g. rAABABB ...). Alternatively, systematic alternation of treatments within pairs may follow a single, initial randomisation (e.g. rABABAB ...). However, the latter design is more vulnerable to carryover effects and inadvertent unblinding.[15]

Randomisation is usually performed at the beginning of each new treatment period/cycle, but can be done at each point where treatment is to change.

Double-blind treatment allocation

Both the clinician and the patient are 'blind' to the random treatment allocation, whenever possible.

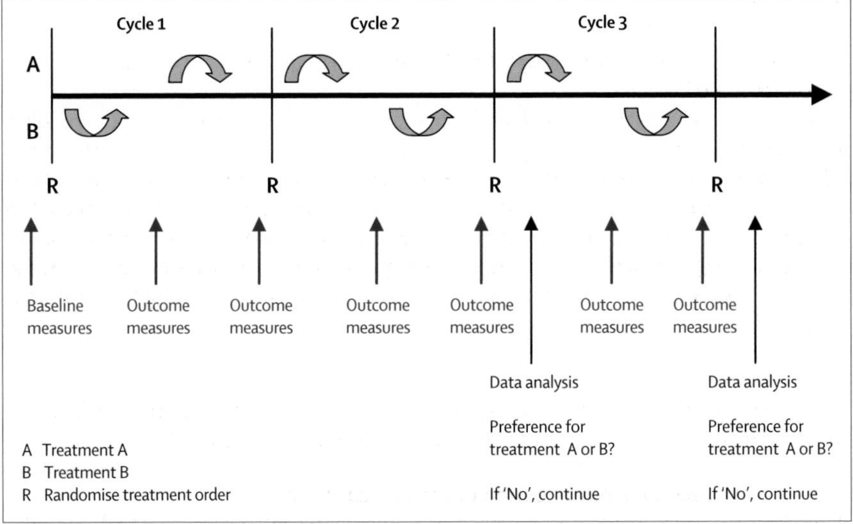

***Figure* 15.1: Schema of an *n*-of-1 trial design.**

A collaborating pharmacist or pharmacy service who/which can (i) prepare placebos that are as close as possible (or feasible) to the active medication in appearance, taste and texture, (ii) package the active medication and placebo in identical forms, (iii) label and fill the medication containers with appropriate medication or placebo, (iv) dispense the medication to the patient, and (v) prepare and keep the randomisation code, allows the clinician and patient to remain blind to the treatment allocation.[12]

Treatment intervals

The treatment intervals allow for known delays in onset of drug action or for washout periods.

Treatment periods (cycles)

A treatment period (cycle) includes an exposure to the experimental treatment and the comparator treatment (placebo or alternative). The order is determined by random allocation (see figure 15.1).

Outcome measures (treatment targets)

Outcome measures are predefined and valid (i.e. they measure what they are supposed to measure), reliable (i.e. they are reproducible), sensitive to clinically important change, and communicable measures of the treatment target(s).

The nature of the outcomes/treatment targets are more subtle than the 'hard' clinical outcomes of large RCTs (e.g. death or stroke). They are usually patient generated and derived from a minimum of three, and maximum of seven, of the patient's most troubling symptoms and problems caused by the illness and/or the drug.[12, 19] These symptoms or problems can be palliated, but not removed.

The most common outcomes/treatment targets are symptoms and measures of the patient's quality of life and well-being. The latter usually comprise multiple indirect measures of quality of life and well-being, such as physical signs (e.g. blood pressure, tremor or rigidity), laboratory tests (e.g. erythrocyte sedimentation rate or nerve conduction velocity) and functional outcomes (e.g. timed 10 m walk or exercise tolerance). Although sometimes qualitative (e.g. cessation of pain following analgesia, or recurrence of migraine or epileptic seizures), most are quantitative, and graded from absent to severe in order to increase sensitivity and statistical power. Where possible, the measures are converted into a single-page assessment form that can be self-administered as a questionnaire or diary.

In addition to measures of outcome/treatment targets, it may be useful to record information about drug compliance (e.g. pill return and plasma drug concentrations) and, when two alternative treatments are being compared, to record economic data to enable an estimate to be made of the cost-effectiveness of the treatments in that individual.[20]

Follow-up and outcome evaluation

The treatment targets/outcome measures are monitored, by means of the patient diary/questionnaire or repeated outpatient assessments, to document the potential effect of the treatment currently being applied. The treatment targets/outcome measures are assessed at set time intervals, appropriate to the different treatment periods, and not necessarily restricted to the end of each treatment period. Otherwise, ill effects from stopping and starting treatments may be missed.

In most *n*-of-1 trials, the patient completes the diary/questionnaire or undergoes assessment at least twice during each treatment period (see figure 15.1).

Replication

Pairs of treatment periods are commonly replicated until the clinician and patient are convinced that the two treatments are clearly different or not different. The advantage of not specifying the required number of pairs of treatment periods in advance is that the clinician and patient can stop the trial at any time, when both are convinced that the treatment periods within each pair are exhibiting important differences in the treatment targets/outcome measures. The trial can then be stopped, the code broken and a decision made whether the experimental treatment should be continued indefinitely or ceased.[19]

However, if the clinician is wanting to conduct a formal statistical analysis of the data or publish the results, the analysis is stronger if the number of pairs of treatment periods is specified in advance. The number of periods may be predetermined by convenience or by a power calculation. More pairs are required when a reliable conclusion is needed, or when the treatment effect is expected to be modest in comparison with the underlying fluctuation of the condition or the sensitivity of the outcome measures. For example, within a trial consisting of a series of three pairs and where outcome is assessed only *qualitatively* (e.g. as 'better' or 'worse'), a consistent preference for treatment over placebo will occur by chance alone with a probability of one in eight (i.e. $1/2^3 = 0.125$). *Quantitative* evaluation (e.g. grades from 'absent' to 'severe') by multiple series enhances the sensitivity (power) of a trial.

Alternatively, comparisons may be continued under the guidance of an independent unblinded data-monitoring committee, which terminates the trial only when it is possible reliably to conclude that one treatment is more effective or harmful than the other, or that there is no clinically important difference.[15]

Irrespective of whether the number of treatment periods is prespecified or not, a general rule of thumb is that at least two, and preferably three or more, replications (treatment periods) should be performed before breaking the code, in order to reduce the chance that non-drug-related trends have led to false (positive or negative) conclusions (see figure 15.1).

Analysis

Following multiple crossover periods, the outcomes obtained for the two (or more) drugs are compared. However, there is no consensus on how the results are best analysed.[14, 21–23]

Visual assessment

Informal visual assessment ('eyeball') of raw or graphical data is simple and appealing.[24] It also has face validity in demonstrating clinically meaningful benefit.[15, 25] However, it does not quantify the likelihood of a false-positive result (type I error), and is open to bias and poor reproducibility in the consistency and interpretation of the results. In order to avoid false-positive and false-negative interpretations, it is appropriate to carry out some sort of statistical analysis.

The sign test

The simplest form of statistical analysis of an *n*-of-1 trial with a paired design is to determine qualitatively the outcome from the experimental treatment in each treatment pair (e.g. as 'positive' or 'negative', or 'better' or 'worse') and analyse the results by means of the 'sign test'.[19, 26] This is akin to analysing the results of repeatedly tossing a coin. It begins by assuming the null hypothesis (i.e. that a particular result, e.g. 'positive', in the trial, or 'heads' with coin tossing, is due to chance) and calculating the probability that during each treatment pair the occurrence of a particular result (e.g. 'positive', or 'heads' with coin tossing) was by chance alone. Therefore, the probability of a particular response (e.g. 'positive') to treatment by chance alone is 1/2 for each treatment pair. If four treatment pairs are undertaken, and if the patient responds positively to treatment compared with placebo in all four pairs, then the probability of a positive response during all four pairs of treatment by chance alone is $1/2 \times 1/2 \times 1/2 \times 1/2 = 1/16 = 0.0625$. As this result is close to statistical significance at the 0.05 level, it is reasonably convincing evidence that the patient's positive response is attributable to the treatment.

If the results are less striking and more likely due to chance, the sign test is insufficient, because it lacks statistical power and may lead to erroneous conclusions of a false-negative result (i.e. that no treatment effect exists when it may).

The Student's paired t-*test*

The Student's paired *t*-test is a more powerful statistical test, which utilises all the degrees of symptom severity incorporated in the questionnaire or diary. It is called a 'paired' *t*-test because the observations from the treatment and control groups arise from the same patient(s), rather than from different groups of patients (in which case an 'unpaired' *t*-test would be appropriate).[19]

A potential limitation of the *t*-test is that it assumes that the observations are independent of one another (e.g. that a patient is equally likely to have a symptom or not, or exacerbation or not, on a particular day or week, irrespective of whether he or she had a symptom or not, or exacerbation or not, the day or week before). Some autocorrelation (data that are not independent) is likely to exist in many *n*-of-1 trials, but any adverse impact on the analysis can be reduced by conducting the analysis based on the average of all measurements in a given period rather than individual measurements.

The analysis by means of the Student *t*-test begins by calculating the difference (d_i) between the average symptom scores for placebo and active treatment during each pair of treatment periods. The differences (d_i values) are averaged to generate an overall mean difference ($\bar{d}$). The squared differences between each d_i value and the overall mean difference ($\bar{d}$) are added. This sum is divided by the number of degrees of freedom (df; i.e. the number of treatment periods minus 1), and the square root of the dividend is taken. The resulting *t* statistic is compared with the critical *t*-value (obtained from statistical tables) for the relevant degrees of freedom. If the calculated t value is greater than the corresponding critical t value, the risk of drawing the false-negative conclusion that the patient fared no differently on active treatment than placebo is less than 0.05.

Bayesian statistics

Although data from *n*-of-1 trials often violate strict assumptions underlying parametric tests (e.g. the *t*-test), it is usually not to a degree that threatens validity.[12, 14] However, fewer assumptions are made in applying non-parametric methods.

Bayesian methods of analysis are attractive because they use available data from previous experience and studies to assume a 'prior' distribution for the treatment effect, and they adjust this distribution using the results of another study to produce a 'posterior' distribution.[27, 28] In the context of *n*-of-1 trials, Bayesian methods enable the clinician to build in his or her and the patient's preconceived notions of the likelihood that active treatment is more effective and, if it is, reach a definitive answer sooner than would be the case using other approaches, such as the sign test. The use of a fully parametric Bayesian method for analysing *n*-of-1 trials based on the notion of treatment 'preference' has been recently described.[29]

Ethics

Because the raison d'être of *n*-of-1 trials is to improve the treatment of a consenting and participating patient, one view is that their prime role is to contribute to optimal clinical care rather than to research in a conventional sense, despite using some of the tools developed for research.[30, 31] Indeed, it may be argued that they should be part of routine clinical practice because it is obligatory to find out if a patient is a responder to a treatment known to be of benefit to only a proportion of those who receive it, and to avoid the potential costs of not identifying, and treating inappropriately, a patient who is a non-responder.[15]

As in all clinical practice, it is necessary to obtain informed consent from the participating patient, and the principles of partnership in care and individualised evidence-based medicine are integral to the ethical conduct of *n*-of-1 trials. Furthermore, a written protocol of the trial must be available, which includes explicit data-monitoring procedures to initiate unblinding of the trial.

What are the strengths of an *n*-of-1 trial?

In contrast to centre-based RCTs, which estimate the average treatment effectiveness for the study population, the *n*-of-1 study can provide a reliable estimate of the effectiveness, ineffectiveness or harm of a treatment for an individual patient, which is not confounded by the responses of other patients to the treatment(s) in question.[14] It therefore has the potential to avoid the costs of ineffective and harmful treatment. These potential benefits are greater for treatments that are expensive, prolonged and associated with adverse effects.[15] In addition, *n*-of-1 trials can also help determine whether the occurrence of an adverse effect following exposure to a treatment is causal or coincidental.[32]

Outcomes that are important to individuals, but which are difficult to evaluate practically and accurately in large RCTs (e.g. quality of life, well-being and pain) and elements of functional status scores can be measured in *n*-of-1 trials.[33]

Participation in *n*-of-1 trials can also realise indirect rewards for patients and carers. Patients have reported increased knowledge, awareness and understanding of their condition,[17] which may be attributed to them collecting information about their condition and participating actively in therapeutic decision-making at the end of the trial period.

Given their utility and potential for integration with normal clinical practice, it is perhaps surprising that *n*-of-1 trials are not used more often.[34]

What are the limitations of an *n*-of-1 trial?

The limitations of *n*-of-1 trials are that they are applicable only to assessments of symptomatic treatments of chronic diseases and to therapies that have a rapid onset and offset of action that allow for independent period measurements (see below and panel 15.1).[12, 21]

In addition, it can be difficult, if not impossible, successfully to blind patients and outcome observers if matching drug and control formulations cannot be obtained. However, even when these can be obtained, blinding may be compromised in placebo-controlled trials of drugs with noticeable adverse effects (e.g. dry mouth due to donepezil), even though these effects may not be confined to the active treatment.[32]

Trials of the *n*-of-1 type are much more time consuming for the clinician and patient (and pharmacist and statistician, if used) than is a simple 'trial of therapy'.

The results of *n*-of-1 trials (e.g. evidence of lack of efficacy) may not have any practical significance in changing firmly held beliefs about the efficacy of a treatment. In a recent set of *n*-of-1 trials, patients did not clearly benefit from treatment but still elected to continue using the treatment.[17] Consequently, if *n*-of-1 trials do not shift patients off ineffective treatments, their worth might be questionable.[18]

Finally, the results of an *n*-of-1 trial cannot be generalised confidently beyond the particular patient to other such patients. Perhaps this is a reason why the results of *n*-of-1 trials are often not published and the potential effectiveness and safety of the treatment in a wider range of individual patients and practice settings is not shared with the outside world.[34]

In what situations are *n*-of-1 trials of any practical value to clinicians and researchers?

RCTs of the *n*-of-1 type (*n*-of-1 trials) are best reserved for situations characterised by all of the points listed in panel 15.1 and described in more detail below.[12, 19, 30]

Panel 15.1: **Criteria for deciding whether an *n*-of-1 RCT is likely to be of practical value to clinicians and patients**

The patient
- The patient is keen to consent and collaborate in designing and carrying out an *n*-of-1 RCT
- The patient is ready to change their behaviour (i.e. continue or cease the treatment) according to the results of an *n*-of-1 RCT

The disease
- The disease is chronic and relatively stable, or frequently recurring, so that modest but clinically important treatment or preventive effects can be detected

The treatment
- The effectiveness of the treatment in the particular patient is uncertain
- The potential exists for important treatment benefit or harm
- Prolonged or expensive drug treatment is being considered
- The effect of the treatment is quickly apparent
- The effect of the treatment diminishes quickly after it is discontinued

The trial design
- An unblinded run-in period can be conducted
- An optimal treatment duration is feasible
- Clinically relevant treatment targets (clinical outcomes) can be measured
- Sensible criteria for stopping the trial can be established

The clinician
- The clinician has adequate time and expertise, or has access to a trials support service

Support services
- A pharmacist or pharmacy service is available and willing to collaborate
- Strategies for the statistical analysis and interpretation of the trial data are in place

Ethics
- The *n*-of-1 RCT is ethical

The patient

- *The patient is keen to consent and collaborate in designing and carrying out an* n-*of-1 RCT*. The *n*-of-1 RCT is a cooperative venture between the clinician and patient and requires a fully informed and enthusiastic patient who is likely to comply through a sufficiently prolonged trial.

The disease

- *The disease is chronic and relatively stable, or frequently recurring, so that modest but clinically important treatment or preventive effects can be detected.* Many such conditions lend themselves to *n*-of-1 trials because maintenance therapy is likely to be continued over long periods of time (e.g. Parkinson's disease, asthma, osteoarthritis, attention deficit hyperactivity disorder, chronic inflammatory demyelinating polyradiculoneuropathy, diabetes, fibromyalgia, migraine, epilepsy and hypertension).[21, 24, 30, 35, 36]

The treatment

- *The effectiveness of the treatment in the particular patient is uncertain*:
  - the clinician and the patient are uncertain whether a current treatment is really beneficial
  - the clinician and the patient are uncertain whether a proposed treatment is likely to work in that patient
  - the clinician and the patient are uncertain of the optimal dose of a medication or replacement therapy
  - the patient insists, despite the clinician's best efforts, to take a treatment that the clinician considers ineffective or potentially harmful[17]
  - the patient is experiencing symptoms that both patient and clinician suspect represent an adverse effect of a current (and otherwise beneficial) treatment, but neither the clinician nor the patient is certain.
- *The potential exists for important treatment benefit or harm.*
- *Prolonged or expensive drug treatment is being considered.*
- *The effect of the treatment is quickly apparent.* The more rapidly the treatment manifests its effectiveness (e.g. within hours to days, rather than weeks to months), the quicker and more feasible it is to complete an *n*-of-1 RCT.
- *The effect of the treatment diminishes quickly after it is discontinued.* The more rapidly the effectiveness of the treatment resolves when it is withdrawn (e.g. within hours to a few days, rather than several days to weeks or months), the shorter the wash-out period and the greater the likelihood of no interaction or blunting of the effect.

The trial design

- *An unblinded run-in period can be conducted.* An unblinded run-in is advisable to ensure that there is at least a hint of a response to treatment and that no intolerable adverse effects occur. It may also help determine the optimal dose of active medication for the trial.
- *An optimal treatment duration is feasible.* Treatment periods need to be short enough to make *n*-of-1 RCTs feasible, yet long enough to make them valid. For example, even when the active treatment takes less than a few days to achieve its full effect and less than a few days to cease acting after the treatment is stopped, treatment periods of at least 10 days are required to allow the drug to equilibrate or wash out and to provide sufficient time thereafter to monitor the patient's response to treatment. When peak effects and washout periods are even more delayed, substantially longer treatment periods are required.

  When the treatment target is to prevent or reduce exacerbations of the disease (e.g. recurrent seizures or migraine), the treatment periods need to be long enough to include one or more exacerbations if one is going to occur. If an exacerbation is expected to occur, on average, once every y days, about $3y$ days need to be observed to have 95% confidence of observing, at least one exacerbation.[19] The clinician and patient need to determine whether the exacerbations are sufficiently frequent to make an *n*-of-1 RCT feasible.
- *Clinically relevant treatment targets (clinical outcomes) can be measured.* The most common outcomes/treatment targets are symptoms and indirect measures of the patient's quality of life and well-being (see outcome measures/treatment targets in the section on methods, above).

- *Sensible criteria for stopping the trial can be established.* The criteria for stopping the trial should be prespecified as a certain number (at least three pairs) of treatment periods, or whenever the clinician and patient are certain that the treatment periods within each pair are associated with noticeable and important differences in the treatment targets.

The clinician

- *The clinician has adequate time and expertise, or has access to a trials support service.*

Support services

- *A pharmacist or pharmacy service is available and willing to collaborate.* Pharmacy support is helpful in design, preparation of placebo, supply and packaging, and holding the randomisation code to maintain blinding.[12]
- *Strategies for the statistical analysis and interpretation of the trial data are in place.* In the event that the results are not striking, and may be due to chance, a collaborating statistician or statistical service allows for appropriate statistical analysis and interpretation of the trial data (see the section on analysis, above).

Ethics

- *The* n-*of-1 trial is ethical.* If the spirit in which an *n*-of-1 trial is conducted is as a clinical act, designed to improve the quality of care for an individual patient, it can be considered a part of routine clinical practice, and thereby ethical. This is provided that the patient has given informed consent by participating in the design of the trial and, in collaboration with the clinician, decides when the trial should start and stop. Like any medical innovation, however, the *n*-of-1 trial demands adequate documentation, scrutiny and study.

Clinical examples in which *n*-of-1 trials may be of practical value

The elderly

There is very little evidence from large RCTs about the effectiveness and safety of interventions in old people because they have been excluded from large RCTs at the level of study inclusion criteria, ethics committee approval[37] and publication.[38] Increasing age is also associated with increasing variance in physiological and psychological functioning, and so the choice of drugs and their appropriate doses are likely to be more critical for older than for younger people. Trials of the *n*-of-1 type can be used to compare the therapeutic and adverse effects of drugs, drug doses and drug combinations, and to determine the optimal treatment for individual older patients with chronic, multiple and interacting illnesses taking multiple and interacting medications.[14]

Uncertainty about drug-induced adverse effects

In situations where an effect (favourable or adverse) coincides with an intervention, an *n*-of-1 trial can determine the causality of the association. For example, Price and Grimley Evans[32] described an *n*-of-1 trial in which a significant symptom that might have led to the discontinuation of an active treatment was found later to have occurred during a placebo phase.

Research examples in which *n*-of-1 trials may be of practical value

Improving treatment compliance in large RCTs

Withdrawal of participants from large RCTs can occur because of symptoms thought to be related to the study medicine, but the causal relationship between the study medicine and the symptoms is often not clear. Trials of the *n*-of-1 type can be embedded within larger placebo-controlled trials for participants who consider withdrawing because they believe the study medication is causing them adverse effects.[39]

Refining estimates of treatment effectiveness in populations and individuals

A hierarchical, Bayesian, random-effects model has been used to combine the results of multiple *n*-of-1 trials to obtain an overall estimate of treatment effectiveness for the population, which takes into account the direction and magnitude of the effects and the extent of patient response heterogeneity.[40] This approach has been used to study valerian for chronic insomnia.[41]

The information acquired from other patients' responses in *n*-of-1 trials can also be used to aid in the interpretation of an individual patient's *n*-of-1 trial results.[40]

References

1 Rothwell PM, Metha Z, Howard SC, et al. From subgroups to individuals: general principles and the example of carotid endarterectomy. *Lancet* 2005; **365:** 256–65.

2 Cochrane AL. *Effectiveness and Efficiency: Random Reflections on Health Services.* London: Nuffield Provincial Hospitals Trust, 1972.

3 Majumdar SR, McAlister FA, Furberg CD. From knowledge to practice in chronic cardiovascular disease: a long and winding road. *J Am Coll Cardiol* 2004; **43:** 1738–42.

4 Rothwell PM. External validity of randomised controlled trials: 'To whom do the results of this trial apply?' *Lancet* 2005; **365:** 82–93.

5 Rothwell PM. Subgroup analysis in randomised controlled trials: importance, indications, and interpretation. *Lancet* 2005; **365:** 176–86.

6 Wolf CR, Smith G, Smith RL. Science, medicine, and the future: pharmacogenetics. *BMJ* 2000; **320:** 987–90.

7 Davey Smith G, Ebrahim S, Lewis S, et al. Genetic epidemiology and public health: hope, hype, and future prospects. *Lancet* 2005; **366:** 1484–98.

8 Benson H, McCallie DP. Angina pectoris and the placebo effect. *N Engl J Med* 1979; **300:** 1424–29.

9 Hrobjartsson A, Gotzsche PC. Is the placebo powerless? An analysis of clinical trials comparing placebo with no treatment. *N Engl J Med* 2001; **344:** 1594–602.

10 Barlow DH, Hersen M. *Single Case Study Experimental Designs: Strategies for Studying Behavioural Change,* 2nd edn. Oxford: Pergamon, 1984.

11 Louis TA, Lavori PW, Bailaar JC, Polansky M. Crossover and self-controlled designs in clinical research. *N Engl J Med* 1984; **310:** 24–31.

12 Guyatt G, Sackett D, Taylor DW, et al. Determining optimal therapy – randomised trials in individual patients. *N Engl J Med* 1986; **314:** 889–92.

13 Larson EB. *N*-of-1 clinical trials: a technique for improving medical therapeutics. *West J Med* 1990; **152:** 52–56.

14 Guyatt GH, Heyting A, Jaeschke R, et al. *N* of 1 randomised trials for investigating new drugs. *Control Clin Trials* 1990; **11:** 88–100.

15 Price JD, Grimley Evans J. *N*-of-1 randomized controlled trials ('*N*-of-1 trials'): singularly useful in geriatric medicine. *Age Ageing* 2002; **31:** 227–32.

16 Prochaska JO, DiClemente CC, Norcross JC. In search of how people change. *Am Psychol* 1992; **47:** 1102–04.

17 Woodfield R, Goodyear-Smith F, Arrol B. *N*-of-1 trials of quinine efficacy in skeletal muscle cramps of the leg. *Br J Gen Pract* 2005; **55:** 181–85.

18 Jull A, Bennett D. Do *n*-of-1 trials really tailor treatment? *Lancet* 2005; **365:** 1992–94.
19 Sackett DL, Haynes RB, Guyatt GH, Tugwell P. *Clinical Epidemiology: A Basic Science for Clinical Medicine*, 2nd edn. Boston, MA: Little, Brown, 1991.
20 Karnon J, Qizilbash N. Economic evaluation alongside *n*-of-1 trials: getting closer to the margin. *Health Econ* 2001; **10:** 79–82.
21 Edgington ES. Statistics and single case analysis. *Prog Behav Modif* 1984; **16:** 83–119.
22 Spiegelhalter DJ. Statistical issues in studies of individual response. *Scand J Gastroenterol* 1988; **23:** 40–45.
23 Guyatt GH, Keller JL, Jaeschke R, et al. The *n*-of-1 randomised controlled trial: clinical usefulness. Our three year experience. *Ann Intern Med* 1990; **112:** 293–99.
24 Hankey GJ, Todd AA, Yap PL, Warlow CP. An '*n* of 1' trial of intravenous immunoglobulin treatment for chronic inflammatory demyelinating polyneuropathy. *J Neurol Neurosurg Psychiatry* 1994; **57:** 1137.
25 Bobrovitz CD, Ottenbacher KJ. Comparison of visual inspection and statistical analysis of single-subject data in rehabilitation research. *Am J Phys Med Rehabil* 1998; **77:** 94–102.
26 Conover WJ. *Practical Nonparametric Statistics.* New York: Wiley, 1971: 121.
27 Spiegelhalter DJ, Freedma LS, Parmar MK. Applying Bayesian ideas in drug development and clinical trials. *Stat Med* 1993; **12:** 1501–11.
28 Diamond GA, Kaul S. Prior convictions: Bayesian approaches to the analysis and interpretation of clinical megatrials. *J Am Coll Cardiol* 2004; **43:** 1929–39.
29 Schluter PJ, Ware RS. Single patient (*n*-of-1) trials with binary treatment preference. *Stat Med* 2005; **24:** 2625–36.
30 Guyatt G, Sackett D, Adachi J, et al. A clinician's guide for conducting randomised trials in individual patients. *Can Med Assoc J* 1988; **139:** 497–503.
31 Irwig L, Glasziou P, March L. Ethics of *N*-of-1 trials. *Lancet* 1995; **345:** 469.
32 Price JD, Grimley Evans J. An *N*-of-1 randomised controlled trial ('*N*-of-1 trial') of donepezil in the treatment of non-progressive amnestic syndrome. *Age Ageing* 2002; **31:** 307–09.
33 Kane RI, Rockwook T, Philp I, Finch M. Differences in valuation of functional status components among consumers and professionals in Europe and the United States. *J Clin Epidemiol* 1998; **51:** 657–66.
34 Porta M, Bolumar F, Hernandez I, Vioque J. *N* of 1 trials. Research is needed on why such trials are not more widely used. *BMJ* 1996; **313:** 427.
35 Duggan CM, Mitchell G, Nikles CJ, et al. Managing ADHD in general practice. *N* of 1 trials can help! *Aust Fam Physician* 2000; **29:** 1205–09.
36 Nikles CJ, Clavarino AM, Del Mar CB. Using *n*-of-1 trials as a clinical tool to improve prescribing. *Br J Gen Pract* 2005; **55:** 175–80.
37 Bayer A, Tadd W. Unjustified exclusion of elderly people from studies submitted to research ethics committee for approval: descriptive study. *BMJ* 2000; **321:** 992–93.
38 Bugeja G, Kumar A, Banerjee AK. Exclusion of elderly people from clinical research: a descriptive study of published reports. *BMJ* 1997; **315:** 1059.
39 Avins AL, Bent S, Neuhaus JM. Use of an embedded *N*-of-1 trial to improve adherence and increase information from a clinical study. *Contemp Clin Trials* 2005; **26:** 397–401.
40 Zucker DR, Schmid CH, McIntosh MW, et al. Combined single patient (*N*-of-1) trials to estimate population treatment effects and to evaluate individual patients responses to treatment. *J Clin Epidemiol* 1997; **50:** 401–10.
41 Coexeter PD, Schluter PJ, Eastwood HL, et al. Valerian does not appear to reduce symptoms for patients with chronic insomnia in general practice using series of *n*-of-1 trials. *Complement Ther Med* 2003; **11:** 215–22.

Section 4

Targeting of treatment in routine practice

16

Primary prevention of cardiovascular disease: the absolute-risk-based approach

Rod Jackson

Introduction

For decades the major risk factors for cardiovascular disease have been treated in isolation from each other because of their apparent independent effects on cardiovascular risk. This single risk factor approach to treatment is reflected in the numerous management guidelines still being written about specific risk factors.[1–3] However, the concept of independence of effect of single factors on cardiovascular risk is only relevant in aetiological terms and has little clinical relevance.

From a clinical perspective the only meaningful measure of cardiovascular risk is absolute or global risk, which is the probability that a person will have an event during a defined period. No single cardiovascular risk factor has an independent effect on absolute cardiovascular risk, and this observation was the reason for Geoffrey Rose's often quoted statement that:

> *All policy* [including treatment] *decisions should be based on absolute measures of risk, relative risk is strictly for researchers only.*[4] [Present author's addition.]

A person's absolute risk of cardiovascular disease is determined by the interaction of all risk factors present for that person, and it is not possible to determine the clinical importance of a single factor in isolation from all other risk factors.[5] More importantly, the absolute benefits of interventions to modify single or multiple risk factors have been shown to be directly proportional to a person's pretreatment absolute cardiovascular risk.[6–8]

These observations have major implications for clinical practice. Firstly, some people with, for example, average or below average levels of blood pressure, but who are at high absolute cardiovascular risk, would gain a greater absolute benefit from blood pressure lowering than other people with higher levels of blood pressure but lower absolute cardiovascular risk. Secondly, to determine the benefits of modifying a single risk factor, whatever the level of that factor, an assessment must be made of the person's pretreatment absolute cardiovascular risk. While an absolute-risk-based approach to managing cardiovascular risk has been advocated for at least a decade,[9, 10] and is well supported by both observational and trial evidence, many clinicians still initiate treatment based primarily on levels of single risk factors.

This chapter addresses the key implications of an absolute-risk-based approach to the primary prevention of cardiovascular disease in clinical practice, under the headings:

- What is the influence of multiple risk factors on absolute cardiovascular risk?
- What is the influence of absolute cardiovascular risk on treatment benefits?
- How can absolute cardiovascular risk be estimated in a clinical setting?
- Are absolute-risk-based approaches to cardiovascular risk management appropriate, practical and effective in a clinical setting?

The chapter uses examples mainly on the management of raised blood pressure and blood cholesterol, as these are the most common pharmacologically managed cardiovascular risk factors.

What is the influence of multiple risk factors on absolute cardiovascular risk?

For a given increase in blood pressure or blood cholesterol, there is a remarkably constant relative increase in cardiovascular risk, across a wide range of levels of these risk factors[11–14] (figure 16.1). Based on these 'relative' risk data, clinicians have traditionally targeted treatment to people with high levels of a risk factor, regardless of the presence or absence of other risk factors. However, the clinically relevant 'absolute' cardiovascular risk can vary dramatically in people with the same blood pressure or cholesterol levels (figures 16.2 and 16.3), and some people with high blood pressure or high blood cholesterol can be at much lower absolute cardiovascular risk than other people with lower blood pressure or blood cholesterol levels.[15, 16] Figure 16.2 shows the effect on 5-year absolute cardiovascular risk of successively adding other risk factors to people with systolic blood pressure levels of 110, 120, 130, 140, 150, 160, 170 and 180 mmHg, and figure 16.3 shows a similar pattern of effects of additional risk factors in people with

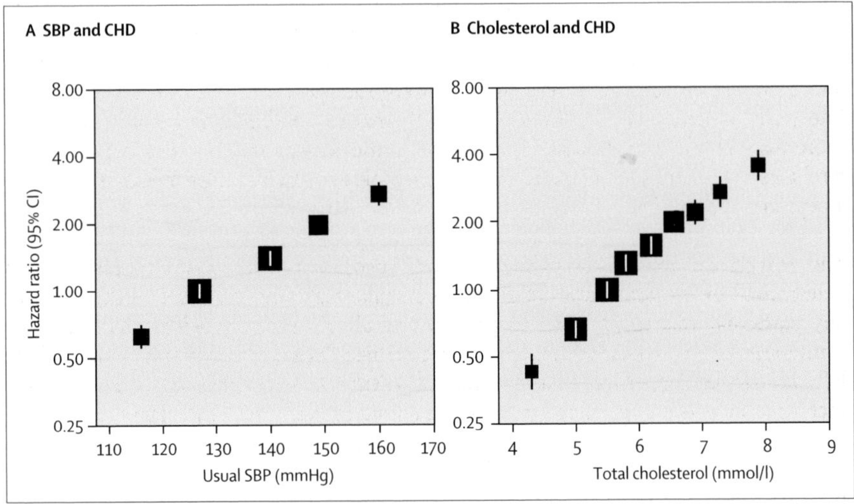

Figure 16.1: **Relative risk of coronary heart disease (CHD) by (A) systolic blood pressure (SBP) and (B) cholesterol level.**

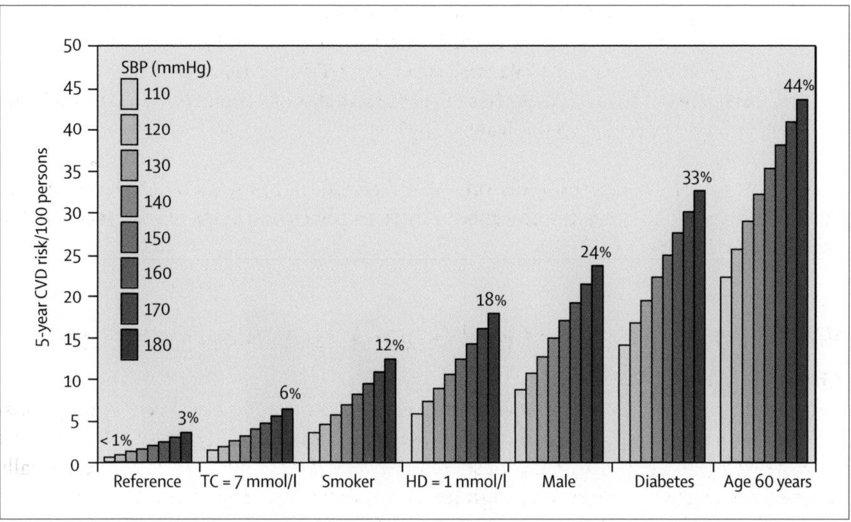

***Figure** 16.2:* **Absolute risk of cardiovascular disease over 5 years in patients by systolic blood pressure (SBP) at specified levels of other risk factors. The reference category is a 50-year-old woman with a total cholesterol (TC) of 4.0 mmol/l, a high density lipoprotein cholesterol (HDL) of 1.6 mmol/l, with no diabetes and a non-smoker. Risks are given for SBP levels of 110, 120, 130, 140, 150, 160, 170 and 180 mmHg. In each of the other categories additional risk factors are added consecutively; for example, the diabetes category is a 50-year-old man with TC = 7 mmol/l, HDL = 1 mmol/l, diabetes and a smoker.**

blood cholesterol levels in the range 4.0–8.0 mmol/l.[16] For any given blood pressure or cholesterol level shown in these two figures, the 5-year cardiovascular risk varies up to 20-fold, depending on the combination of other risk factors present. If more extreme values of some risk factors (e.g. older age) or additional powerful risk factors (e.g. previous symptomatic cardiovascular disease) were included, the potential range of absolute cardiovascular risk for the same blood pressure or cholesterol levels could vary more than 30-fold (not shown). Similarly, the same change in blood pressure or cholesterol levels can have very different effects on absolute cardiovascular risk, depending on a person's risk profile.

The reason for these observations is that absolute cardiovascular disease risk is determined by the interaction of all cardiovascular risk factors present rather than by any particular risk factor.[5] The most powerful absolute risk predictors are previous symptomatic cardiovascular disease and pathophysiological changes such as increasing left ventricular hypertrophy and renal impairment, but numerous other factors, including increasing age, blood pressure and lipid levels, number of cigarettes smoked and male sex, interact multiplicatively to influence risk.[17] Single risk factors, such as high blood pressure or high blood cholesterol, will have a minor influence on a person's absolute risk in the absence of other risk factors, but a major impact in the presence of multiple risk factors.

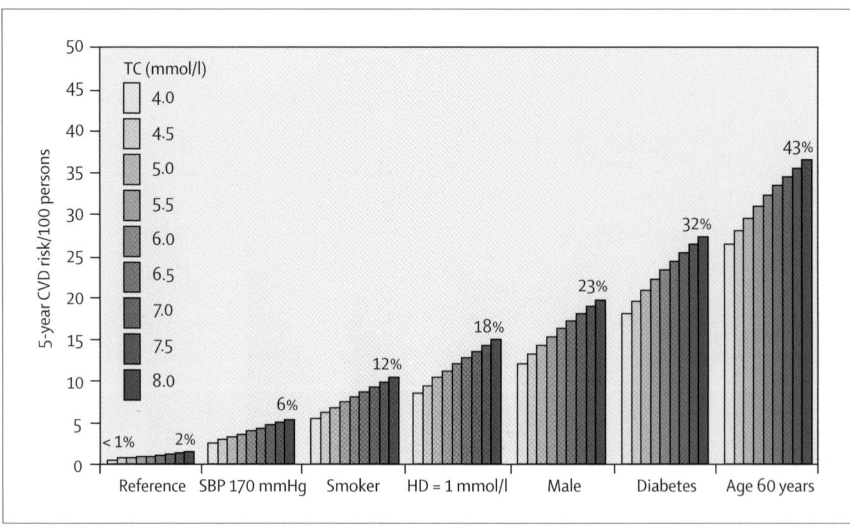

***Figure 16.3:* Absolute risk of cardiovascular disease over 5 years in patients by blood total cholesterol (TC) at specified levels of other risk factors The reference category is a 50-year-old woman with a systolic blood pressure (SBP) of 110 mmHg, a high density lipoprotein cholesterol (HDL) of 1.6 mmol/l, no diabetes and a non-smoker. Risks are given for TC levels of 4.0, 4.5, 5.0, 5.5, 6.0, 6.5, 7.0, 7.5 and 8.0 mmol/l. In each of the other categories additional risk factors are added consecutively; for example, the 60 years category is a 60-year-old man with SBP = 170 mmHg, HDL = 1 mmol/l, diabetes and a smoker.**

What is the influence of absolute cardiovascular risk on treatment benefits?

The absolute cardiovascular risk reductions observed in clinical trials of blood pressure or cholesterol lowering are consistent with the expected absolute benefits predicted from prospective observational studies.[11, 15, 16] For a given reduction in either blood pressure or blood cholesterol, randomised trials show that the absolute cardiovascular treatment benefit is directly proportional to the pretreatment absolute risk.[7, 8, 11, 18] This is illustrated for blood pressure lowering and stroke in figure 16.4. The figure is based on a recent meta-analyses of randomised trials,[19] and shows similar relative reductions in risk whether or not the trials included people with previous stroke. In contrast, the absolute differences in benefit vary approximately two- to three-fold, with a greater absolute benefit in people with previous cardiovascular disease. These differences in benefit are not as great as the 10- to 20-fold differences in risk shown in figures 16.2 and 16.3, because low-risk participants have not generally been included in trials. Of note, there was a more than 10-fold greater absolute treatment benefit for total mortality in older participants (age 60–69 years) compared with younger participants (age 30–49 years) in the Hypertension Detection Follow-up Program,[20] a randomised trial of blood pressure lowering conducted in the 1970s, when the inclusion of low-risk participants in trials was more common.

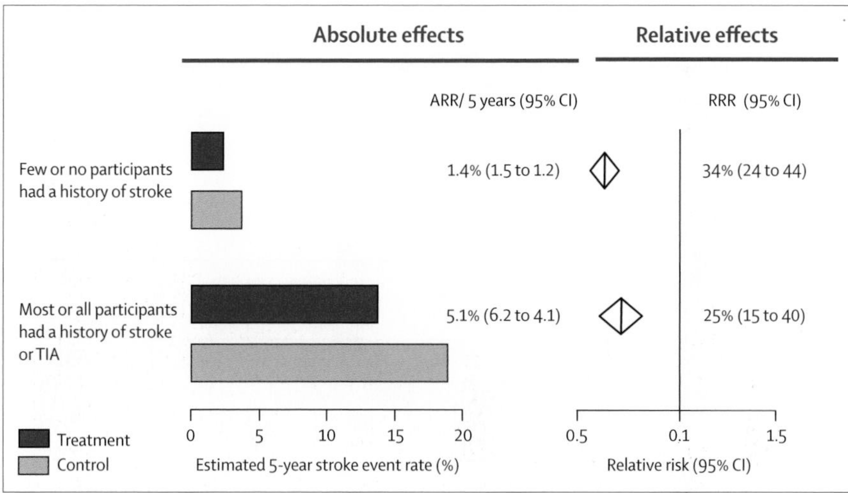

***Figure* 16.4: Absolute and relative treatment effects on stroke in blood pressure lowering trials, by prior history of stroke. CI, confidence interval; TIA, transient ischaemic attack.**

How can absolute cardiovascular risk be estimated in a clinical setting?

Given the wide variation in absolute cardiovascular risk among people with similar blood pressure or blood cholesterol levels, accurate risk assessment is fundamental to effective and efficient clinical management of cardiovascular risk factors. An American study examining clinicians' ability to quantify cardiovascular risk and treatment benefits suggests that their skills in quantifying absolute risk and absolute treatment benefits are poor.[21] Clinicians generally had inflated perceptions of both absolute cardiovascular risk and the absolute benefits of treatment. When given a scenario of a person with raised blood cholesterol, family physicians and general internists overestimated 5-year risk of myocardial infarction more than three-fold and absolute treatment benefits by a greater margin. Studies done in the UK[22] and in Canada[23] report similar results.

Fortunately, a number of paper-based and electronic cardiovascular risk prediction scores are now available to help clinicians quantify risks and treatment benefits. Three commonly used risk prediction charts are illustrated in figures 16.5 to 16.7,[24–26] and these can also be downloaded from the BMJ website.[27] While the degree of uptake of routine quantitative risk prediction by general practitioners is uncertain, an increasing body of research has shown that risk prediction scores can be incorporated in routine general practice.[28, 29]

Many of the available scores are derived from the Framingham Heart Study, a cohort study of approximately 5000 white Americans, established over 50 years ago and replenished by offspring of the original cohort.[30] The risk prediction charts shown in figures 16.5 to 16.7 were all derived from the Framingham Study. Each chart takes a

16 Absolute-risk-based approach in cardiovascular disease

INSTRUCTIONS

- Choose table for men or women.
- **Hypertension** means SBP ≥ 140 or DBP ≥ 90 or on antihypertensive treatment.
- Identify correct column for hypertension, smoking, and diabetes.
- Identify row showing age.
- Read off total:HDL-C ratios at intersection of column and row. If there is an entry, **measure serum cholesterol:HDL ratio**. If no entry, lipids need not be measured unless familial hyperlipidaemia suspected.
- If total:HDL-C ratio confers CHD risk of 15%, consider treatment of **mild hypertension** (SBP 140–159 or DBP 90–99) and with **aspirin**.
- If total:HD-C ratio confers CHD risk of 30%, consider **statin** if serum choesterol ≥ 5.0 mmol/l.
- Decisions on statin at CHD risk between 15% and 30% depend on local policy.
- The table can be used to assess CHD risk at an older age.

Men Total:HDL cholesterol ratio

Hypertension	Yes		No		Yes		Yes		No		No		Yes		No	
Smoking	Yes		Yes		Yes		No		Yes		No		No		No	
Diabetes	Yes		Yes		No		Yes		No		Yes		No		No	
CHD risk	15%	30%	15%	30%	15%	30%	15%	30%	15%	30%	15%	30%	15%	30%	15%	30%
Age 70	2.0	3.0	2.0	3.6	2.1	3.8	2.4	4.4	2.5	4.6	2.9	5.3	3.1	5.6	3.7	6.7
68	2.0	3.2	2.1	3.8	2.2	4.1	2.6	4.7	2.7	4.8	3.0	5.6	3.3	6.0	3.9	7.1
66	2.0	3.4	2.2	4.0	2.4	4.3	2.7	5.0	2.8	5.2	3.2	5.9	3.5	6.3	4.1	7.6
64	2.0	3.6	2.4	4.3	2.5	4.6	2.9	5.3	3.0	5.5	3.5	6.3	3.7	6.8	4.4	8.1
62	2.1	3.8	2.5	4.6	2.7	4.9	3.1	5.6	3.2	5.9	3.7	6.7	3.9	7.2	4.7	8.6
60	2.2	4.1	2.7	4.9	2.9	5.2	3.3	6.0	3.4	6.3	3.9	7.2	4.2	7.7	5.0	9.2
58	2.4	4.4	2.9	5.3	3.1	5.6	3.5	6.5	3.7	6.7	4.2	7.7	4.5	8.3	5.4	9.9
56	2.6	4.7	3.1	5.7	3.3	6.0	3.8	7.0	4.0	7.2	4.6	8.3	4.9	8.9	5.8	10.6
54	2.8	5.1	3.3	6.1	3.6	6.5	4.1	7.5	4.3	7.6	4.9	9.0	5.2	9.6	6.3	-
52	3.0	5.5	3.6	6.6	3.9	7.0	4.4	8.1	4.6	8.4	5.3	9.7	5.7	10.4	6.8	-
50	3.3	6.0	3.9	7.1	4.2	7.6	4.8	8.8	5.0	9.1	5.7	10.5	6.1	-	7.3	-
48	3.6	6.5	4.3	7.8	4.5	8.3	5.2	9.6	5.4	9.9	6.3	-	6.7	-	8.0	-
46	3.9	7.1	4.6	8.5	5.0	9.1	5.7	10.4	5.9	10.8	6.8	-	7.3	-	8.7	-
44	4.3	7.8	5.1	9.3	5.4	9.9	6.3	-	6.5	-	7.5	-	8.0	-	9.6	-
42	4.7	8.6	5.6	10.2	6.0	10.9	6.9	-	7.2	-	8.2	-	8.8	-	10.5	-
40	5.2	9.5	6.2	-	6.6	-	7.6	-	7.9	-	9.1	-	9.7	-		
38	5.8	10.5	6.9	-	7.3	-	8.5	-	8.8	-	10.1	-	10.8	-		
36	6.4	-	7.7	-	8.2	-	9.5	-	9.8	-						
34	7.2	-	8.6	-	9.2	-	10.6	-								
32	8.2	-	9.8	-	10.5	-										
30	9.4	-														
28	10.8	-														

Women	Total:HDL cholesterol ratio															
Hypertension	Yes		No		Yes		Yes		No		No		Yes		No	
Smoking	Yes		Yes		No		Yes		No		Yes		No		No	
Diabetes	Yes		Yes		Yes		No		Yes		No		No		No	
CHD risk	15%	30%	15%	30%	15%	30%	15%	30%	15%	30%	15%	30%	15%	30%	15%	30%
Age 70	2.3	4.1	2.7	4.9	3.3	6.1	3.8	7.0	4.0	7.2	4.6	8.3	5.6	10.2	6.7	-
68	2.3	4.2	2.7	5.0	3.4	6.1	3.9	7.0	4.0	7.3	4.6	8.4	5.7	-	6.8	-
66	2.3	4.2	2.8	5.1	3.4	6.2	3.9	7.1	4.1	7.4	4.7	8.5	5.7	-	6.9	-
64	2.4	4.3	2.8	5.2	3.5	6.4	4.0	7.3	4.2	7.6	4.8	8.7	5.9	-	7.0	-
62	2.4	4.4	2.9	5.3	3.6	6.5	4.1	7.5	4.3	7.8	4.9	9.0	6.0	-	7.2	-
60	2.5	4.6	3.0	5.5	3.7	6.7	4.2	7.7	4.4	8.1	5.1	9.3	6.2	-	7.4	-
58	2.6	4.8	3.1	5.7	3.8	7.0	4.4	8.0	4.6	8.4	5.3	9.6	6.5	-	7.8	-
56	2.7	5.0	3.3	6.0	4.0	7.4	4.6	8.4	4.8	8.8	5.5	10.1	6.8	-	8.1	-
54	2.9	5.3	3.5	6.3	4.3	7.8	4.9	8.9	5.1	9.3	5.8	-	7.2	-	8.6	-
52	3.1	5.6	3.7	6.8	4.5	8.3	5.2	9.5	5.4	9.9	6.2	-	7.7	-	9.2	-
50	3.3	6.1	4.0	7.3	4.9	9.0	5.6	-	5.9	-	6.7	-	8.3	-	9.9	-
48	3.6	6.6	4.3	7.9	5.3	9.8	6.1	-	6.4	-	7.3	-	9.0	-		
46	4.0	7.3	4.8	8.8	5.9	-	6.8	-	7.1	-	8.1	-	10.0	-		
44	4.5	8.2	5.4	9.8	6.6	-	7.6	-	7.9	-	9.1	-				
42	5.1	9.4	6.1	-	7.5	-	8.6	-	9.0	-	10.3	-				
40	5.9	-	7.1	-	8.7	-	10.0	-								
38	7.0	-	8.4	-												
36	8.5	-	10.2	-												

READ BEFORE USING TABLE

- **Do not use for secondary prevention**: patients with MI, angina, PVD, non-haemorrhagic stroke, TIA, or diabetes with microvascular complications have high CHD risk. Treat mild hypertension: treat with aspirin; and treat with statin if serum cholesterol ≥ 5.0 mmol/l.
- **Treat hypertension above mild range** (average ≥ 160 or ≥ 100).
- **Treat mild hypertension** (140–159 or 90–99) with **target organ damage** (LVH, proteinuria, renal impairment) or with diabetes (type 1 or 2).
- Consider drug treatment only **after** 6 months of appropriate advice on smoking, diet, and repeated BP measurements.
- Use **average** of repeated total:HDL-C measurements. If HDL-C not available, assume 1.2 mmol/l.
- Those with total:HDL-C ratio ≥ 8.0 may have familial hyperlipidaemia.
- The table underestimates CHD risk in:
  - LVH on ECG (risk doubled – add 20 years to age)
  - family history of premature CHD (add 6 years)
  - familial hyperlipidaemia
  - British Asians.
- See instructions above table.

Figure 16.5: **Sheffield table for primary prevention of cardiovascular disease. Figures are serum total:HDL cholesterol ratios conferring an estimated risk of coronary heart disease events of 15% and 30% over 10 years.**

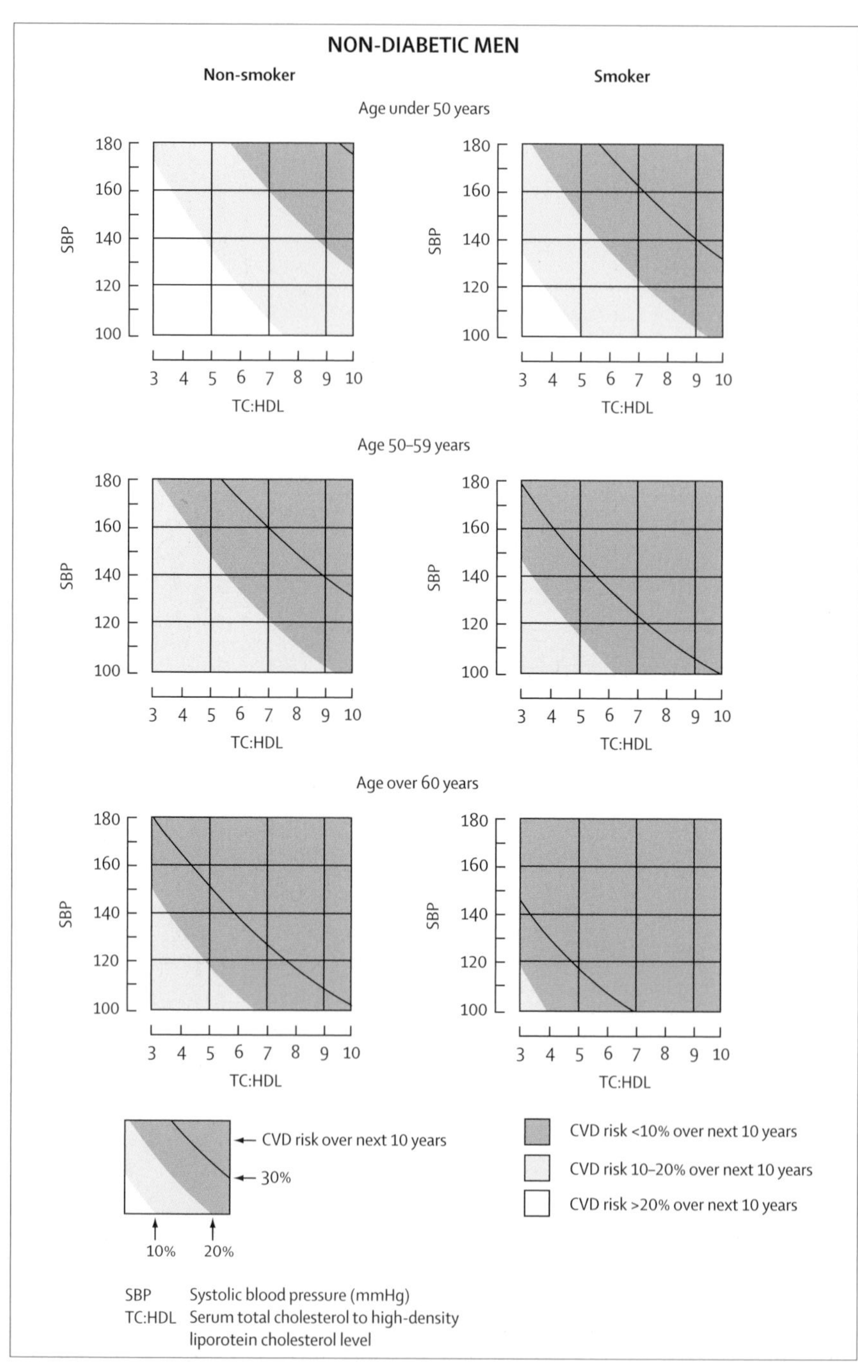

***Figure** 16.6:* **Joint British Societies coronary risk prediction charts.**[25]

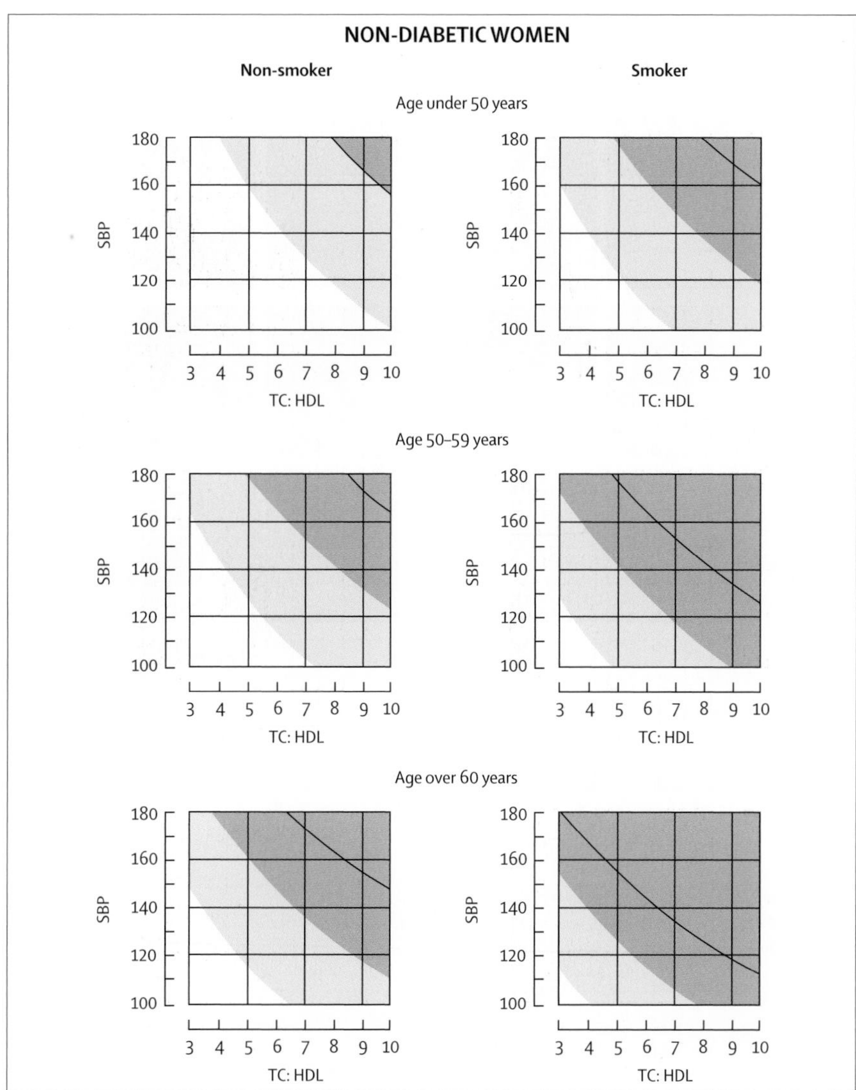

Figure 16.6: Continued.

slightly different approach to risk assessment, and there is conflicting evidence as to which one is the easiest to use and most likely to be interpreted correctly.[22, 29, 31] This is not surprising, as each chart has its strengths and weaknesses; nevertheless, all perform reasonably well. Moreover, there is increasing evidence demonstrating that absolute-risk-based approaches to cardiovascular disease management improve practice.[28, 32]

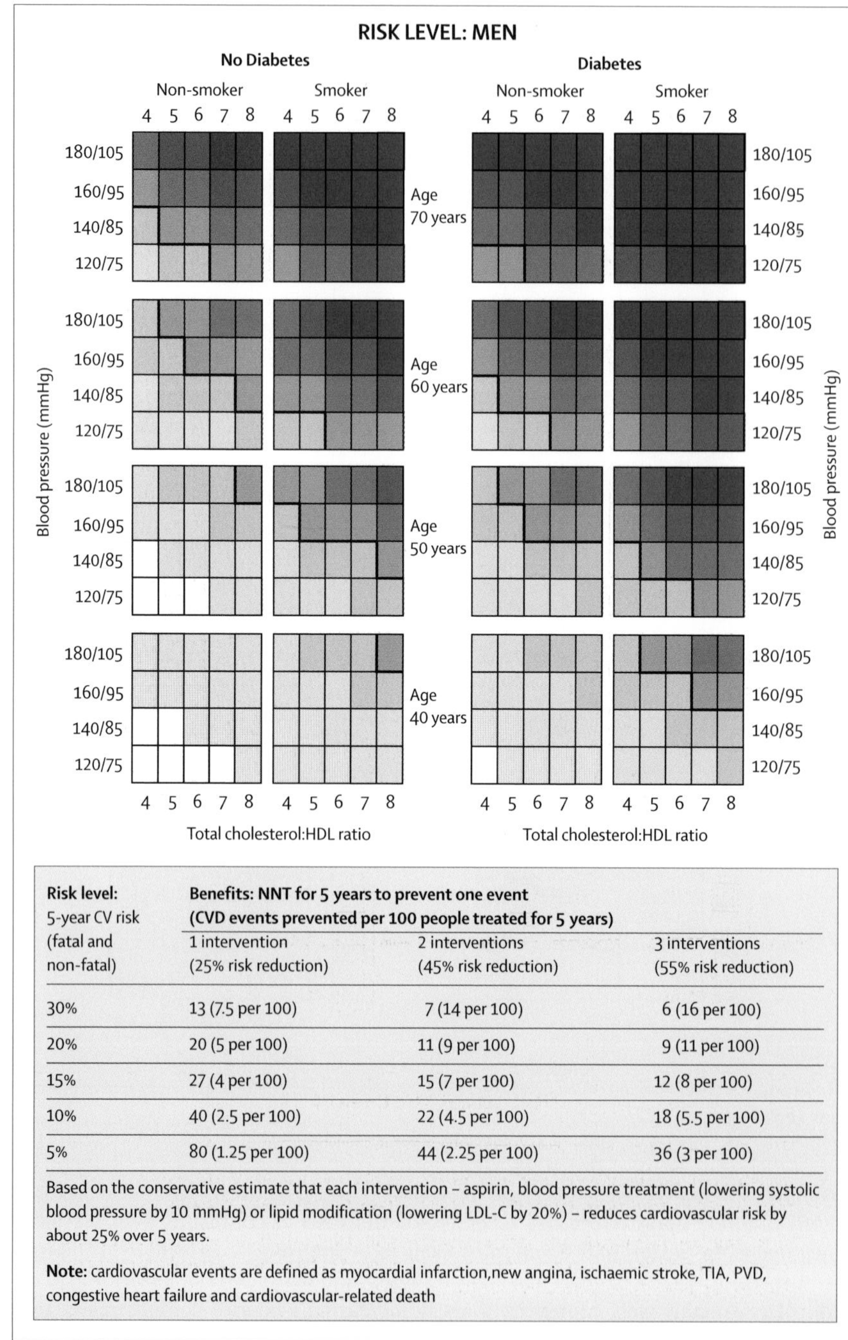

Risk level: 5-year CV risk (fatal and non-fatal)	Benefits: NNT for 5 years to prevent one event (CVD events prevented per 100 people treated for 5 years)		
	1 intervention (25% risk reduction)	2 interventions (45% risk reduction)	3 interventions (55% risk reduction)
30%	13 (7.5 per 100)	7 (14 per 100)	6 (16 per 100)
20%	20 (5 per 100)	11 (9 per 100)	9 (11 per 100)
15%	27 (4 per 100)	15 (7 per 100)	12 (8 per 100)
10%	40 (2.5 per 100)	22 (4.5 per 100)	18 (5.5 per 100)
5%	80 (1.25 per 100)	44 (2.25 per 100)	36 (3 per 100)

Based on the conservative estimate that each intervention – aspirin, blood pressure treatment (lowering systolic blood pressure by 10 mmHg) or lipid modification (lowering LDL-C by 20%) – reduces cardiovascular risk by about 25% over 5 years.

Note: cardiovascular events are defined as myocardial infarction,new angina, ischaemic stroke, TIA, PVD, congestive heart failure and cardiovascular-related death

Figure 16.7: **New Zealand cardiovascular risk prediction charts.**

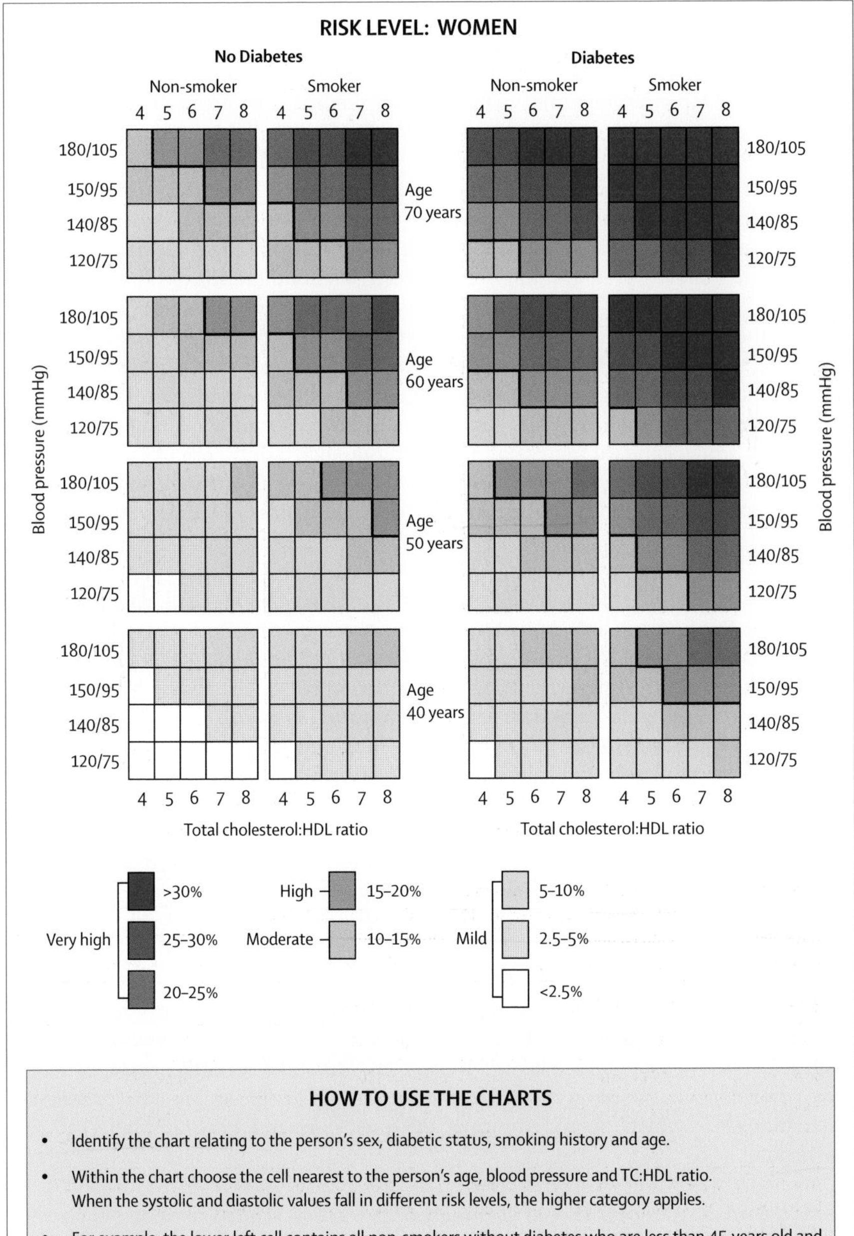

HOW TO USE THE CHARTS

- Identify the chart relating to the person's sex, diabetic status, smoking history and age.
- Within the chart choose the cell nearest to the person's age, blood pressure and TC:HDL ratio. When the systolic and diastolic values fall in different risk levels, the higher category applies.
- For example, the lower left cell contains all non-smokers without diabetes who are less than 45 years old and have a TC:HDL ratio less than 4.5 and a blood pressure less than 130/80 mmHg. People who fall exactly on a threshold between cells are paced in the cell indicating higher risk.

Figure 16.7: Continued.

A number of other cardiovascular risk prediction scores have been developed or are currently under development. One of the best known is based on the Prospective Cardiovascular Munster (PROCAM) Study, a working population in northern Germany, initiated in 1979.[33] More recent scores include one for predicting coronary heart disease and stroke risk in people with diabetes, based on about 5000 diabetics from the UK Prospective Diabetes Study,[34] and another for predicting cardiovascular mortality, based on 47 088 adults with raised blood pressure from eight European and North American trials.[35] A European research group has recently been established to generate risk charts specific to European populations (the SCORE Project) by pooling multiple European cohorts; the group has already produced interim Northern and Southern European risk charts.[36]

Most of the scores described above were developed using regression-based statistical modelling, although the PROCAM investigators have recently described a neural-network-based score.[37] This neural network model predicted about 75% of all cohort cardiovascular events over 10 years within a high-risk subgroup including only 7.9% of the cohort, while standard regression modelling predicted only 46% of events in 8.4% of the same cohort. However, the investigators have yet to validate their model in independent populations, and neural network models are typically less generalisable than regression models.

Numerous validation studies have been carried out on the Framingham prediction scores, but the findings are conflicting. Framingham investigators and others report that the Framingham risk scores perform reasonably well in populations with coronary rates similar to North American rates and that the scores can be recalibrated for other populations.[38–40] Other investigators report less favourable results for both the discriminatory power and generalisability of predictive functions from the Framingham Heart Study.[41, 42] Unfortunately, validation studies generally report relative measures of validity, such as relative risks or the area under receiver–operator characteristic curves. These relative measures of validity fail to capture the more clinically relevant absolute predictive validity of the tools, such as the positive predictive and negative predictive values of risk assessment in different clinical populations, or the proportion of all events that can be predicted using different cut-off levels of calculated risk.

Scores including a greater range of risk factors[34, 37] tend to be more predictive than those with fewer factors,[16] suggesting there is potential to improve on the predictive validity of current models, and the usefulness of recently identified predictive factors such as C-reactive protein[43] are being investigated. Moreover, recently developed scores have generally been based on much greater numbers of people and in a wider range of populations,[35, 36] which should improve the precision and generalisability of risk prediction.

Primary care practitioners should ideally chose prediction scores based on people with similar risk profiles and cardiovascular event rates to their practice populations. At a regional or national level, the proportions of people in a population who are likely to be classified at different absolute risk levels using the chosen risk score should be estimated so that practical and financially sustainable treatment thresholds can be set.[39, 42] Prediction models should ideally be developed nationally, but if international scores are used they should be validated nationally.[40] With the increasing use of electronic medical records it is now theoretically possible to link risk-factor profiles with disease-event data in large numbers of people.[44, 45] These recent developments in information technology will enable new cardiovascular risk prediction scores to be generated rapidly as part of routine clinical practice.

Are absolute-risk-based approaches to cardiovascular risk management appropriate, practical and effective in the clinical setting?

The potential health impacts of an absolute-risk-based treatment strategy for managing raised blood pressure in primary care has been investigated in New Zealand using data from a large cross-sectional survey of cardiovascular risk factors conducted in 1993–1994.[46] The survey was undertaken just prior to the introduction of national absolute-risk-based guidelines for managing raised blood pressure.[47] Approximately 12% of the population aged 35–79 years were estimated to be taking blood pressure lowering medication at the time of the survey. It was estimated that an absolute-risk-based strategy targeting treatment to those with raised blood pressure if they also had a calculated 5-year cardiovascular risk of greater than 15% could have averted almost 40% more cardiovascular events than the observed practice, despite a less than 10% increase in the total numbers requiring drug treatment.

While the potential benefits of targeting treatment are impressive, the costs of the comprehensive risk assessment required to identify those at risk must also be considered. General practitioners have questioned whether the ambitious recommendations described in the recent UK National Service Framework for cardiovascular disease are either realistic or appropriate given the major workload implications yet modest benefits.[48, 49] The UK framework endorses joint British recommendations on preventing coronary heart disease which state that primary health teams should assess absolute cardiovascular risk in adult patients every 5 years and treat those with a 10-year coronary heart disease risk of greater than 15%.[50]

Marshall and Rouse[51] recently assessed the likely resource implications and health benefits of the non-targeted risk assessment strategy recommended in the UK National Service Framework, and compared it to an alternative targeted risk assessment strategy. They modelled both a targeted strategy of preselection of people for full risk assessments, based on a proxy risk assessment using risk factors typically documented by general practitioners (i.e. age, gender, smoking and diabetes status, and assuming standard population average blood lipid and blood pressure levels), and the UK National Framework assessment strategy. They compared the resources required and events averted, and concluded that a targeted strategy would not only prevent more cardiovascular events but would be cheaper and have less impact on general practice workloads.

These modelling studies[46, 51] provide support for targeted absolute-risk-based screening and treatment in primary care and, as discussed in a previous section, there is substantial evidence from randomised trials that the absolute benefits of treating cardiovascular risk factors are directly proportional to person's pretreatment absolute risk. A recent Cochrane Systematic Review of multiple risk factor intervention trials was unable to demonstrate any effect on mortality,[52] but multiple risk factor interventions should not be confused with interventions targeting people at high absolute risk identified through multiple risk factor assessment. The majority of participants in the trials included in the Cochrane Review were at low absolute cardiovascular risk before the interventions, and therefore even effective interventions could have at most a very modest impact. A novel multiple risk factor intervention approach involving a 'polypill' incorporating a diuretic, beta-blocker, angiotensin-converting enzyme (ACE) inhibitor, statin, aspirin and folic acid, has been estimated to be able to reduce cardiovascular risk by about 80%.[53] Wald and Law[53] state that: 'one third of people taking this pill from age 55 would benefit, gaining on average about 11 years of life free from an IHD event or stroke.' The key determinant of the large estimated absolute benefit of the polypill is the targeting of treatment to high-risk people rather than the large relative benefit of the intervention.

It is this author's opinion that there is sufficient evidence of both effectiveness and efficiency to endorse highly targeted absolute-risk-based screening and treatment strategies for managing cardiovascular risk in general practice. However, current national and international guidelines are not sufficiently targeted to be sustainable without substantial injections of new funding.[48, 49, 51] Priority should be given to identifying and treating those people likely to be at very high risk. In the first instance, general practitioners should establish systems to identify and treat all people with a personal history of cardiovascular disease, who are the patient group at highest risk. The next priority for assessment should be older people (men over about 55 years and women over about 65 years), who experience the majority of new cardiovascular events. Intensive treatment should be targeted at those with cardiovascular disease or with a calculated risk similar to that for people with cardiovascular disease (above about 20% 5-year cardiovascular risk using the New Zealand risk charts shown in figure 16.7). Younger people with these levels of risk are likely to be already known to their general practitioners, because they would have diabetes or be smokers with high blood pressure. Neither systematic nor opportunistic screening and treatment of other people should be considered a priority until general practitioners have demonstrated that they have the ability and capacity to identify and manage the high-risk people described above.

Summary

- From a clinical perspective, the only meaningful measure of cardiovascular risk is absolute or global risk, which is the probability that a person will have an event during a defined period.
- The absolute benefits of interventions to modify single or multiple risk factors have been shown to be directly proportional to the pretreatment absolute cardiovascular risk.
- Some people with, for example, average or below average levels of blood pressure or blood cholesterol, but who are at high absolute cardiovascular risk, would gain a greater absolute benefit from blood pressure or lipid lowering than other people with higher levels of these risk factors but lower absolute cardiovascular risk.

- It is not possible to determine the benefits of modifying a single risk factor, whatever the level of that factor, without initially assessing a person's pretreatment absolute cardiovascular risk.
- Clinicians' ability to quantify absolute cardiovascular risk and treatment benefits in their heads is poor.
- Paper-based and electronic cardiovascular risk prediction scores are now readily available to help clinicians quantify risks and treatment benefits.
- There is evidence demonstrating that absolute-risk-based approaches to cardiovascular disease management using risk prediction scores improve practice.
- Multiple risk factor interventions should not be confused with interventions targeting people at high absolute risk identified through multiple risk factor assessment.
- Current national and international guidelines on cardiovascular risk assessment and treatment are not sufficiently targeted to be cost-effective or sustainable.
- Highly targeted absolute-risk-based screening and treatment strategies need to be developed for effectively and efficiently managing cardiovascular risk in clinical practice.

References

1 Chobanian AV, Bakris GL, Black HR, et al. The Seventh Report of the Joint National Committee on Prevention, Detection, Evaluation, and Treatment of High Blood Pressure: the JNC 7 report. *JAMA* 2003; **289:** 2560–72.

2 Expert Panel on Detection Evaluation Treatment of High Blood Cholesterol in Adults. Executive Summary of The Third Report of The National Cholesterol Education Program (NCEP) Expert Panel on Detection, Evaluation, and Treatment of High Blood Cholesterol In Adults (Adult Treatment Panel III). *JAMA* 2001; **285:** 2486–97.

3 Guidelines Subcommittee. 1999 World Health Organization–International Society of Hypertension Guidelines for the Management of Hypertension. *J Hypertens* 1999; **17:** 151–83.

4 Rose G. Sick individuals and sick populations. *Int J Epidemiol* 2001; **30:** 427–32.

5 Kannel WB. Some lessons in cardiovascular epidemiology from Framingham. *Am J Cardiol* 1976; **37:** 269–82.

6 Mulrow CD, Cornell JA, Herrera CR, et al. Hypertension in the elderly. Implications and generalizability of randomised trials. *JAMA* 1994; **272:** 1932–38.

7 Rodgers A, Neal B, MacMahon S. The effects of blood pressure lowering in cerebrovascular disease. *Neurol Rev Int* 1997; **2:** 12–15.

8 West of Scotland Coronary Prevention Group. West of Scotland Coronary Prevention Study: identification of high-risk groups and comparison with other cardiovascular intervention trials. *Lancet* 1996; **348:** 1339–42.

9 Alderman MH. Blood pressure management: individualised treatment based on absolute risk and the potential for benefit. *Ann Intern Med* 1993; **119:** 329–35.

10 Jackson R, Barham P, Maling T, et al. The management of raised blood pressure in New Zealand. *BMJ* 1993; **307:** 107–10.

11 Law MR, Wald NJ. Risk factor thresholds: their existence under scrutiny. *BMJ* 2002; **324:** 1570–76.

12 Lewington S, Clarke R, Qizilbash N, et al., for the Prospective Studies C. Age-specific relevance of usual blood pressure to vascular mortality: a meta-analysis of individual data for one million adults in 61 prospective studies. *Lancet.* 2002; **360:** 1903–13.

13 Eastern Stroke and Coronary Heart Disease Collaborative Research Group. Blood pressure, cholesterol, and stroke in eastern Asia. *Lancet* 1998; **352:** 1801–07.

14 Neal B, MacMahon S, Chapman N. Effects of ACE inhibitors, calcium antagonists, and other blood-pressure-lowering drugs: results of prospectively designed overviews of randomised trials. Blood Pressure Lowering Treatment Trialists' Collaboration. *Lancet* 2000; **356:** 1955–64.

15 Neaton JD, Wentworth D, for the Multiple Risk Factor Intervention Trial Research G. Serum cholesterol, blood pressure, cigarette smoking, and death from coronary heart disease. Overall findings and differences by age for 316,099 white men. *Arch Intern Med* 1992; **152:** 56–64.

16 Anderson KV, Odell PM, Wilson PWF, Kannel WB. Cardiovascular disease risk profiles. *Am Heart J* 1991; **121:** 293–98.

17 D'Agostino RB, Russell MW, Huse DM, et al. Primary and subsequent coronary risk appraisal: new results from the Framingham study. *Am Heart J* 2000; **139**: 272–81.

18 Lawes C, Bennett D, Lewington S, Rodgers A. Blood pressure and coronary heart disease: a review of the evidence. *Semin Vasc Med* 2002; **2**: 355–68.

19 Lawes C. Assessing the impact of different blood pressure lowering strategies to lower the global burden of cardiovascular disease. PhD thesis, University of Auckland, 2003.

20 Hypertension Detection and Follow-up Program Cooperative Group. Five year findings of the Hypertension Detection and Follow-up Program. 1. Reduction in mortality in persons with high blood pressure, including mild hypertension. *JAMA* 1979; **242**: 2562–71.

21 Friedmann PD, Brett AS, Mayo-Smith MF. Differences in generalists' and cardiologists' perceptions of cardiovascular risk and the outcomes of preventive therapy in cardiovascular disease. *Ann Intern Med* 1996; **124**: 414–21.

22 McManus RJ, Mant J, Meulendijks CF, et al. Comparison of estimates and calculations of risk of coronary heart disease by doctors and nurses using different calculation tools in general practice: cross sectional study. *BMJ* 2002; **324**: 459–64.

23 Grover SA, Lowensteyn I, Esrey KL, et al. Do doctors accurately assess coronary risk in their patients? Preliminary results of the coronary health assessment study. *BMJ* 1995; **310**: 975–78.

24 Wallis EJ, Ramsay LE, Haq IU, et al. Coronary and cardiovascular risk estimation for primary prevention: validation of a new Sheffield table in the 1995 Scottish Health Survey population. *BMJ* 2000; **320**: 671–76.

25 HEART UK, Primary Care Cardiovascular Society, The Stroke Association, British Cardiac Society, British Hypertension Society, Diabetes UK. JBS 2: Joint British Societies' guidelines on prevention of cardiovascular disease in clinical practice. *Heart* 2005; **91**: 1–52.

26 Jackson R. Updated New Zealand cardiovascular disease risk-benefit prediction guide. *BMJ* 2000; **320**: 709–10.

27 BMJ. Available at: http://bmj.com (accessed February 2007).

28 Montgomery AA, Fahey T, Peters TJ, et al. Evaluation of computer based clinical decision support system and risk chart for management of hypertension in primary care: randomised controlled trial. *BMJ* 2000; **320**: 686–89.

29 Isles CG, Ritchie LD, Murchie P, Norrie J. Risk assessment in primary prevention of coronary heart disease: randomised comparison of three scoring methods. *BMJ* 2000; **320**: 690–91.

30 Kannel WB. The Framingham Study: its 50-year legacy and future promise. *J Atherosler Thromb* 2000; **6**: 60–6.

31 Haq IU, Ramsay LE, Jackson PR, Wallis EJ. Prediction of coronary risk for primary prevention of coronary heart disease: a comparison of methods. *Q J Med* 1999; **92**: 379–85.

32 Hall LML, Jung RT, Leese GP. Controlled trial of effect of documented cardiovascular risk scores on prescribing. *BMJ* 2003; **326**: 251–52.

33 Assmann G, Cullen P, Schulte H. Simple scoring scheme for calculating the risk of acute coronary events based on the 10-year follow-up of the prospective cardiovascular Munster (PROCAM) study. *Circulation* 2002; **105**: 310–15.

34 Stevens RJ, Kothari V, Adler AI, et al. The UKPDS risk engine: a model for the risk of coronary heart disease in type II diabetes (UKPDS 56). *Clin Sci* 2001; **101**: 671–79.

35 Pocock SJ, McCormack V, Gueyffier F, et al. A score for predicting risk of death from cardiovascular disease in adults with raised blood pressure, based on individual patient data from randomised controlled trials. *BMJ* 2001; **323**: 75–81.

36 Menotti A, Lanti M, Puddu PE, Kromhout D. Coronary heart disease incidence in northern and southern European populations: a reanalysis of the seven countries study for a European coronary risk chart. *Heart* 2000; **84**: 238–44.

37 Voss R, Cullen P, Schulte H, Assmann G. Prediction of risk of coronary events in middle-aged men in the Prospective Cardiovascular Munster Study (PROCAM) using neural networks. *Int J Epidemiol* 2002; **31**: 1253–62.

38 D'Agostino RB Sr, Grundy S, Sullivan LM, Wilson P. Validation of the Framingham coronary heart disease prediction scores: results of a multiple ethnic groups investigation. *JAMA* 2001; **286**: 180–87.

39 Cappuccio FP, Oakeshott P, Strazzullo P, Kerry SM. Application of Framingham risk estimates to ethnic minorities in United Kingdom and implications for primary prevention of heart disease in general practice: cross sectional population based study. *BMJ* 2002; **325**: 1271.

40 Ramachandran S, French JM, Vanderpump MPJ, et al. Using the Framingham model to predict heart disease in the United Kingdom: retrospective study. *BMJ* 2000; **320**: 676–77.

41 Diverse Populations Collaborative G. Prediction of mortality from coronary heart disease among diverse populations: is there a common predictive function? *Heart* 2002; **88**: 222–28.

42 Hense HW, Schulte H, Lowel H, et al. Framingham risk function overestimates risk of coronary heart disease in men and women from Germany – results from the MONICA Augsburg and the PROCAM cohorts. *Eur Heart J* 2003; **24:** 937–45.

43 Pearson TA, Mensah GA, Alexander RW, et al. Markers of inflammation and cardiovascular disease: application to clinical and public health practice: A statement for healthcare professionals from the Centers for Disease Control and Prevention and the American Heart Association. *Circulation* 2003; **107:** 499–511.

44 Black N. Using clinical databases in practice. *BMJ* 2003; **326:** 2–3.

45 Lundin J, Lundin M, Isola J, Joensuu H. A web-based system for individualised survival estimation in breast cancer. *BMJ* 2003; **326:** 29.

46 Baker S, Priest P, Jackson R. Targeting blood pressure-lowering therapy in a primary care setting; the influence of absolute risk-based treatment thresholds on recommendations for therapy, and cardiovascular disease events averted by therapy. *BMJ* 2000; **320:** 680–85.

47 Core Services Committee. Guidelines for the Management of Mildly Raised Blood Pressure in New Zealand. Wellington, 1995.

48 Toop L, Richards D. Preventing cardiovascular disease in primary care. *BMJ* 2001; **323:** 246–47.

49 Hippisley-Cox J, Pringle M. General practice workload implications of the national service framework for coronary heart disease: cross sectional survey. *BMJ* 2001; **323:** 269–70.

50 Wood D, Durrington P, Poulter N, et al. Joint British recommendations on prevention of coronary heart disease in clinical practice. *Heart* 1998; **80** (suppl 2): S1–29.

51 Marshall T, Rouse A. Resource implications and health benefits of primary prevention strategies for cardiovascular disease in people aged 30 to 74: mathematical modelling study. *BMJ* 2002; **325:** 197.

52 Ebrahim S, Davey Smith G. Multiple risk factor interventions for primary prevention of coronary heart disease. *Cochrane Database Systematic Review* 2000(2): CD001561.

53 Wald NJ, Law MR. A strategy to reduce cardiovascular disease by more than 80%. *BMJ* 2003; **326:** 1419. Errata: *BMJ* 2003; **327:** 586, and 2006; **60:** 823.

Antithrombotic therapy to prevent stroke in patients with atrial fibrillation

Robert G. Hart

Introduction

Atrial fibrillation is a common cardiac dysrhythmia that predisposes to brain infarction via embolism of stasis-precipitated thrombi forming in the left atrial appendage. There is indisputable evidence from consistent results of randomised clinical trials (RCTs) that treatment with adjusted-dose warfarin sharply reduces the risk of stroke nearly to the levels of age-matched people without atrial fibrillation. From pooled results of RCTs comparing warfarin to control (2900 participants in six trials), stroke is reduced by 62% (95% confidence interval (CI) 48 to 72).[1] Comparing adjusted-dose warfarin to antiplatelet therapy (10 969 participants in nine trials), stroke is reduced by 36% (95% CI 20 to 45).[1,2] These relative risk reductions by anticoagulation apply to all subgroups of atrial fibrillation patients in which it has been assessed.[3–5]

The management implication at first seems straightforward: all patients with atrial fibrillation who can safely receive adjusted-dose warfarin should be anticoagulated. This uncomplicated approach has been endorsed, in essence, by several guidelines that would withhold anticoagulation only for a small fraction of relatively young atrial fibrillation patients without cardiovascular comorbidities.[6,7] But we can do better for atrial fibrillation patients by individualising therapy using solid clinical evidence emerging from these same RCTs.

Does cardioversion to sinus rhythm reduce the stroke risk for patients with atrial fibrillation?

We still do not know for sure. In the only large RCT comparing rate control with cardioversion/antiarrhythmic therapy (Atrial Fibrillation Follow-up Investigation of Rhythm Management, AFFIRM),[8] investigators were encouraged to anticoagulate participants in both treatment arms, but it was permitted to stop warfarin at the physician's discretion after 4–12 weeks of sustained sinus rhythm. Sinus rhythm was present in 82%, 73% and 63% of patients assigned to rhythm control after 1, 3 and 5 years of follow-up, respectively. All-cause mortality was the primary outcome, and it was marginally lower (2.5% absolute reduction in death, $p = 0.06$) in those assigned to *rate control* during the mean follow-up of about 3.5 years.[8] The numbers and types of stroke were nearly identical (table 17.1).[9] Fewer participants in the rhythm-control arm were anticoagulated during follow-up compared to those assigned rate control (~70% versus ~90%, respectively), and the equal numbers of strokes with fewer anticoagulated patients may offer some support to the proposal that rhythm control reduces stroke. However, strokes widely overlapped, and withdrawal of anticoagulation was likely more frequent in younger, healthier participants whose stroke rates are inherently low.

	Rate control (n = 2027)	Rhythm control (n =2033)
All strokes	105	106
Ischaemic stroke	77	80
Fatal or disabling	35	38
(presumed cardioembolic)	(41)	(44)
Intracerebral haemorrhages	18	16
Subdural haematomas	11	13
All deaths	310	356
Anticoagulated during follow-up	~90%	~70%

*AFFIRM trial randomising recent-onset atrial fibrillation patients with one additional stroke risk factor to rate control versus cardioversion/antiarrhythmic drug therapy.[9] Investigators were encouraged to anticoagulate participants in both treatment arms, but it was permitted to stop warfarin after 4–12 weeks of sinus rhythm.

***Table 17.1:* Strokes in the AFFIRM trial[9] ***

In short, in the wake of several RCTs testing rhythm versus rate control in atrial fibrillation patients, the value of cardioversion in reducing stroke risk and (perhaps) the need for anticoagulation has not been convincingly established, in part due to confounding protocol stipulations encouraging anticoagulation of all participants. While long-term restoration of sinus rhythm should logically decrease formation and embolism of left atrial appendage thrombi, solid clinical evidence is lacking and cardioversion/antiarrhythmic drug therapy cannot be recommended with confidence to reduce stroke (particularly given the trend toward increased mortality seen in the AFFIRM trial).

Is there anything as efficacious as adjusted-dose warfarin for preventing stroke in atrial fibrillation patients?

As noted above, RCTs have firmly established the value of antithrombotic therapies for reducing stroke in patients with atrial fibrillation.[1] To date, 27 RCTs have compared different anticoagulant and antiplatelet agents with placebo/control and with each other in over 27 000 participants. Stroke risk (considering both ischaemic and haemorrhagic stroke) is reduced by approximately 60% with adjusted-dose warfarin and by about 20% with aspirin.[1] Adjusted-dose warfarin reduces stroke by about 40%, as compared with antiplatelet therapy.[2] Aspirin appears to have its major effect on the non-disabling, non-cardioembolic strokes from which elderly, often hypertensive, atrial fibrillation patients are not immune.[10] Both the benefits and risks of anticoagulation appear greater in very elderly atrial fibrillation patients, and the ongoing primary-care-based Birmingham (UK) Atrial Fibrillation Trial in the Aged (BAFTA) is comparing adjusted-dose warfarin with aspirin in those over 75 years old, with results anticipated in late 2007.

The novel direct thrombin inhibitor ximelagatran was compared with high-quality, adjusted-dose warfarin in two large RCTs involving 7329 moderate-risk atrial fibrillation patients.[11, 12] The dose of ximelagatran (36 mg twice daily) did not require adjustment in patients with normal renal function, and no coagulation monitoring was required. By pooled analysis, the rates of stroke and death were equal for those assigned to ximelagatran (93 strokes, 201 deaths) versus adjusted-dose warfarin (102 strokes, 205 deaths), with a suggestion of reduced serious haemorrhage with ximelagatran. However, about 6% of those given ximelagatran developed elevations of liver function tests between 1 and 4 months after initiation; these elevations were usually transient but appeared to have serious consequences in two or three participants. Because of concerns about hepatic toxicity, differing trends in the open-label versus double-blind trial and inadequate numbers of strokes to establish convincingly clinical equivalence with warfarin, the US Food and Drug Administration (FDA) declined to approve the use of ximelagatran. In early 2006, ximelagatran was withdrawn from the market worldwide, due to continuing concerns about hepatotoxicity.

The combination of clopidogrel and aspirin was compared with high-quality anticoagulation in 6706 atrial fibrillation patients in the large ACTIVE-W clinical trial.[2] Warfarin was more efficacious, and the relative risk reduction with warfarin, compared to clopidogrel plus aspirin (38%), was similar to that seen from pooled analysis of aspirin alone (36%).[1, 2] Whether the combination of clopidogrel plus aspirin offers advantages over aspirin alone in low-risk atrial fibrillation patients and in those who cannot/will not take warfarin is being tested in the ongoing large ACTIVE-A trial. A multinational trial comparing idraparineux, a long-acting parenteral factor Xa inhibitor, to adjusted-dose warfarin (AMADEUS), was recently stopped due to excessive bleeding in patients in the experimental treatment arm, but no specific results have yet been published.

The therapeutic window bounded by beneficial antithrombotic effects and adverse bleeding is relatively narrow for the use of anticoagulants in elderly atrial fibrillation patients. Warfarin has been used clinically for more than 50 years (and even longer for other purposes; figure 17.1), and its optimal dosing has been carefully assessed over this interval (see below). Doses of novel anticoagulants are determined by small pilot trials, sometimes involving different patient populations, putting these novel agents at a distinct disadvantage in direct randomised comparisons with warfarin.

Left atrial appendage occlusion devices that can be implanted percutaneously have been used in several hundred atrial fibrillation patients to date, most of whom had bleeding contraindications to warfarin use.[13] Available clinical case series suggest feasibility and relative safety; efficacy is impossible to assess meaningfully. RCTs are getting underway.

In short, adjusted-dose warfarin remains the most efficacious available prophylaxis for atrial fibrillation patients at high (and for many at moderate) risk of stroke. Ongoing clinical trials are attempting to identify novel antithrombotic agents that are more efficacious than antiplatelet therapy and that are easier and safer to use than warfarin, but results appear to be several years away.

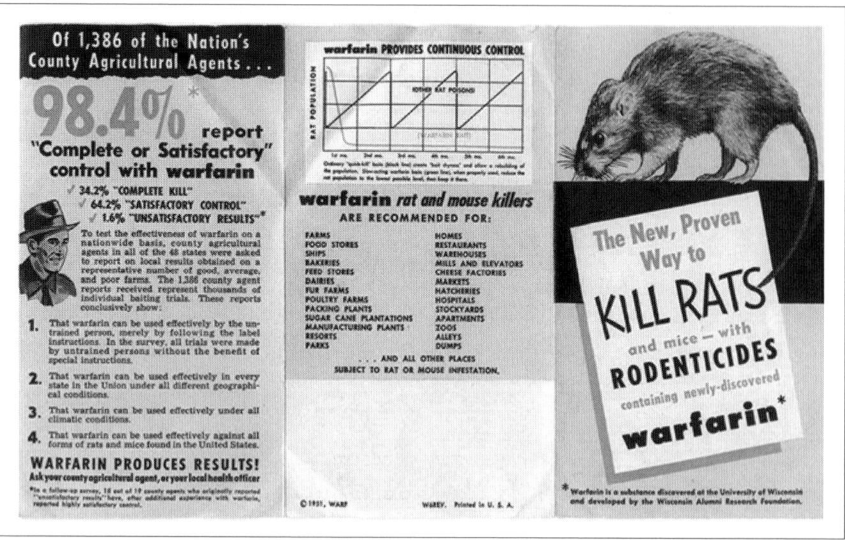

Figure 17.1: **Advertisement for the use of warfarin as a rodenticide following its introduction in 1951. (Image supplied by Bo Norrving, MD, Lund, Sweden.)**

What is the optimal target intensity of anticoagulation for elderly atrial fibrillation patients?

The optimal international normalised ratio (INR) for primary prevention of stroke (and perhaps death) in elderly atrial fibrillation patients appears to be 2.0–2.5 in my view.[14] There is a pervasive misimpression that INRs less than 2.0 are not efficacious in preventing stroke in atrial fibrillation patients. Four studies have shown that INRs of 1.6–1.7 provide 80–90% of the protection against stroke afforded by more intensive anticoagulation (table 17.2, figure 17.2).[15–18] The slopes of the intensity–efficacy curves are notable: there is rapid fall-off with INRs below 1.6 (see figure 17.2). Indirect compari-

Study	Design	Maximal protection (%)
Massachusetts General Hospital[15]	Case–control	91
Stroke Prevention in Atrial Fibrillation III[17]	Clinical trial	90
Anticoagulation and Risk Factors in Atrial Fibrillation (ATRIA) study[16]	Prospective cohort	80
Hong Kong[18]	Case series	91

*See figure 17.2 for plots of the relationship between achieved INRs and ischaemic stroke.

Table 17.2*: Estimated percentage of the maximum protection with achieved INRs of 1.6–1.7

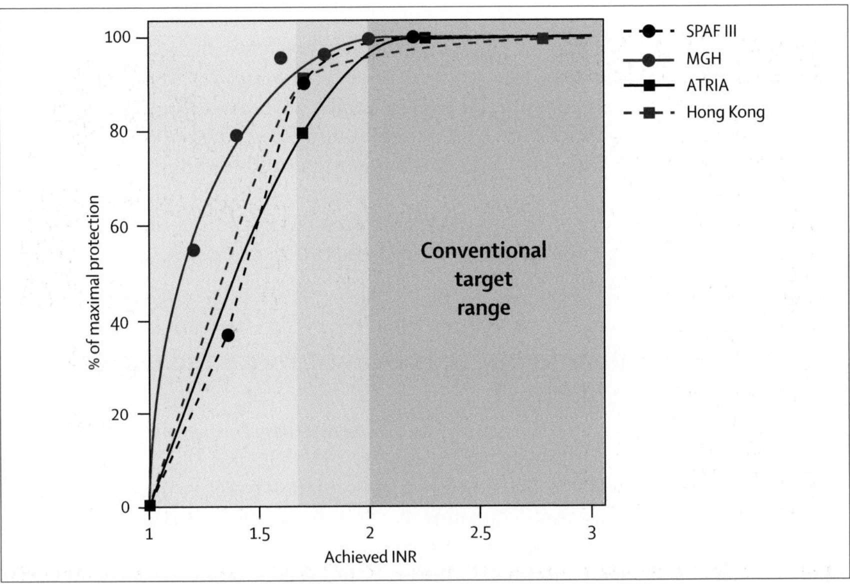

Figure 17.2: **Relationship between achieved INRs and ischaemic stroke rates in four studies: the Stroke Prevention in Atrial Fibrillation (SPAF) III clinical trial,[17] the Massachusetts General Hospital (MGH) case–control series,[15] the Anticoagulation and Risk Factors in Atrial Fibrillation (ATRIA) prospective cohort[16] and the Hong Kong series.[18]**

sons of relative risk reductions from RCTs confirm that achieved INRs of about 2.0 are efficacious (table 17.3).[19–23] The absolute rate of intracerebral haemorrhage is not substantially increased by warfarin until the INR exceeds 3.5.[16, 24] Consequently, a

Trial	PTR target	INR target	Mean achieved INR (estimated)	No. of ischaemic strokes	Relative risk reduction (%)
AFASAK I[22]	–	2.8–4.2	2.5	27	58
SPAF I[21]	1.3–1.8	(2.0–4.5)	(2.6)	23	65
BAATAF[19]	1.2–1.5	(1.5–2.7)	(2.1)	15	86
SPINAF[20]	1.2–1.5	(1.4–2.8)	(2.0)	29	74
CAFA[23]	–	2.0–3.0	2.4	14	44

INR, international normalised ratio; PTR, prothrombin time ratio. *Patients with prior stroke made up 4–8% of the trial cohorts. For trials measuring PTRs, INRs are those estimated by the investigators. Note that the relatively small numbers of stroke events make point estimates relatively imprecise.

Table 17.3: **Anticoagulation intensity and ischaemic stroke reduction in five RCTs of primary prevention***

practical target INR range for anticoagulation intensity for primary stroke prevention appears to be 1.6–3.0 (aiming for 2.2). Available data are fewer for secondary prevention; in the two largest trials, mean achieved INRs of 2.5 and 2.9 were highly efficacious.[4, 17, 25] Current management guidelines generally advocate a target INR range of 2.0–3.0,[6, 7] with one prominent guideline suggesting a lower target of 1.6–2.5 as an option for those over 75 years old,[6] who have higher rates of bleeding.[26, 27]

Self-monitoring of warfarin anticoagulation increases the fraction of time spent in the desired therapeutic range, reduces thromboembolic events and death,[28] and should be offered to suitable candidates.[29]

Which atrial fibrillation patients benefit most and least from life-long anticoagulation?

In assessing the potential benefits of antithrombotic therapy of individual patients, it is the absolute risk reduction, rather than the relative risk reduction, that is relevant. The absolute risk of stroke varies 20-fold among atrial fibrillation patients, depending on age and associated vascular diseases. Estimating an individual's stroke risk is the initial step in decisions regarding antithrombotic prophylaxis. More than ten stroke risk stratification schemes have been published in the English language literature;[6, 7, 30–37] most are quite similar, but their differences are important for individual patient management. The CHADS2 scheme awards one point each for congestive heart failure, hypertension, age ≥75 years and diabetes mellitus, and two points for prior stroke or transient ischaemic attack (TIA), and has been validated in three separate cohorts that involved hospital discharge follow-ups,[33] outpatients[3] and participants in clinical trials given aspirin[38] (table 17.4). Based on 5089 atrial fibrillation outpatients followed for 2.2 years, a CHADS2 score of 0 (22% of the cohort) had a low risk of stroke, averaging 0.5% per year, while those with a CHADS2 score of 1 (an additional 32%) had a stroke rate of 1.5% per year.[3] In each of the validation studies, those with CHADS2 scores of 0 or 1 had stroke rates of ≤ 2.5% per year (see table 17.4). The wider range of stroke rates with CHADS2 scores ≥ 2 in these studies is likely explained by the differing fractions of atrial fibrillation patients with prior stroke or TIA, the most potent risk predictor (4% in the outpatient-based study[3] versus 25% in the hospital discharge cohort[33]).

For the infrequent atrial fibrillation patients with prior stroke or TIA who have no other risk factors, a CHADS2 score of 2 yields an estimated stroke risk of 2.5–4.5% per year (see table 17.4), which is too low and represents a limitation of the CHADS2 scheme, in my view. All atrial fibrillation patients with prior stroke or TIA, recent or remote, should be considered high risk. Consequently, the estimated stroke risk associated with a CHADS2 score of 2 is a misleading pooling of a few high-risk secondary prevention patients combined with a larger number of low- to moderate-risk primary prevention patients. In short, the stroke risk associated with a CHADS2 score of 2 is very different in terms of primary versus secondary prevention. The use of a CHAD score (i.e. dropping 'S2') for primary prevention or a CHADS3 score for secondary prevention appears to fit the available data better. If precordial echocardiographic data are available, the Stroke Prevention in Atrial Fibrillation (SPAF) III risk stratification scheme has also been validated in several, albeit smaller, cohorts.[39]

	Hospital discharge cohort[33]	HMO outpatients[3]	Aspirin-treated clinical trial participants[38]
No. of patients	1733	5089	2580
Prior stroke (%)	25	4	22
Overall stroke rate	4.4[†]	2.0	4.2
CHADS2 score	**Stroke + TIA rate (estimated INR)**	**Stroke + non-CNS rate (estimated INR)**	**Stroke rate (estimated INR)**
0[‡]	1.9 (1.2–3.0)[†]	0.5 (0.3–0.8)	0.8 (0.4–1.7)
1[§]	2.8 (2.0–3.8)[†]	1.5 (1.2–1.9)	2.2 (1.6–3.1)
2**	4.0 (3.1–5.1)[†]	2.5 (2.0–3.2)	4.5 (3.5–5.9)[††]
3	5.9 (4.6–7.3)[†]	5.3 (4.2–6.7)	8.6 (6.8–11.0)
4	8.5 (6.3–11)[†]	6.0 (3.9–9.3)	10.9 (7.8–15.2)
5–6	> 12%/year[†]	6.9 (3.4–13.8)	> 12%/year

CNS, central nervous system; HMO, health maintenance organisation; INR, international normalised ratio, estimated values from studies that used the prothombin time ratio; TIA, transient ischaemic attack. *The CHADS2 score is based on congestive heart failure, hypertension, age ≥ 75 years, diabetes conferring one point for each, while prior stroke or TIA confers two points.[33] [†]24% of outcome events were TIAs, so the stroke rates averaged ~25% lower. This inpatient cohort was a decade older than most cohorts, and 56% had heart failure; the 30-day mortality rate was remarkably high, being 27% for outcome events.[33] [‡]Among 705 atrial fibrillation patients in the Framingham Heart Study cohort, the stroke rate for a CHADS2 score of 0 (10% of atrial fibrillation patients) was reported as 1.7% per year, but this was based on 3–5 events with wide confidence intervals that were not reported.[36] [§]The observed stroke rate among participants with a CHADS2 score of 1 given aspirin plus clopidogrel in the ACTIVE-W trial[2] was 1.3% per year (S. Connolly, personal communication, 6 December 2005). **The infrequent atrial fibrillation patients with a CHADS2 score of 2 due to prior stroke or TIA are at high risk (see text). [††]Observed rate for primary prevention (i.e. a CHADS2 score of 2 without prior stroke or TIA) was 3.6% (95%CI 2.6 to 5.0) (B. F. Gage, personal communication, 14 June 2005).

Table 17.4*: Assessment of the CHADS2 stroke risk stratification scheme

Risk of bleeding during anticoagulation

Bleeding associated with warfarin therapy is a serious issue, both for the direct morbidity in those suffering haemorrhage, and because physicians' fear of inducing bleeding (often exaggerated) contributes to underuse of anticoagulation in atrial fibrillation patients at high risk of stroke.[40] The experience of having a patient bleed during anticoagulation (with the associated 'chagrin factor') has a larger influence on physician prescribing patterns than does a thromboembolic event occurring in an untreated patient.[41] Major haemorrhage occurred at a rate of about 2% per year among atrial fibrillation patients anticoagulated in large RCTs, but the rate varies considerably in different reports due to the differing criteria used for diagnosis.[1, 2, 11, 12, 42] Patient-related predictors of major haemorrhage in anticoagulated atrial fibrillation patients include increasing age, heart failure and multiple associated medical conditions.[26, 42, 43] Stratification of bleeding risks into high versus low absolute risks has been proposed,[44] but not studied or validated as extensively as schemes for stroke risk stratification.

Intracerebral haemorrhage occurs at a rate of 0.3–0.8% per year in anticoagulated atrial fibrillation patients.[1,2,42,45,46] Consistent patient-related risk factors for intracerebral haemorrhage during anticoagulation are patient age, prior stroke and uncontrolled hypertension.[24,46] In a recent analysis of a large administrative database, physicians' subjective recording of a 'tendency for falls' was an independent predictor of intracranial haemorrhage in anticoagulated atrial fibrillation patients, but age was not (although the two variables were directly related).[47]

Microvascular abnormalities predisposing to bleeding can be detected by magnetic resonance imaging (MRI). 'Leukoaraiosis' and asymptomatic cerebral microbleeds have been correlated with intracranial haemorrhage during anticoagulation and aspirin therapy.[47,48] However, these MRI lesions suffer from non-standardised definition, acquisition techniques and interpretation; the positive and negative predictive values are inadequately defined to permit application to individual patient management. A recent comprehensive review of the clinical implications of MRI-detected microbleeds concluded that 'recommendations to guide antithrombotic treatment based on detection of cerebral microbleeds are presently not justified.'[47] With additional research, MRI-detected microbleeds should soon become a useful clinical tool.

Can antiplatelet therapy be safely combined with adjusted-dose warfarin in elderly atrial fibrillation patients?

The combination of antiplatelet therapy (typically low-dose aspirin) with adjusted-dose warfarin is often used in patients with prosthetic cardiac valves, and appears to be well tolerated based on studies involving those whose average age is the early 60s.[49] Whether safety can be extrapolated to more elderly atrial fibrillation patients with a higher frequency of systolic hypertension and age-related predisposition to intracerebral haemorrhage is of concern. About one in six anticoagulated patients with atrial fibrillation also takes regular aspirin, these mainly being patients with concomitant coronary artery disease.[24,50] Adding aspirin to anticoagulation likely increases centra nervous system (CNS) bleeding. A meta-analysis of five randomised trials in which aspirin was added to equal intensities of anticoagulation showed a relative risk (RR) of 2.6 (95% CI 1.3 to 5.4, $p = 0.009$), albeit involving several older studies in which CNS bleeding was not documented by neuroimaging.[51] A retrospective study of a hospital discharge cohort of 10 093 atrial fibrillation patients found that use of antiplatelet therapy was associated with a three-fold increase in intracranial haemorrhage (RR = 3.0, 95% CI 1.6 to 5.5, bivariate analysis).[50] In contrast, two case–control studies did not identify concomitant aspirin use as a predictor of intracerebral haemorrhage during anticoagulation.[24,52] A recent case–control study from the UK General Practice Research Database identified the combined use of warfarin and aspirin in elderly atrial fibrillation patients as being independently associated with bleeding that was fatal or required hospitalisation (RR = 4.5, 95% CI 1.1 to 18).[53]

Available data are not consistent, but some accentuation of CNS haemorrhage appears probable with combination anticoagulant–antiplatelet therapy, and an increase in serious non-CNS haemorrhage is certain. Whether combination therapy is of overall benefit for elderly atrial fibrillation patients with manifest coronary artery disease is not settled, although it is endorsed by one international guideline.[6] CNS bleeding during antithrombotic therapy is exquisitely sensitive to blood pressure control.[54] In atrial fibrillation patients receiving anticoagulation plus antiplatelet therapy, special efforts to control hypertension are particularly important, as discussed below.

What absolute threshold of benefit warrants anticoagulation? Who decides?

Many current management guidelines and expert opinions advocate life-long anticoagulation for atrial fibrillation patients with 'one or more additional risk factors' (i.e. CHADS2 scores of ≥ 1).[6, 7, 55] About 30% of atrial fibrillation patients (~800 000 people in the USA) have a CHADS2 score of 1,[3] and consequently have stroke rates of 1.5–2.5% (see table 17.4). For these patients, treatment with adjusted-dose warfarin over aspirin would be predicted to reduce stroke by 0.8% per year (number needed to treat with warfarin for 1 year to prevent one additional stroke of 125). Physician expert panels that generate guidelines may not reflect the views of general physicians or the values of the broad spectrum of patients. Reliable quantitative data about patient preference are sparse and difficult to acquire; they indicate (not surprisingly) a wide range of patient values and preferences, influenced by factors that are not often considered by physician expert panels.[56, 57] The lack of complete concordance between recommendations of physician expert guideline authors and the views of general physicians and patients explains, in part, the underuse of warfarin.

There is no single threshold of stroke risk that warrants anticoagulation therapy. Patient preferences and values, access to high-quality anticoagulation monitoring and estimated bleeding risk during anticoagulation are key issues. Considerable progress in developing patient decision aids for atrial fibrillation patients has been made.[58–60]

What are the benefits of blood pressure control for atrial fibrillation patients?

Intracerebral haemorrhage is the most devastating complication of antithrombotic therapy. The risk of intracranial haemorrhage is increased two to three times by adjusted-dose warfarin (INR 2–3) and by about 40% with aspirin use.[46] Modest reduction in blood pressure profoundly lowers the risk of intracranial haemorrhage, including patients taking antiplatelet therapy.[54, 61, 62] In the randomised PROGRESS trial involving patients with prior stroke or TIA, haemorrhagic stroke was reduced by 50% (95% CI 26 to 67) by a mean 9 mmHg reduction in systolic blood pressure, and by 76% (95% CI 55 to 87) by a 12 mmHg reduction (absolute rates of 0.6% per year to 0.3% per year and 0.2% per year, respectively).[54] In addition, ischaemic strokes in atrial fibrillation patients are reduced by blood pressure lowering,[63] this probably being mediated by the effects on left atrial stasis and thrombus formation.[64, 65] Hence, management of blood pressure in elderly atrial fibrillation patients on antithrombotic therapy is *doubly* important, reducing both ischaemic stroke and CNS bleeding. The optimal target levels are not clear, but modest lowering of blood pressure using safe, well-tolerated agents (e.g. diuretics, angiotensin-converting enzyme (ACE) inhibitors) is probably sensible for all atrial fibrillation patients who have systolic blood pressures consistently exceeding 120 mmHg. In my view, vigorous efforts should be made to keep the systolic blood pressure below 140 mmHg in anticoagulated atrial fibrillation patients.

Obstacles to individualising treatment

> *Everything should be made as simple as it is, but not simpler.*
> (A. Einstein, 1879–1955)

Adjusted-dose warfarin is highly efficacious for stroke prevention in atrial fibrillation patients. Some have argued that the issues discussed above (panel 17.1) make treatment too complicated for general physicians, and that the nuances of individualising therapy distract from making anticoagulation widely used, widely available and as safe as possible. 'Warfarin all around' for atrial fibrillation patients has the advantage of simplicity, but it results in anticoagulation of those for whom the benefits are very small.

If anticoagulation were inexpensive, easy to administer and safe, such an approach would be reasonable. Stroke risk stratification schemes are multiple and relatively complicated, management guidelines conflict and determining individual patient preferences is time consuming. Can a general physician be expected to provide optimal individualised stroke prophylaxis for atrial fibrillation patients? This remains a formid-

Panel 17.1: Individualising treatment to prevent stroke in atrial fibrillation patients

- There is no solid evidence that cardioversion and/or antiarrhythmic drug therapy importantly reduces stroke.
- There is nothing superior to adjusted-dose warfarin. Ximelagatran may be comparable, clopidogrel combined with aspirin is less efficacious, and the value of left atrial occlusion devices remains to be established.
- Achieved INRs between 1.6 and 3.0 offer substantial protection against stroke and are relatively safe. The optimal INR is probably between 2.0 and 2.5 for primary prevention in most atrial fibrillation patients.
- Estimating the individual patient's absolute stroke risk is an important initial step in antithrombotic prophylaxis. The CHADS2 scheme appears the best available.
- Patient preferences and values are infrequently incorporated in management guidelines and explain the apparent underuse of anticoagulation.
- Modest blood pressure control importantly reduces ischaemic and haemorrhagic stroke for atrial fibrillation patients.
- Elderly patients receiving combined antithrombotic therapy with aspirin and adjusted-dose warfarin have an increased risk of CNS bleeding, and vigorous control of blood pressure is especially important.
- Individualised treatment is inherently challenging, requiring availability of high-quality data, an informed doctor and time.

able challenge that involves developing effective systems to make the relevant knowledge available at the point of patient care.

References

1 Hart RG, Benavente O, McBride R, Pearce LA. Antithrombotic therapy to prevent stroke in patients with atrial fibrillation: a meta-analysis. *Ann Intern Med* 1999; **131:** 492–501.

2 ACTIVE Writing Group, on behalf of the ACTIVE Investigators. Clopidogrel plus aspirin versus oral anticoagulation for atrial fibrillation in the Atrial Fibrillation Clopidogrel Trial with Irbesartan for Prevention of Vascular Events (ACTIVE W). *Lancet* 2006; **367:** 1903–12.

3 Go AS, Hylek EM, Chang Y, et al. Anticoagulation therapy for stroke prevention in atrial fibrillation. How well do randomized trials translate into clinical practice? *JAMA* 2003; **290:** 2685–92.

4 Hart RG, Pearce LA, Koudstaal PJ. Transient ischemic attacks in patients with atrial fibrillation. Implications for secondary prevention. *Stroke* 2004; **35:** 948–51.

5 van Walraven C, Hart RG, Singer DE, et al. Oral anticoagulants vs. aspirin in nonvalvular atrial fibrillation. An individual patient meta-analysis. *JAMA* 2002; **288:** 2441–48.

6 Fuster V, Ryden LE, Asinger RW, et al. ACC/AHA/ESC guidelines for the management of patients with atrial fibrillation: executive summary. *Circulation* 2001; **104:** 2118–50.

7 Singer DE, Albers GW, Dalen JE, et al. Antithrombotic therapy in atrial fibrillation. The Seventh ACCP Conference. *Chest* 2004; **126** (suppl): 429S–56S.

8 Atrial Fibrillation Follow-up Investigation of Rhythm Management (AFFIRM) Investigators. A comparison of rate control and rhythm control in patients with atrial fibrillation. *N Engl J Med* 2002; **347:** 1825–33.

9 Sherman DG, Kim SG, Boop BS, et al., and the NHLBI AFFIRM Investigators. The occurrence and characteristics of stroke events in the AFFIRM study. *Arch Intern Med* 2005; **165:** 1185–91.

10 Hart RG, Pearce LA, Miller VT, et al. Cardioembolic vs. noncardioembolic stroke in atrial fibrillation: frequency and effect of antithrombotic agents. *Cerebrovasc Dis* 2000; **10:** 39–43.

11 Olsson SB, Executive Steering Committee on behalf of the SPORTIF III Investigators. Stroke prevention with the oral direct thrombin inhibitor ximegalatran compared with warfarin in patients with non-valvular atrial fibrillation: randomized controlled trial. *Lancet* 2003; **362:** 1691–98.

12 SPORTIF Executive Steering Committee for the SPORTIF V Investigators. Ximelagatran vs. warfarin for stroke prevention in patients with nonvalvular atrial fibrillation. *JAMA* 2005; **293:** 690–98.

13 Ostermayer SH, Reisman M, Kramer PH, et al. Percutaneous left atrial appendage transcatheter occlusion (PLAATO system) to prevent stroke in high-risk patients with nonrheumatic atrial fibrillation: results from the international multi-center feasibility trials. *J Am Coll Cardiol* 2005; **46:** 9–14.

14 Oden A, Fahlen M, Hart RG. Optimal INR for prevention of stroke and mortality in atrial fibrillation: a critical appraisal. *Thromb Res* 2006; **117:** 493–99.

15 Hylek EM, Skates SJ, Sheehan MA, Singer DE. An analysis of the lowest effective intensity of prophylactic anticoagulation for patients with nonrheumatic atrial fibrillation. *N Engl J Med* 1996; **335:** 540–46.

16 Hylek EM, Go AS, Chang Y, et al. Effect of intensity of oral anticoagulation on stroke severity and mortality in atrial fibrillation. *N Engl J Med* 2003; **349:** 1019–26.

17 Stroke Prevention in Atrial Fibrillation Investigators. Adjusted-dose warfarin versus low-intensity, fixed-dose warfarin plus aspirin for high-risk patients with atrial fibrillation: the Stroke Prevention in Atrial Fibrillation III randomized clinical trial. *Lancet* 1996; **348:** 633–38.

18 Cheung C-M, Tsoi T-H, Huang C-Y. The lowest effective intensity of prophylactic anticoagulation for patients with atrial fibrillation. *Cerebrovasc Dis* 2005; **20:** 114–19.

19 Boston Area Anticoagulation Trial for Atrial Fibrillation Investigators. The effect of low-dose warfarin on the risk of stroke in nonrheumatic atrial fibrillation. *N Engl J Med* 1990; **323:** 1505–11.

20 Ezekowitz MD, Bridgers SL, James KE, et al. Warfarin in the prevention of stroke associated with nonrheumatic atrial fibrillation. Veterans Affairs Stroke Prevention in Nonrheumatic Atrial Fibrillation Investigators. *N Engl J Med* 1992; **327:** 1406–12.

21 Stroke Prevention in Atrial Fibrillation Investigators. The Stroke Prevention in Atrial Fibrillation Study: final results. *Circulation* 1991; **84:** 527–39.

22 Petersen P, Boysen G, Godtfredsen J, et al. Placebo-controlled, randomized trial of warfarin and aspirin for prevention of thromboembolic complications in chronic atrial fibrillation. The Copenhagen AFASAK study. *Lancet* 1989; **1:** 175–79.

23 Connolly SJ, Laupacis A, Gent M, et al. Canadian Atrial Fibrillation Anticoagulation (CAFA) Study. *J Am Coll Cardiol* 1991; **18:** 349–55.

24 Fang MC, Chang Y, Hylek EM, et al. Advanced age, anticoagulation intensity, and risk for intracranial hemorrhage among patients taking warfarin for atrial fibrillation. *Ann Intern Med* 2004; **141:** 745–52.

25 European Atrial Fibrillation Trial Study Group. Secondary prevention in non-rheumatic atrial fibrillation after transient ischemic attack or minor stroke. *Lancet* 1993; **342:** 1255–62.

26 Stroke Prevention in Atrial Fibrillation Investigators. Bleeding during antithrombotic therapy in atrial fibrillation. *Arch Intern Med* 1996; **156:** 409–16.

27 Johnson CE, Lim WK, Workman BS. People aged over 75 in atrial fibrillation on warfarin: the rate of major hemorrhage and stroke in more than 500 patient-years of follow-up. *J Am Geriatr Soc* 2005; **53:** 655–59.

28 Heneghan C, Alonso-Coello P, Garcia-Alamino JM, et al. Self-monitoring of oral anticoagulation: a systematic review and meta-analysis. *Lancet* 2006; **367:** 404–11.

29 Ansell J, Jacobson A, Levy J, et al. Guidelines for implementation of patient self-testing and patient self-management of oral anticoagulation. International consensus guidelines prepared by the International Self-Monitoring Association for Oral Anticoagulation. *Int J Cardiol* 2005; **99:** 37–45.

30 Atrial Fibrillation Investigators. Risk factors for stroke and efficacy of antithrombotic therapy in atrial fibrillation. Analysis of pooled data from five randomized controlled trials. *Arch Intern Med* 1994; **154:** 1449–57.

31 Stroke Prevention in Atrial Fibrillation Investigators. Risk factors for thromboembolism during aspirin therapy in patients with atrial fibrillation: the Stroke Prevention in Atrial Fibrillation Study. *J Stroke Cerebrovasc Dis* 1995; **5:** 147–57.

32 Hart RG, Pearce LA, McBride R, et al. Factors associated with ischemic stroke during aspirin therapy in atrial fibrillation: analysis of 2012 participants in the SPAF I-III clinical trials. The Stroke Prevention in Atrial Fibrillation (SPAF) Investigators. *Stroke* 1999; **30:** 1223–29.

33 Gage BF, Waterman AD, Shannon W, et al. Validation of clinical classification schemes for predicting stroke: results of the National Registry of Atrial Fibrillation. *JAMA* 2001; **285:** 2864–70.

34 Albers GW, Dalen JE, Laupacis A, et al. Antithrombotic therapy in atrial fibrillation. *Chest* 2001; **119:** 194S–206S.

35 van Walraven C, Hart RG, Wells GA, et al. A clinical prediction rule to identify patients with atrial fibrillation and a low risk for stroke while taking aspirin. *Arch Intern Med* 2003; **163:** 936–43.

36 Wang TJ, Massaro JM, Levy D, et al. A risk score for predicting stroke or death in individuals with new-onset atrial fibrillation in the community. The Framingham Study. *JAMA* 2003; **290:** 1049–56.

37 Lip GY, Boos C. Antithrombotic therapy for atrial fibrillation. *Heart* 2006; **92:** 155–61.

38 Gage BF, van Walraven C, Pearce LA, et al. Selecting patients with atrial fibrillation for anticoagulation. Stroke risk stratification in patients taking aspirin. *Circulation* 2004; **110:** 2287–92.

39 Hart RG, Halperin JL, Pearce LA, et al. Lessons from the Stroke Prevention in Atrial Fibrillation trials. *Ann Intern Med* 2003; **138:** 831–38.

40 Man-Son-Hing M, Laupacis A. Anticoagulant-related bleeding in older persons with atrial fibrillation: physicians' fears often unfounded. *Arch Intern Med* 2003; **163:** 1580–86.

41 Choudhry NK, Anderson GM, Laupacis A, et al. Impact of adverse events on prescribing warfarin in patients with atrial fibrillation: matched pair analysis. *BMJ* 2006; **332:** 141–45.

42 DiMarco JP, Flaker G, Waldo AL, et al. Factors affecting bleeding risk during anticoagulant therapy in patients with atrial fibrillation: observations from the Atrial Fibrillation Follow-up Investigation of Rhythm Management (AFFIRM) Study. *Am Heart J* 2005; **149:** 650–56.

43 Wehinger C, Stollberger C, Langer T, et al. Evaluation of risk factors for stroke/embolism and of complications due to anticoagulant therapy in atrial fibrillation. *Stroke* 2001; **32:** 2246–52.

44 Aspinall SL, DeSanzo BE, Trilli LE, Good CB. Bleeding risk index in an anticoagulation clinic. Assessment by indication and implications for care. *J Gen Intern Med* 2005; **20:** 1008–13.

45 Gage BF, Birman-Deych E, Kerzner R, et al. Incidence of intracranial hemorrhage in patients with atrial fibrillation who are prone to fall. *Am J Med* 2005; **118:** 612.

46 Hart RG, Tonarelli SB, Pearce LA. Avoiding CNS bleeding during antithrombotic therapy. Recent data and ideas. *Stroke* 2005; **36:** 1588–93.

47 Koennecke H-C. Cerebral microbleeds on MRI. Prevalence, associations, and potential clinical implications. *Neurology* 2006; **66:** 165–72.

48 Viswanathan A, Chabriat H. Cerebral microhemorrhage. *Stroke* 2006; **37:** 550–55.

49 Turpie AGG, Gent M, Laupacis A, et al. A comparison of aspirin with placebo in patients treated with warfarin and heart valve replacement. *N Engl J Med* 1993; **329:** 524–49.

50 Shireman TI, Howard PA, Kresowik TF, Ellerbeck EF. Combined anticoagulant–antiplatelet use and major bleeding events in elderly atrial fibrillation patients. *Stroke* 2004; **35:** 2362–67.

51 Hart RG, Benavente O, Pearce LA. Increased risk of intracranial hemorrhage when aspirin is combined with warfarin: a meta-analysis and hypothesis. *Cerebrovasc Dis* 1999; **9:** 215–17.

52 Berwaerts J, Webster J. Analysis of risk factors involved in oral-anticoagulant-related intracranial hemorrhages. *Q J Med* 2000; **93:** 513–21.

53 Gasse C, Hollowell J, Meier CR, Haefeli WE. Drug interactions and risk of acute bleeding leading to hospitalization or death in patients with chronic atrial fibrillation treated with warfarin. *Blood Coagul Fibrinol Cell Haemost* 2005; **94:** 537–43.

54 Chapman N, Huxley R, Anderson C, et al. Effects of a peindopril-based blood pressure-lowering regimen on the risk of recurrent stroke according to stroke subtype and medical history. The PROGRESS Trial. *Stroke* 2004; **35:** 116–21.

55 Nattel S, Opie L. Controversies in atrial fibrillation. *Lancet* 2006; **367:** 262–72.

56 Howitt A, Armstrong D. Implementing evidence-based medicine in general practice: audit and quantitative study of antithrombotic therapy for atrial fibrillation. *BMJ* 1999; **318:** 1324–27.

57 Fuller R, Dudley N, Blacktop J. Avoidance hierarchies and preferences for anticoagulation – semi-qualitative analysis of older patients' views about stroke prevention and the use of warfarin. *Age Ageing* 2004; **33:** 608–11.

58 Man-Son-Hing M, Laupacis A, O'Connor AM, et al. Development of a decision aid for patients with atrial fibrillation who are considering antithrombotic therapy. *J Gen Intern Med* 2000; **15:** 723–30.

59 Man-Son-Hing M, Laupacis A, O'Connor AM, et al. A patient decision aid regarding antithrombotic therapy for stroke prevention in atrial fibrillation: a randomized controlled trial. *JAMA* 1999; **282:** 737–43.

60 McAlister FA, Man-Son-Hing M, Straus SE, et al. Decision Aid in Atrial Fibrillation (DAAFI) Investigators. Impact of a patient decision aid on care among patients with nonvalvular atrial fibrillation: a cluster randomized trial. *Can Med Assoc J* 2005; **17:** 496–501.

61 PROGRESS Collaborative Group. Randomised trial of a perindopril-based blood-pressure-lowering regimen among 6,105 individuals with previous stroke or transient ischemic attack. *Lancet* 2001; **358:** 1033–41.

62 Perry H, Davis B, Price T, et al. Effects of treating isolated systolic hypertension on the risk of developing various types and subtypes of stroke. *JAMA* 2000; **284:** 465–71.

63 Arima H, Hart RG, Colman S, et al. Perindopril-based blood pressure lowering reduces major vascular events in patients with atrial fibrillation and prior stroke or TIA. *Stroke* 2005; **36:** 2164–69.

64 Goldman ME, Pearce LA, Hart RG, et al. Pathophysiologic correlates of thromboembolism in nonvalvular atrial fibrillation: Reduced flow velocity in the left appendage. *J Am Soc Echo* 1999; **12:** 1080–87.

65 Zabalgoitia M, Halperin JL, Pearce LA, et al. Transesophageal echocardiographic correlates of clinical risk of thromboembolism in nonvalvular atrial fibrillation. *J Am Coll Cardiol* 1998; **31:** 1622–26.

Reperfusion therapies in acute cardiovascular and cerebrovascular syndromes

David M. Kent

Introduction

Readers of previous chapters will not be surprised by the theme of this chapter: overall results of a clinical trial do not generally apply to all patients in the trial.[1–6] Indeed, the average results may not even apply to a typical patient in the clinical trial, as these results may be especially influenced by a relatively small group of (typically high-risk) patients who account for most of the outcome risk and treatment effect.[5,7] Thus, even when a therapy is beneficial on average, it may be highly unlikely to benefit patients with a risk–benefit treatment profile typical of trial participants, and it may be more apt to harm than benefit others who meet the inclusion criteria of a trial.[5,6,8,9] Conversely, there are other trials with overall 'negative' results that include important subgroups of patients – identifiable on the basis of pretreatment characteristics – who get substantial benefit.[5,10] Furthermore, these subgroups with clinically relevant differences in treatment effect frequently cannot be identified on the basis of conventional (one variable at a time) subgroup analyses, which are also prone to showing spurious treatment differences between subgroups, but can be identified when multiple clinical characteristics are considered simultaneously.[4,5,11]

In this chapter I review examples in the treatment of acute coronary syndromes and acute ischaemic stroke in which independently derived risk models are useful in distinguishing patients likely to benefit from therapy from those highly unlikely to benefit, or likely to be harmed, with an emphasis on thrombolytic therapy.

Acute coronary syndromes

Background

The dramatic improvement due to therapeutic innovations in outcomes in acute coronary syndromes generally, and acute myocardial infarction (AMI) in particular, has led to a state of 'diminishing returns' for increasingly intensive therapies.[12] Even a cursory review of therapeutic innovations in AMI serves to show that new improvements in acute cardiac care can not possibly match our previous successes in terms of improvements in case fatality rates. As reviewed by Antman and Braunwald,[13] in the era before coronary care units, case fatality rates were approximately 30%. With the close monitoring and the prompt treatment of potentially fatal arrhythmias that coronary care units permitted, these rates were cut virtually in half. The addition of beta-blockers, aspirin and thrombolytic therapy led to further decreases in mortality. The acute mortality rate found in most clinical trials in the period since the introduction of thrombolytic therapy have been roughly in the 6% range. Somehow, new agents, or new combinations of agents, must have sufficient incremental impact on this group of patients with a relatively low overall mortality to warrant their costs and their risks. This is getting progressively more difficult, and therefore 30-day mortality has been replaced as the primary outcome in clinical trials by composite outcome measures, which aggregate less consequential clinical outcomes, such as the need for target vessel revascularisation and non-fatal reinfarction, together with mortality.

This account of the average results of AMI trials over time obscures the fact that patients with AMI, even those with ST-segment-elevation AMI, are not a homogeneous group. Indeed, for most patients – particularly otherwise healthy patients with small or inferior-wall acute infarcts and stable vital signs – the risk of mortality is much lower than even the overall average. However, for other patients – especially older patients, with comorbid conditions such as diabetes, with large or anterior-wall infarcts and possibly unstable vital signs – the risk of mortality and, more generally, a poor outcome can be several-fold higher than average.

A number of models have been developed to stratify patients according to their risk of adverse outcomes from acute coronary syndromes generally, and ST-segment-elevation AMI in particular.[14–18] One such model is the thrombolytic predictive instrument (TPI).[18] The TPI predicts patient-specific outcomes for patients with ST-segment-elevation AMI based on easily obtainable clinical and electrocardiographic variables, using a logistic regression model derived from a combined database of 4911 patients with ST-segment-elevation AMI from 13 clinical trials and registries testing thrombolytic therapy. The variables used are shown in panel 18.1. The TPI equations have been programmed into commercially available electrocardiographic equipment, and predictions for various outcomes, including 30-day mortality (with and without thrombolytic therapy), appear on the top margin of a conventional electrocardiogram.

Panel 18.1: Variables used in the TPI prediction of 30-day mortality for patients with ST-segment-elevation AMI

- Age (years): truncated from 40 to 75
- Systolic blood pressure: interacted with AMI location
- Diabetes
- Heart rate (beats/min) – 70: truncated from 0 to 50
- Infarct size: defined as the number of contiguous leads involved plus the sum of the ST-segment elevation in these leads
- Anterior wall location
- Right bundle branch block
- Effect of time from symptom onset to presentation: a complex variable derived by piece-wise linear regression
- Effect of thrombolytic therapy: the variable for the effects of treatment with thrombolytic agents interacted with reported time from symptom onset to presentation, as well as electrocardiographic signs of earliness

Figure 18.1 shows the distribution of TPI predictions of 30-day mortality in 1058 consecutive patients receiving reperfusion therapy for ST-segment-elevation AMI in a community-based sample of 22 hospitals.[19] The average expected mortality rate in this sample was 6.0% overall, based on the pretreatment variables listed in panel 18.1. However, the overall rate obscures a large degree of individual patient variation in risk; in the quartile of patients at the highest risk, the predicted 30-day mortality is 16.3%, but in the quartile at lowest risk the predicted 30-day mortality is only 1.0%. Moreover, the average mortality risk of the lower risk two-thirds of patients is about 2%. These large differences in outcome risk may make some therapies appropriate only for high-risk patients, especially if the therapies are risky or costly, as outcomes for other patients are already quite good and they may be very unlikely to get additional benefit from increasingly intense therapy.

A reanalysis of the GUSTO Trial

These considerations led us to reanalyse the results obtained in the GUSTO trial.[20] This landmark 1993 trial tested two forms of thrombolytic therapy, 'accelerated' tissue plasminogen activator (tPA) and streptokinase, and found a decrease in mortality among those treated with accelerated tPA compared with those treated with streptokinase (mortality 6.3% versus 7.3%, $p = 0.001$), despite a small increase in the risk of intracranial haemorrhage (ICH) (0.72% versus 0.52%, $p = 0.03$).[20] Despite these favourable results, use of tPA was not immediately adopted universally, largely because the costs of tPA were considerably more than for streptokinase. (At the time of GUSTO, the average wholesale price of tPA in the USA was $2750 compared with $320 for streptokinase). A cost-effectiveness analysis, published in 1995, found that the mortality benefit of tPA warranted the extra costs; the average cost-effectiveness was approximately $33 000 per year of life saved, which compared favourably with other accepted

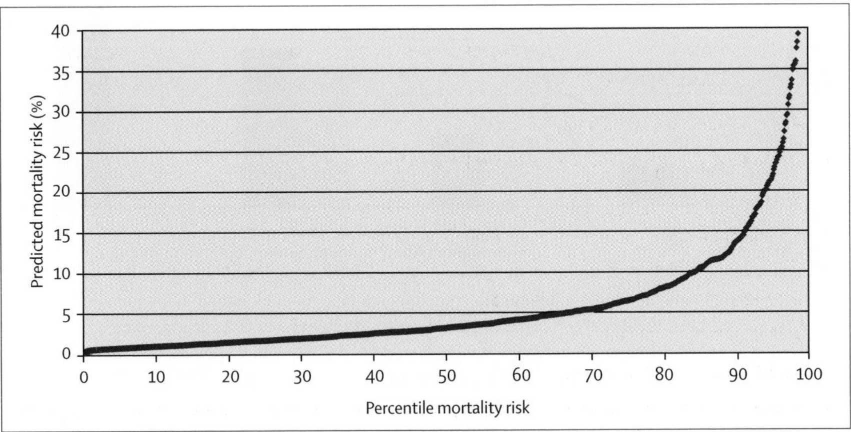

Figure 18.1: **The distribution of mortality risk in patients who received reperfusion therapy for AMI. The predicted mortality with thrombolytic therapy in 1058 consecutive patients who were treated for ST-segment-elevation AMI, using individual patient characteristics and the TPI. The area under the curve represents the mortality burden. Most patients are at relatively low risk of mortality. The highest quartile of risk (at the right of the graph) accounts for roughly 70% of all expected deaths.**

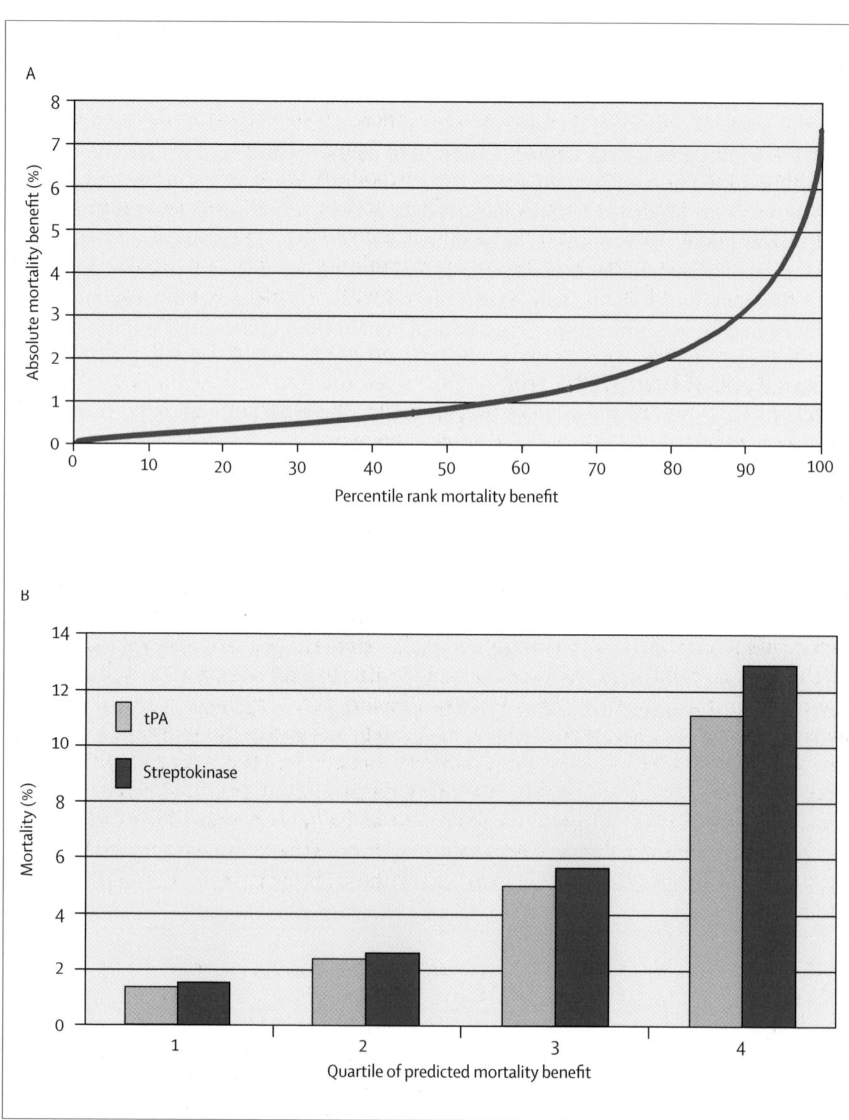

Figure.18.2: **Predicted and observed distribution of mortality benefit of tPA compared to streptokinase. (A) The difference between the predicted 30-day mortality (not including intracranial haemorrhage) if treated with tPA versus if treated with streptokinase for 24 146 patients in the GUSTO trial, from those with the lowest predicted benefit (percentile 0) to those with the highest predicted benefit (percentile 100). This was obtained by using the TPI predictions of benefit for thrombolytic therapy and standardising to yield an average benefit of 1%. The upper quartile was predicted to account for 61% of the total benefit, and the upper half to account for 84% of the total benefit. (B) When the actual outcomes were examined in each quartile, the upper quartile accounted for 59% of the total benefit and the upper half for 87%. Patients in the lower two quartiles obtained very little additional mortality benefit from the more potent and expensive thrombolytic agent.**

therapies.[21] Indeed, following the trial and the economic study, tPA (or related agents) has become the thrombolytic of choice in the USA and much of the developed world.

However, we hypothesised that the average efficacy (and, therefore, the average cost-effectiveness) is unlikely to apply to all patients. Specifically, with a distribution of risk roughly similar to that seen in figure 18.1, we hypothesised that most of the incremental benefit of tPA relative to streptokinase is likely to be captured by a subgroup of high-risk (high benefit) patients, and that many patients, on the basis of pretreatment variables, are likely to have excellent outcomes regardless of which thrombolytic agent they receive, and thus will be cost-ineffective to treat with the more expensive agent.

To test this hypothesis, we obtained predictions on 24 146 patients from the GUSTO trial using a TPI-based mortality model.[9] We assumed that the incremental benefit of tPA compared to streptokinase would be proportional to the expected benefit of thrombolytic therapy generally (i.e. predicted 30-day mortality without thrombolytic therapy minus predicted 30-day mortality with thrombolytic therapy). Thus, to estimate this incremental benefit of tPA, we simply standardised the TPI-predicted benefit to yield an overall average benefit of 1% using a multiplicative constant (figure 18.2(A)). Since, in the predictive model, the effect of thrombolytic therapy does not interact with any variable apart from time from symptom onset (i.e. thrombolytic therapy has the same odds ratio for all patients treated at a given time), the absolute benefit of thrombolytic therapy is essentially proportional to the baseline mortality risk, and the shape of the distribution of the predicted incremental benefits was similar to that seen for mortality risk in figure 18.1. Although the average predicted absolute mortality benefit from tPA across all patients was 1%, some patients were predicted to be much more likely to benefit than this average, yet most patients were less likely to benefit than the overall results suggest. According to the model, more than 60% of all the benefit was predicted to accrue to just the highest risk 25% of patients and about 85% of the benefit to the highest risk half of patients. When the actual mortality outcomes of these patients were examined by quartile, the results corresponded almost precisely to these independently derived predictions (figure 18.2(B)).

Furthermore, the more potent tPA also carries some incremental risk of thrombolytic-related ICH compared to streptokinase. Again, much as there is heterogeneity in mortality risk, there is also heterogeneity in the risk of ICH. To include this risk in our predictions, we used an independently derived model that predicts the likelihood of thrombolytic-related ICH (developed on a registry database of 71 073 patients treated for AMI with tPA), based on a patient's age, gender, race, systolic blood pressure, diastolic blood pressure and history of prior stroke.[22] When the incremental risk of tPA-related ICH was included in model predictions of composite benefit (mortality or thrombolytic-related ICH), predictions of benefit were even more skewed, with 90% of the incremental benefit of tPA predicted to go to half the patients (figure 18.3(A)). Indeed, some patients were more likely to be harmed than to benefit from tPA, specifically patients with lower risk AMIs (e.g. patients with smaller or inferior-wall AMIs and stable vital signs) who were also not at low risk for thrombolytic-related ICH (e.g. if they had higher blood pressure and/or a prior stroke). Again, when the actual outcomes were examined, they corresponded well to model predictions (figure 18.3(B)).

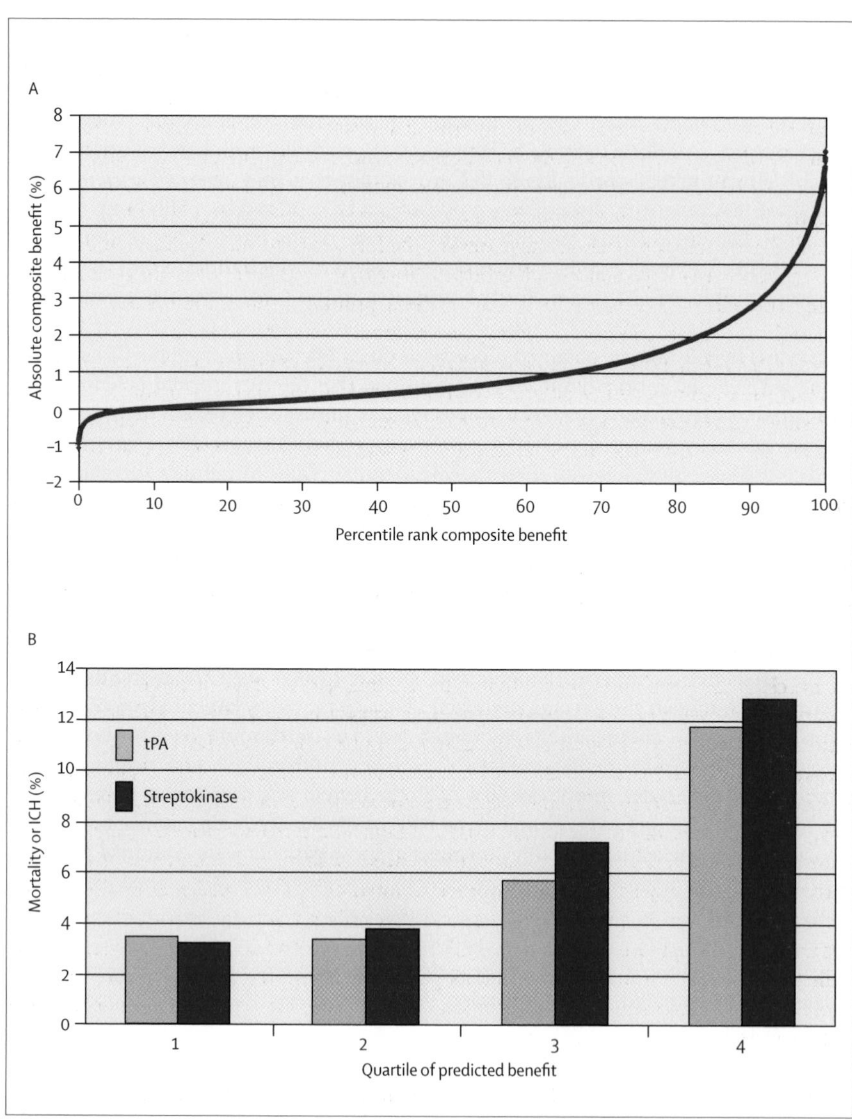

Figure 18.3: **Predicted and observed distribution of composite (mortality and ICH) benefit of tPA compared to streptokinase. (A) The difference between the predicted 30-day composite benefit if treated with tPA versus if treated with streptokinase for 24 146 patients in the GUSTO trial, from those with the lowest predicted benefit (percentile 0) to those with the highest predicted benefit (percentile 100). Compared to figure 18.2(A), this graph is even more skewed, and shows that some patients are, on the basis of pretreatment variables, more likely to be harmed by tPA compared to streptokinase. These are patients with low-risk myocardial infarctions, who may be at somewhat greater than average risk for a thrombolytic-related ICH. (B) The observed outcomes by quartiles agree closely with predictions. As predicted, 90% of the benefit of population-wide tPA use could be obtained by treating only 50% of patients.**

The skewed distribution of benefits led to estimates of the cost-effectiveness of tPA that were also skewed. Although the average cost-effectiveness was about $33 000 per life-year saved, more than half of patients had an estimated cost-effectiveness ratio of greater than $50 000 and a third of patients had a cost-effectiveness ratio of more than $100 000. When we examined the distribution of incremental benefits we would expect, in a non-trial, community-based population receiving thrombolytic therapy (i.e. the patients in figure 18.1), we found that the distribution was shifted to include more low-benefit/harm patients, such as those toward the left of figure 18.3(A). Thus, if one uses the frequently employed (although arbitrary) threshold of $50 000 per life-year saved to define cost-effective interventions, our analysis produced the paradoxical result that, although tPA is cost-effective on average compared to streptokinase, it may not be cost-effective for the typical (i.e. median) patient.[23] In our community-based sample, treating just the high-risk half of patients with tPA would result in near-identical outcomes and substantial cost savings compared to tPA for all (and would have been both cost- and life-saving compared to the allocation that was actually observed in that sample).[23]

Our model was based on a set of complex equations that we have incorporated into computer programmes (for the web link see reference 24). Although it is the only independently derived model evaluated directly on the GUSTO data, others have proposed similar risk models, which are available in the form of nomograms.[25, 26]

Primary coronary intervention compared to thrombolytic therapy

In much of the developed world, thrombolytic therapy is being displaced by primary coronary intervention (PCI) as the preferred reperfusion method, which has been shown to be superior to thrombolysis in reducing mortality, non-fatal reinfarction and stroke.[27, 28] Despite the superiority of PCI in clinical trials, most hospitals do not have the facilities to perform PCI, and many are not staffed to perform it on a 24-hours-a-day, 7-days-a-week basis. Thus, in most settings, thrombolytic therapy remains the standard of care, and physicians are often faced with a choice between immediate thrombolytic therapy or PCI, with some additional delay for transfer to a PCI-capable centre. Indeed, recent registry data suggest that only a minority of patients receiving reperfusion therapy are treated with PCI.[29, 30] Because of this, there have been recent calls to regionalise cardiac care so that all patients with ST-segment-elevation AMI can receive the superior form of reperfusion therapy.[31, 32] This would require a massive reorganisation of cardiac services.

Given our prior results modelling thrombolytic therapy, we hypothesised that many patients are at such low risk of mortality with thrombolysis that they are extremely unlikely to obtain any additional benefit from PCI (at least in terms of mortality), such that routinely bypassing community hospitals, or transferring all AMI patients to regional centres, may not be justified. To explore this hypothesis, we initially performed meta-regression on the results of ten published trials, and this suggested that trials enrolling higher risk patients were more likely to show benefit than were trials enrolling low-risk patients.[19] This 'control-rate metaregression' (so-called because it uses the rate of the outcome in the control group as a surrogate marker for population risk profile) suggested that trials in which the average risk was less than about 2–3% were highly unlikely to demonstrate any mortality benefit for PCI compared to thrombolytic therapy

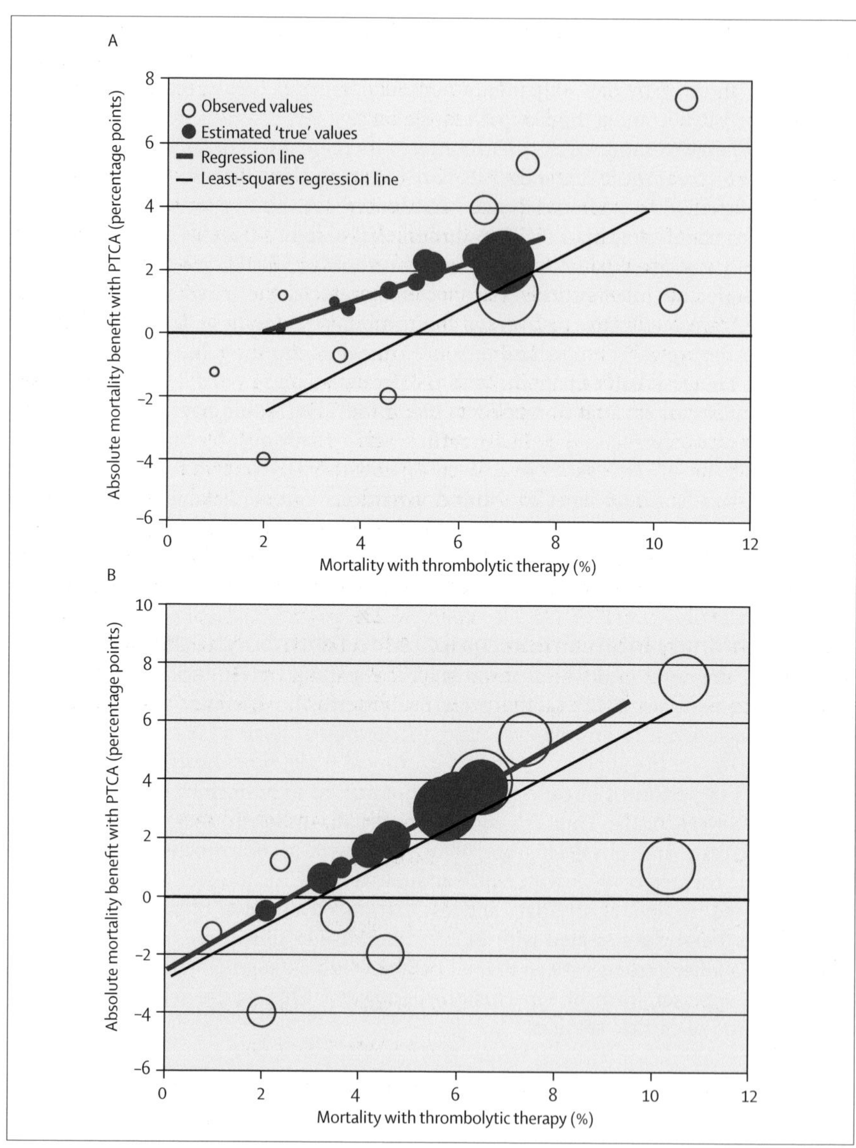

Figure 18.4: **Control rate meta-regression: the absolute benefit of primary angioplasty (PTCA) relative to thrombolytic therapy observed in trials with different baseline mortality rates. Observed values from the reported trials and estimated 'true' values; the size of the circles reflects the relative size of the trials. (A) The slope of the regression line is 0.56 and the x-axis intercept is 2.0%, indicating that populations at mortality risks below this level are unlikely to demonstrate benefit from PTCA over thrombolytic therapy, and may show harm. The simple weighted least-squares regression is shown for purposes of comparison only. (B) When the influential GUSTO IIb trial is removed, the slope of the regression line increases greatly, while the mortality risk at which the treatments yield equivalent outcomes increases to 2.6%.**

(figure 18.4). From our modelling in typical AMI populations (see figure 18.1), we knew that the average mortality of the low-risk two-thirds of patients was in this range, suggesting that similar mortality rates to population-wide PCI might be achieved by treatment of patients in the highest risk tertile only.

Indeed, a recent reanalysis of the DANAMI-2 trial showed results consistent with these findings.[33] Briefly, the DANAMI-2 trial randomised 1572 patients with acute ST-segment-elevation AMI to either PCI or thrombolysis with intravenous alteplase, and recruited most of their patients from referral hospitals without invasive treatment facilities. The overall results of this trial showed that treatment with PCI was associated with a significant reduction at 30-days of the combined endpoint of death, reinfarction or disabling stroke (6.7% versus 12.3%, $p = 0.05$), although the improvement for death alone did not reach statistical significance (6.6% versus 7.8%, $p = 0.35$).[34] The reanalysis using 3-year outcomes, stratified patients using the TIMI risk score for patients with ST-segment-elevation AMI (table 18.1)[16] into low-risk patients (TIMI risk score < 4) and high-risk patients (TIMI risk score ≥ 5). In the low-risk group (comprising 74% of the sample), there was a non-significant trend toward increased mortality at 3 years with PCI (PCI, 8.0%; thrombolysis, 5.6%; $p = 0.11$). For comparison, this group had a 30-day mortality of 2.5%, which corresponded closely with the low-risk/low-benefit group identified in our analysis. In the high-risk group, there was a significant reduction in mortality at 3 years with PCI (25.3% versus 36.2%, $p = 0.02$). There was a significant treatment-by-risk group interaction ($p = 0.008$), and the differential survival and differential treatment effect are shown graphically in figure 18.5(A). When the composite endpoint of death, reinfarction and disabling stroke was examined, again there

ST-segment-elevation AMI		**Unstable angina/non-ST-segment-elevation AMI**	
Characteristic	No. of points	Characteristic	No. of points
Age 65–74/≥ 75 years	2/3	Age ≥ 65 years	1
Systolic blood pressure < 100	3	≥ 3 risk factors for CAD	1
Heart rate > 100 beats/min	2	Known CAD (stenosis ≥ 50%)	1
Killip II–IV	2	Aspirin use in past 7 days	1
Anterior STE or LBBB	1	Recent (≤ 24 hours) severe angina	1
Diabetes, h/o HTN, or h/o angina	1	ST-segment deviation > 0.5 mm	1
Weight < 67 kg	1	↑ Cardiac markers	1
Time to treatment > 4 hours	1		
Risk score = total points	(0–14)	Risk score = total points	(0–7)

CAD, coronary artery disease; h/o, history of; HTN, hypertension; LBBB, left bundle branch block; STE, ST-segment elevation.

***Table* 18.1: The TIMI risk scores for ST-segment-elevation AMI and unstable angina/non-ST-segment-elevation AMI**

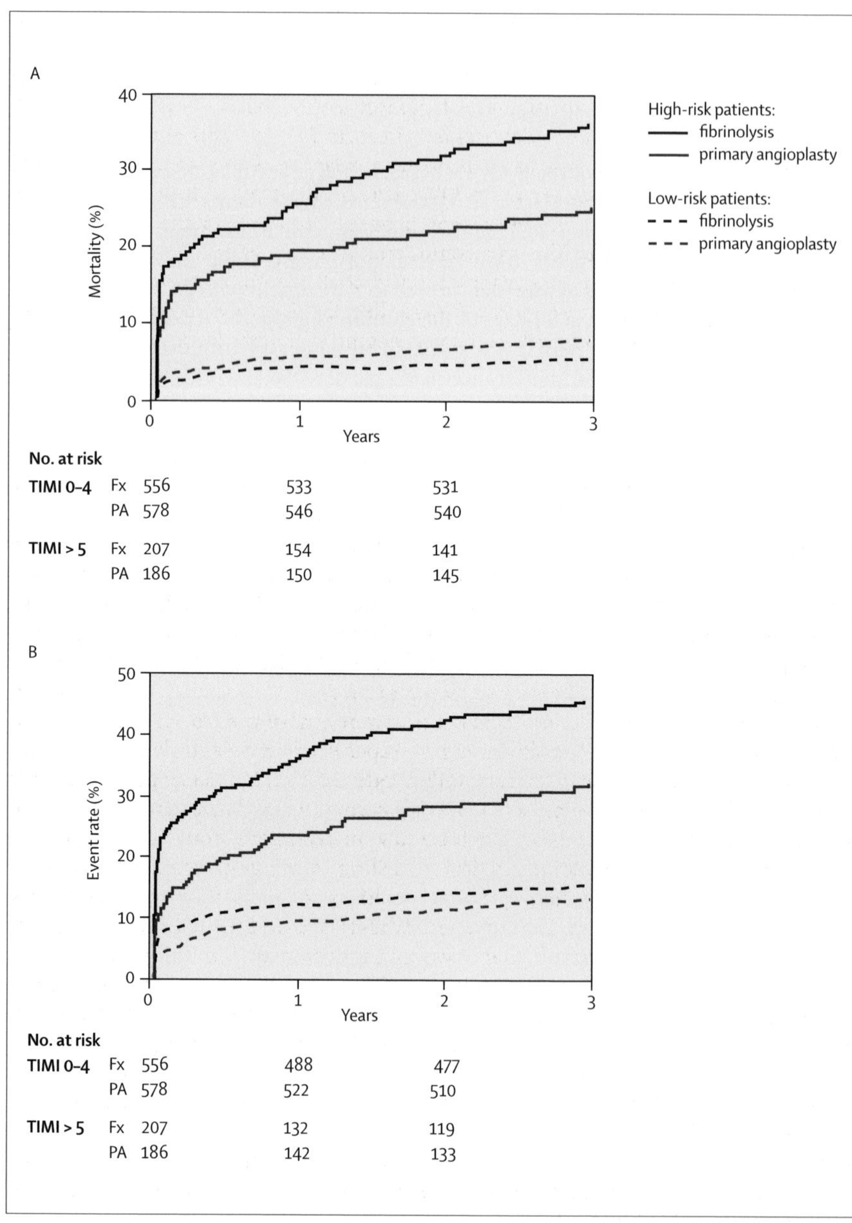

Figure 18.5: **Risk-stratified results of the DANAMI-2 trial: (A) mortality rates and (B) combined event rates, including death reinfarction, or disabling stroke for high-risk and low-risk patients. High-risk patients, comprising a quarter of all subjects, obtain considerable benefit from primary angioplasty, both in terms of mortality and in terms of combined events, while low-risk patients, comprising three-quarters of subjects, do not obtain any mortality benefit, and other adverse events are only marginally reduced.**

was no significant difference in outcomes between PCI and thrombolysis in the low-risk group (13.7% versus 15.7%, $p = 0.30$) but there was for the high-risk group (32.3% versus 45.9%, $p = 0.004$). The interaction for the composite outcome (figure 18.5(B)) was weaker and not statistically significant, in large part because low-risk and high-risk groups appeared to obtain near-identical benefit from PCI in terms of reduced risk of reinfarction. Indeed, in a recent analysis, using a database of combined registries and clinical trials including approximately 3000 patients receiving either PCI or thrombolysis, we have found a similar interaction between baseline mortality risk (as represented by TPI-predicted mortality as a continuous variable) and PCI treatment benefit for the outcome of mortality, suggesting again that all the mortality benefit of PCI is accounted for by the high-risk group.[35] Also, like the DANAMI-2 investigators, we found that the low-risk group still had some degree of benefit from PCI in terms of reduced reinfarction risk.

Unstable angina/non-ST-segment-elevation myocardial infarction

Perhaps across all clinical domains there have been more risk-stratified analyses of clinical trials testing interventions for unstable angina/non-ST-segment-elevation myocardial infarction (UA/NSTEMI). This is not surprising, given the extreme heterogeneity of this presentation. In the TIMI III registry, the rate of mortality was 2.5% and the rate of reinfarction was 2.9%, indicating that the vast majority of patients have excellent outcomes with the extant standard of care;[36] this is true also for clinical trials, although trial participants are at somewhat higher risk. Several risk scores have been developed for UA/NSTEMI.[37–40] The TIMI risk score,[40] which was developed to predict a composite outcome (mortality, new or recurrent myocardial infarction, or severe recurrent ischaemia) in a cohort of 1957 patients who were randomised to the unfractionated heparin arm of the TIMI IIB study (testing enoxaparin) is shown in table 18.1. Although this model was demonstrated to have only moderate discriminatory performance (*c* statistic on the derivation cohort was 0.65), it has consistently been shown to be useful in separating patients likely to benefit from new interventions from those unlikely to benefit. This is consistent with theoretical modelling, which demonstrates that models with even moderate discriminatory power are likely to be useful when relative risk reduction is roughly uniform, and treatment is associated with even a small number of adverse events.[11] Interventions that have been shown in clinical trials to have differential treatment impact depending on TIMI scores, with high-risk patients getting greater absolute and relative risk reductions, include: the low molecular weight heparin enoxaparin (compared to unfractionated heparin),[40] the glycoprotein IIb/IIIa inhibitor tirofiban[41] and an early invasive strategy (compared to a conservative approach).[42] It should be noted, however, that similar treatment-effect modification has been established on the basis of a positive troponin alone,[43–48] suggesting that, while a combination of factors might be better for risk stratification, troponin might be a more specific marker of treatment-modifiable risk, at least for some therapies, compared to other factors included in the TIMI model.

One interesting analysis compared three independently derived models (GRACE,[38] TIMI[40] and PURSUIT[39]) using an independent registry that included patients receiving and not receiving myocardial revascularisation.[49] All three models were able to discriminate between patients who appeared to benefit from myocardial revascularisation and those who did not (figure 18.6), although the treatment allocation was not randomised. However, the model with the best discrimination (the GRACE model) did show the strongest degree of treatment-effect modification, and was able to target treatment most efficiently. In this particular database, assuming comparability of treatment groups, targeting therapy to patients using the GRACE model would have led to the best outcomes, although use of any of these risk models to target therapy would have improved outcomes compared to the observed treatment-allocation strategy.

Acute ischaemic stroke

Background

In 1995, the NINDS trial found that rtPA therapy improved 90-day outcomes in patients with acute ischaemic stroke, in patients treated within 3 hours of symptom onset.[50] Patients receiving the thrombolytic agent had a margin of benefit of 11–15% in their likelihood of a normal or near-normal outcome compared to those receiving placebo, despite a risk of thrombolytic-related symptomatic ICH of about 6% in those treated, a typically catastrophic outcome. Based on these results, use of rtPA for this indication was approved in the USA in 1996. Since this was the first treatment for acute stroke

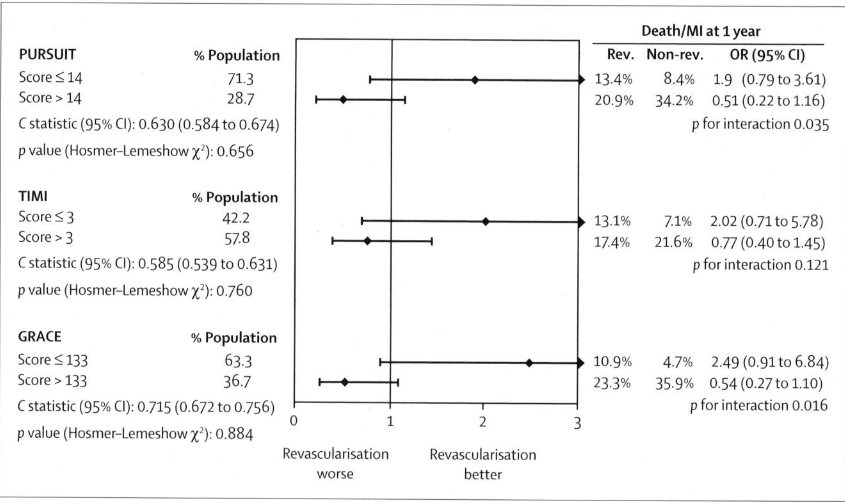

Figure 18.6: **Interaction of prognostic risk score with the impact of myocardial revascularisation. The impact of myocardial revascularisation on 460 consecutive patients admitted to the coronary care unit of Santa Cruz Hospital in Portugal, divided into high- and low-risk patients using three different risk scores (PURSUIT, TIMI and GRACE). Regardless of the risk score used, there is a consistent trend to benefit in high-risk patients and a consistent trend to harm in low-risk patients. The *p* value for the interaction is significant, except for when the TIMI score was used. The *c* statistic and Hosmer–Lemeshow *p* value are shown for each model. Using this database, the GRACE model had the best discrimination and also showed the strongest interaction with treatment effect, indicating the most efficient targeting.**

with proven efficacy, and since the benefits of the treatment were time sensitive, this was expected to revolutionise the care of acute stroke, transforming suspected 'brain attacks' into medical emergencies similar to heart attacks. However, in the years that followed, registry data from the USA show that only about 2% of patients with acute ischaemic stroke are being treated with thrombolytic therapy.[51, 52] The major reason for exclusion from therapy is that patients most typically present too late for treatment, as the therapeutic time window is so narrow. Other clinical trials, including ECASS[53] and ECASS II,[54] and ATLANTIS A[55] and ATLANTIS B,[56] designed to look at therapeutic time windows up to 6 hours after symptom onset, did not find any benefit for rtPA in their primary outcomes.

A reanalysis of the ATLANTIS B trial

The ATLANTIS B trial, performed after the results of NINDS were known, was designed specifically to test whether the therapeutic time window for thrombolysis could be expanded. The trial primarily enrolled patients in the 3–5 hour time window. The results in this trial (figure 18.7(A)), showed no increase in the proportion of patients with a normal or near-normal outcome with rtPA, across four different outcome scales. At the same time, the rate of thrombolytic-related symptomatic ICH was about 7%.

That functional outcomes (as shown in figure 18.7(A)) were essentially identical with and without rtPA, despite a thrombolytic-related ICH rate of about 1/15 patients, suggests that some patients treated during this later time window must be benefiting from rtPA, to compensate for outcomes in those that are harmed. We hypothesised that the overall result obscures the fact that patients at lower risk of thrombolytic-related ICH might benefit from therapy.[10] To test this hypothesis, we applied the same logistic regression model predicting thrombolytic-related ICH (based on age, gender, race, systolic blood pressure, diastolic blood pressure and history of prior stroke),[22] under the assumption that risk factors for this complication in patients receiving tPA for AMI might also put patients at higher risk when receiving rtPA for stroke.

Based on power considerations, patients in the trial were divided into equal-sized tertiles according to their predicted thrombolytic-related ICH risk. Patients in the low-risk tertile had substantially lower ICH risk than did those in the other two tertiles, which showed similar rates for this treatment complication (2.2 versus 9.3, $p = 0.03$). More importantly, when functional outcomes were examined, a consistent benefit of a clinically important magnitude across all four functional outcome scales was noted (from a low of 5 percentage points in the Barthel Index to 12 percentage points on the modified Rankin Score, $p = 0.10$ for the global outcome), and there was a treatment–risk interaction ($p = 0.03$), indicating the presence of a statistically significant treatment effect that varies across this dimension of ICH risk.

Limitations

The particular model used in this study has several limitations. In particular it was derived using data on patients who received thrombolytic therapy for AMI, and is poorly specified for stroke. Secondly, only the risks of therapy are included in the model, and

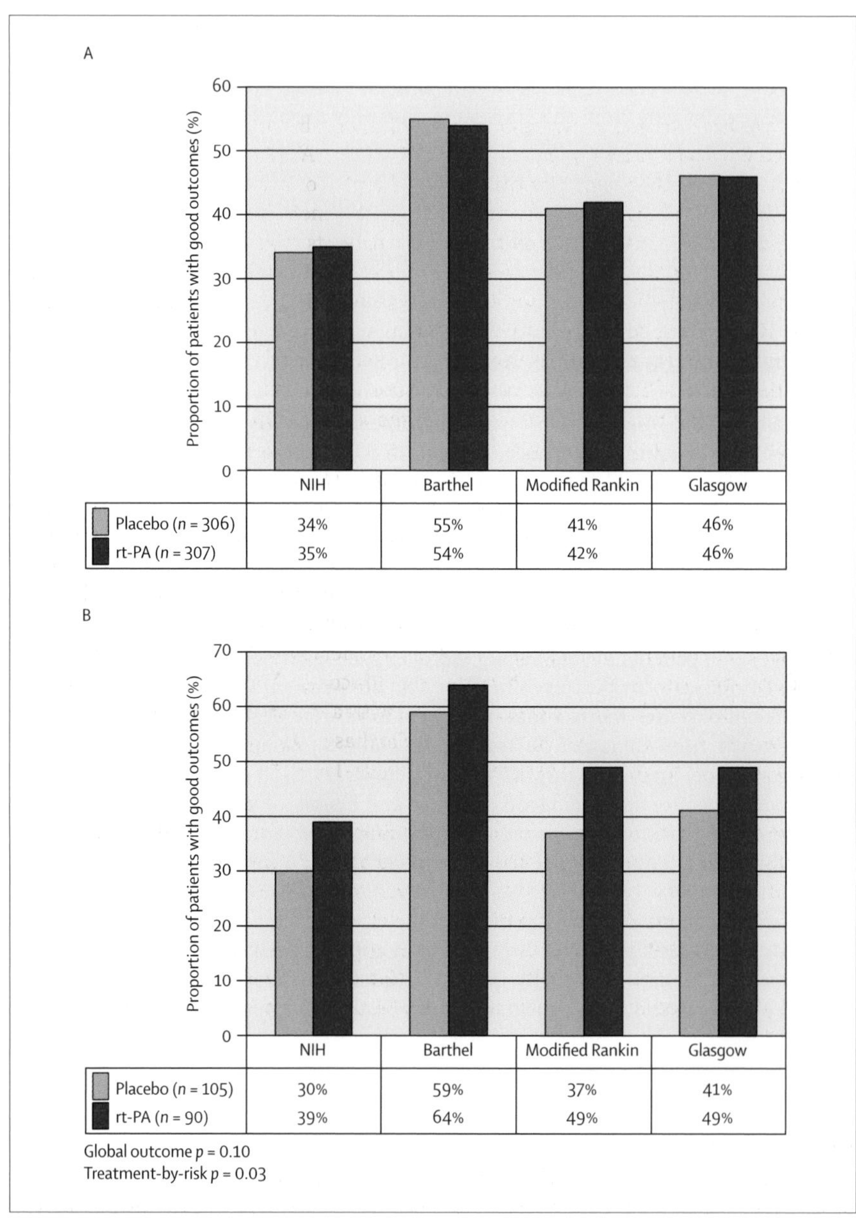

Figure 18.7: Outcomes in the overall ATLANTIS B trial compared with outcomes in the low-risk subgroup. There was no benefit from rtPA therapy in the ATLANTIS B trial overall, with the absolute percentage benefit ranging from –1% to 1% across four different stroke scales. However, for patients identified by the independently derived model for being at relatively low risk of ICH, there was a consistent benefit ranging from 5% to 12% across the four stroke scales. For patients at moderate to high risk, there was a commensurate trend toward harm.

not variables that might alter the benefit of therapy independently of this risk (e.g. time from symptom onset).

Indeed, we have started to address these limitations by modelling directly using a combined database including patients from NINDS,[50] ATLANTIS A,[55] ATLANTIS B[56] and ECASS II.[54] Unlike other domains, such as acute coronary syndromes, where outcome risk is a principal determinant of treatment benefit, this assumption does not appear justified in acute stroke, as higher risk patients (e.g. those with worse stroke severity) who potentially have the most to gain from thrombolytic therapy are typically at higher risk for the main complication of treatment (i.e. thrombolytic-related symptomatic ICH). Thus, stroke severity does not appear to be useful in determining who might and who might not benefit from therapy. Rather, identifying those variables that modify the effects of therapy, and combining these treatment-interaction factors (which are not necessarily risk factors for outcome) into a score, appears to be a more useful approach. Candidate variables are both those that are associated with increased/decreased risk of therapy (e.g. the variables in the ICH risk model used in the ATLANTIS B trial reanalysis), and those associated with increased or decreased benefits (e.g. variables associated with better clot lysis or with enhanced neuronal resistance to ischaemia). Variables that appear to be useful thus far, in predicting less treatment benefit, include: longer symptom onset to treatment time,[57] male gender,[58] higher systolic blood pressure and prior stroke. We have developed a predictive equation that combines these factors, which modify the effect of therapy and other prognostic factors (including age, stroke severity, diabetes and glucose). The equation predicts the likelihood of a normal or near-normal outcome with and without thrombolytic therapy, based on the outcomes in the combined database. The equation and has been incorporated into a computer program, the Stroke-TPI.[24, 59]

The statistical approach used in developing the Stroke-TPI must be distinguished from that using a risk score as a single variable, because combining interaction terms involves testing multiple 'one variable at a time' interactions, increasing the risks of a type I error.[5, 11] Thus, although such modelling has demonstrated promise as a means for selecting 'treatment-favourable' even after the approved 3-hour time window, these analyses should be interpreted with caution. Validation on independent clinical trials is necessary before recommending such models be used for patient selection in clinical practice.[60]

Conclusion

Knowledge of the average results of clinical trials is frequently insufficient to guide physicians in their treatment of individual patients, particularly when treatments are risky or costly. Even when inclusion and exclusion criteria are well defined, there is often wide heterogeneity of outcome risk across patients enrolled in a trial. For some conditions, such as acute coronary syndromes, subgrouping of patients by outcome risk using validated multivariable risk scores is likely to be a useful approach to uncovering heterogeneity in treatment effects, with the objectives of targeting treatments to those most likely to benefit and avoiding therapy in patients who might be harmed. Such a priori subgroup analysis should become a routine part of clinical trials in acute coronary syndromes, including ST-segment-elevation AMI. For other conditions, such as acute stroke, outcome risk may not be a good predictor of treatment benefit, often because the main predictors of outcome risk are also predictors of the main risks of therapy. However, the need to individualise therapies for these conditions is no less important, especially when (as with tPA for stroke) the therapy has considerable risks or costs. In such cases, identification of variables that reliably modify the effects of therapy will be necessary, and will typically require redundancy of clinical trials.

References

1 Rothwell PM. Can overall results of clinical trials be applied to all patients? *Lancet* 1995; **345:** 1616–19.

2 Ioannidis JP, Lau J. Heterogeneity of the baseline risk within patient populations of clinical trials: a proposed evaluation algorithm. *Am J Epidemiol* 1998; **148:** 1117–26.

3 Kravitz RL, Duan N, Braslow J. Evidence-based medicine, heterogeneity of treatment effects, and the trouble with averages. *Milbank Quarterly* 2004; **82:** 661–87.

4 Rothwell PM, Mehta Z, Howard SC, et al. Treating individuals 3: from subgroups to individuals: general principles and the example of carotid endarterectomy. *Lancet* 2005; **365:** 256–65.

5 Hayward RA, Kent DM, Vijan S, Hofer TP. Reporting clinical trial results to inform providers, payers, and consumers. *Health Affairs* 2005; **24:** 1571–81.

6 Kent DM, Hayward RA. When averages hide individual differences in clinical trials. *Am Scientist* 2007; **95:** 60–68.

7 Ioannidis JP, Lau J. The impact of high-risk patients on the results of clinical trials. *J Clin Epidemiol* 1997; **50:** 1089–98.

8 Rothwell PM, Warlow CP. Prediction of benefit from carotid endarterectomy in individual patients: a risk-modeling study. European Carotid Surgery Trialists' Collaborative Group. *Lancet* 1999; **353:** 2105–10.

9 Kent DM, Hayward RA, Griffith JL, et al. An independently-derived model for selecting patients likely to benefit from tissue plasminogen activator: validating with GUSTO. *Am J Med* 2002; **113:** 104–11.

10 Kent DM, Ruthazer R, Selker HP. Are some patients likely to benefit from recombinant tissue-type plasminogen activator for acute ischemic stroke even beyond 3 hours from symptom onset? *Stroke* 2003; **34:** 464–67.

11 Hayward RA, Kent DM, Vijan S, Hofer TP. Multivariable risk prediction can greatly enhance the statistical power of clinical trial subgroup analysis. *BMC Med Res Methodol* 2006; **6:** 18.

12 Kent DM, Langa KM, Selker HP. The potential use of ECG-based prognostic instruments in clinical trials and cost-effectiveness analyses of new therapies in acute cardiac ischemia. *J Electrocardiol* 2000; **33** (suppl): 263–68.

13 Antman EM, Braunwald E. Acute myocardial infarction. In: E Braunwald, DP Zipes, P Libby, eds. *Heart Disease: A Textbook of Cardiovascular Medicine,* 6th edn. Philadelphia, PA: WB Saunders, 2001: 1114–218.

14 Lee KL, Woodlief LH, Topol EJ, et al. Predictors of 30-day mortality in the era of reperfusion for acute myocardial infarction. *Circulation* 1995; **91:** 1659–68.

15 Krumholz HM, Chen J, Wang Y. Comparing AMI mortality among hospitals in patients 65 years of age and older: evaluating methods of risk adjustment. *Circulation* 1999; **99:** 2986–92.

16 Morrow DA, Antman EM, Charlesworth A, et al. TIMI risk score for ST-elevation myocardial infarction: a convenient, bedside, clinical score for risk assessment at presentation. An InTIME II trial substudy. *Circulation* 2000; **102:** 2031–37.

17 Rouleau JL, Talajic M, Sussex B. Myocardial infarction patients in the 1990s – their risk factors, stratification and survival in Canada: the Canadian Assessment of Myocardial Infarction (CAMI) Study. *J Am Coll Cardiol* 1996; **27:** 1119–27.

18 Selker HP, Griffith JL, Beshansky JR, et al. Patient-specific predictions of outcomes in myocardial infarction for real-time emergency use: a thrombolytic predictive instrument. *Ann Intern Med* 1997; **127:** 538–48.

19 Kent DM, Schmid CH, Lau J, Selker HP. Is primary angioplasty for some as good as primary angioplasty for all? Modeling across trials and individual patients. *J Gen Intern Med* 2002; **17:** 887–94.

20 The GUSTO investigators. An international randomized trial comparing four thrombolytic strategies for acute myocardial infarction. *N Engl J Med* 1993; **329:** 673–82.

21 Mark DB, Hlatky MA, Califf RM, et al. Cost effectiveness of thrombolytic therapy with tissue plasminogen activator as compared with streptokinase for acute myocardial infarction. *N Engl J Med* 1995; **332:** 1418–24.

22 Gurwitz JH, Gore JM, Goldberg RJ, et al. Risk for intracranial hemorrhage after tissue plasminogen activator treatment for acute myocardial infarction. *Ann Intern Med* 1998; **129:** 597–604.

23 Kent DM, Vijan S, Hayward RA, et al. Tissue plasminogen activator was cost-effective compared to streptokinase only in selected patients with acute myocardial infarction. *J Clin Epidemiol* 2004; **57:** 843–52.

24 http://www.tufts-nemc.org/icrhps/faculty/fac_respage/KentD_respage.asp

25 Boersma H, van der Vlugt J, Arnold ER, et al. Estimated gain in life expectancy: a simple tool to select optimal reperfusion treatment in individual patients with evolving myocardial infarction. *Eur Heart J* 1996; **17:** 64–75.

26 Califf RL, Woodlief LH, Harrell FE, et al. Selection of thrombolytic therapy for individual patients: development of a clinical model. *Am Heart J* 1997; **133:** 630–39.

27 Weaver W, Simes R, Betriu A, et al. Comparison of primary coronary angioplasty and intravenous thrombolytic therapy for acute myocardial infarction: a quantitative review. *JAMA* 1997; **278:** 2093–98.

28 Keeley EC, Boura JA, Grines CL. Primary angioplasty versus intravenous thrombolytic therapy for acute myocardial infarction: a quantitative review of 23 randomised trials. *Lancet* 2003; **361:** 13–20.

29 Fox KAA, Goodman SG, Anderson FA Jr, et al., for the GRACE Investigators. From guidelines to clinical practice: the impact of hospital and geographical characteristics on temporal trends in the management of acute coronary syndromes. The Global Registry of Acute Coronary Events (GRACE). *Eur Heart J* 2003; **24:** 1414–24.

30 Magid DJ, Wang Y, Herrin J, et al. Relationship between time of day, day of week, timeliness of reperfusion, and in-hospital mortality for patients with acute ST-segment elevation myocardial infarction. *JAMA* 2005; **294:** 803–12.

31 Califf RM, Faxon DP. Need for centers to care for patients with acute coronary syndromes. *Circulation* 2003; **107:** 1467–70.

32 Topol EJ, Kereiakes DJ. Regionalization of care for acute ischemic heart disease: a call for specialized centers. *Circulation* 2003; **107:** 1463–66.

33 Thune JJ, Hoefsten DE, Lindholm MG, et al. Simple risk stratification at admission to identify patients with reduced mortality from primary angioplasty. *Circulation* 2005; **112:** 2017–21.

34 Andersen HR, Nielsen TT, Rasmussen K, et al. A comparison of coronary angioplasty with fibrinolytic therapy in acute myocardial infarction. *N Engl J Med* 2003; **349:** 733–42.

35 Kent DM, Ruthazer R, Griffith JL, et al. Comparison of mortality benefit of immediate thrombolytic therapy versus delayed primary angioplasty. *Am J Cardiol* in press.

36 Sabatine MS, Antman EM. The thrombolysis in myocardial infarction risk score in unstable angina/non-ST-segment elevation myocardial infarction. *J Am Coll Cardiol* 2003; **41:** 89S–95S.

37 Scirica BM, Cannon CP, McCabe CH, et al. Prognosis in the thrombolysis in myocardial ischemia III registry according to the Braunwald unstable angina pectoris classification. *Am J Cardiol* 2002; **90:** 821–26.

38 Jacobs DR Jr, Kroenke C, Crow R, et al. PREDICTA simple risk score for clinical severity and long-term prognosis after hospitalization for acute myocardial infarction or unstable angina: the Minnesota heart survey. *Circulation* 1999; **100:** 599–607.

39 Boersma E, Pieper KS, Steyerberg EW, et al. Predictors of outcome in patients with acute coronary syndromes without persistent ST-segment elevation results from an international trial of 9461 patients. The PURSUIT Investigators. *Circulation* 2000; **101:** 2557–67.

40 Antman EM, Cohen M, Bernink PJ, et al. The TIMI risk score for unstable angina/non-ST elevation MI: a method for prognostication and therapeutic decision making. *JAMA* 2000; **284:** 835–42.

41 Morrow DA, Antman EM, Snapinn SM, et al. An integrated clinical approach to predicting the benefit of tirofiban in non-ST-elevation acute coronary syndromes: application of the TIMI Risk Score for UA/NSTEMI in PRISM-PLUS. *Eur Heart J* 2002; **23:** 223–29.

42 Cannon CP, Weintraub WS, Demopoulos LA, et al. Comparison of coronary syndromes treated with the glycoprotein IIb/IIIa inhibitor tirofiban. *N Engl J Med* 2001; **344:** 1879–87.

43 Newby LK, Goldmann BU, Ohman EM. Troponin: an important prognostic marker and risk-stratification tool in non-ST-segment elevation acute coronary syndromes. *J Am Coll Cardiol* 2003; **41:** 31S–36S.

44 Lindahl B, Venge P, Wallentin L, for the Fragmin in Unstable Coronary Artery Disease (FRISC) Study Group. Troponin T identifies patients with unstable coronary artery disease who benefit from long-term antithrombotic protection. *J Am Coll Cardiol* 1997; **29:** 43–48.

45 Morrow DA, Antman EM, Tanasijevic M, et al. Cardiac troponin I for the stratification or early outcomes and the efficacy of enoxaparin in unstable angina: a TIMI-IIb substudy. *J Am Coll Cardiol* 2000; **36:** 1812–17.

46 The CAPTURE Investigators. Randomised placebo-controlled trial of abciximab before and during coronary intervention in refractory unstable angina: the CAPTURE study. *Lancet* 1997; **349:** 1429–35.

47 Hamm CW, Heeschen C, Goldmann B, et al. Benefit of abciximab in patients with refractory unstable angina in relation to serum troponin T levels. *N Engl J Med* 1999; **340:** 1623–29.

48 Heeschen C, Hamm CW, Goldmann B, et al. Troponin concentrations for stratification of patients with acute coronary syndromes in relation to therapeutic efficacy of tirofiban. *Lancet* 1999; **354:** 1757–62.

49 Gonçalves PA, Ferreira J, Aguiar C, Seabra-Gomes R. TIMI, PURSUIT, and GRACE risk scores: sustained prognostic value and interaction with revascularization in NSTE-ACS. *Eur Heart J* 2005; **26:** 865–72.

50 The NINDS rt-PA Stroke Study Group. Tissue plasminogen activator for acute ischemic stroke. *N Engl J Med* 1995; **333:** 1581–87.

51 Katzan IL, Furlan AJ, Lloyd LE, et al. Use of tissue-type plasminogen activator for acute ischemic stroke: the Cleveland area experience. *JAMA* 2000; **283:** 1151–58.

52 Bravata DM, Kim N, Concato J, et al. Thrombolysis for acute stroke in routine clinical practice. *Arch Intern Med* 2002; **162:** 1994–2001.

53 Hacke W, Kaste M, Fieschi C, et al. Intravenous thrombolysis with recombinant tissue plasminogen activator for acute hemispheric stroke. The European Cooperative Acute Stroke Study (ECASS). *JAMA* 1995; **274:** 1017–25.

54 Hacke W, Kaste M, Fieschi C, et al. Randomised double-blind placebo-controlled trial of thrombolytic therapy with intravenous alteplase in acute ischaemic stroke (ECASS II). Second European–Australasian Acute Stroke Study Investigators. *Lancet* 1998; **352:** 1245–51.

55 Clark WM, Albers GW, Madden KP, Hamilton S. The rtPA (alteplase) 0- to 6-hour acute stroke trial, part A (A0276g): results of a double-blind, placebo-controlled, multicenter study. Thromblytic therapy in acute ischemic stroke study investigators. *Stroke* 2000; **31:** 811–16.

56 Clark WM, Wissman S, Albers GW, et al. Recombinant tissue-type plasminogen activator (alteplase) for ischemic stroke 3 to 5 hours after symptom onset. The ATLANTIS Study: a randomized controlled trial. Alteplase Thrombolysis for Acute Noninterventional Therapy in Ischemic Stroke. *JAMA* 1999; **282:** 2019–26.

57 The ATLANTIS, ECASS, and NINDS rt-PA Study Group Investigators. Association of outcome with early stroke treatment: pooled analysis of ATLANTIS, ECASS, and NINDS rt-PA stroke trials. *Lancet* 2004; **363:** 768–74.

58 Kent DM, Price LL, Ringleb P, et al. Sex-based differences in response to recombinant tissue plasminogen activator in acute ischemic stroke: a pooled analysis of randomized clinical trials. *Stroke* 2005; **36:** 62–65.

59 Kent DM, Selker HP, Ruthazer R, et al. The stroke–thrombolytic predictive instrument: a predictive instrument for intravenous thrombolysis in acute ischemic stroke. *Stroke* 2006; **37:** 2957–62.

60 Kent DM, Selker HP, Ruthazer R, et al. Can multivariable risk–benefit profiling be used to select treatment-favorable patients for thrombolysis in stroke in the 3- to 6-hour time window? *Stroke* 2006; **37:** 2963–69.

19

Choice of agent in treatment of epilepsy

Sanjay M. Sisodiya

Introduction

Epilepsy is the tendency to have recurrent unprovoked seizures, usually diagnosed after the occurrence of at least two such seizures. Ultimately, there is a limited spectrum of clinical phenomena that can be generated by the entire spectrum of brain diseases. It follows that many underlying diseases could result in epileptic seizures as their sole or main manifestation, and thus that 'epilepsy' is a heterogeneous group of conditions, which share some common characteristics, including symptomatic response to a set of drugs ('antiepileptic drugs'), and which it is sometimes appropriate to group under the umbrella term 'epilepsy' or 'the epilepsies'. Most of the drugs currently called 'antiepileptic drugs' (AEDs) are probably in fact 'antiseizure' drugs: given the overwhelming usage of the former term, it will be adopted in this chapter.

An appreciation of the population statistics of the epilepsies sets the treatment of these conditions in context. The cost of epilepsy, estimated at £500 million/year for direct costs in the UK alone,[1] includes about £140 million/year spent on AEDs.[2] Incidence varies both within and between nations: in mature economies it is about 50/100 000 persons/year, being higher in infants and the elderly,[3–5] and in poorer people;[6] in resource-poor countries, the overall incidence is higher, often greater than 100/100 000 persons/year, due to a variety of factors, including poor sanitation and a higher risk of brain infections.[4,7] Patterns of incidence are changing, with a falling childhood incidence and rising elderly incidence in mature economies.[4] The prevalence of epilepsy is between 4 and 10/1000.[4,5] Higher prevalence rates in population isolates[4] should impress upon us the genetic and environmental heterogeneity in disease aetiology. That lifetime prevalence rates are much higher than rates of active epilepsy is partly due to increased mortality,[8] but is predominantly explained by remission.

In mature economies, more than 70% of patients achieve long-term remission, usually within 5 years of diagnosis.[4] The causes of remission are unknown. There are some clinical predictors of good outcome, including age of onset, smaller number of early seizures[9,10] and early response to AEDs.[11] However, even in resource-poor countries, many patients also enter long-term remission, even with a lack of AEDs. Certainly, previous and recent work would suggest that early initiation of AEDs does not affect long-term remission in individuals with single or infrequent seizures, even if it reduces recurrence in the short term.[12–14] Thus, prognosis is thought to be dependent most on cause rather than treatment.[4,15–17] It is also likely that response to AEDs, and hence the choice of AED, will also turn out to be dependent, to some extent, on cause. Up to one-third of people having seizures develop chronic epilepsy, failing to achieve freedom from seizures with currently available AEDs.[17]

19 Choice of agent in treatment of epilepsy

Why is the choice of AED important?

If 70% of patients, at least in mature economies, enter long-term remission, often on low doses of AEDs early in treatment,[18] and the influence of AEDs in this outcome is uncertain, why is the choice of AED important? The choice of drug has important consequences for individual patients in terms of chances of successful treatment (abolition of seizures), absence of adverse effects, speed of achieving control, teratogenicity and risk of seizure exacerbation.

There are about 20 licensed AEDs available in the UK. All may be associated with adverse effects, of varying severity. Some adverse reactions are serious and lead to hospital admission: 6.5% of hospital admissions in one study were due to adverse drug reactions (all drugs),[19] with up to 17% of admissions for adverse reactions to drugs being due to AEDs in an older retrospective study.[20] Rarely, adverse reactions to AEDs prove fatal.[21] Lesser adverse effects impair quality of life.[22]

The teratogenicity of AEDs is perhaps the major consideration in AED choice in clinical practice for women of child-bearing age, who constitute a third of all patients with epilepsy. Data on the teratogenicity of many AEDs, especially more recently licensed AEDs, are lacking:[2] no randomised controlled trials (RCTs) in epilepsy have considered teratogenicity as an outcome in the choice of an AED, and such trials might well be difficult to conduct. Recent retrospective data also suggest that learning disability might be associated with valproate exposure in utero,[23] raising the stakes further, especially as another large study has shown that valproate remains the most efficacious AED in the treatment of idiopathic generalised epilepsies, despite the availability of newer agents.[24] That the risk of learning disability is also increased by the occurrence of five or more generalised tonic–clonic seizures during pregnancy[23] further complicates decision-making in the use of valproate in women of child-bearing age who have an idiopathic generalised epilepsy syndrome.

Some AEDs can aggravate epilepsy.[25–27] Most commonly this is caused by the use of carbamazepine, oxcarbazepine[28] or phenytoin in idiopathic generalised epilepsies that have not received a correct syndromic diagnosis. In some cases, AEDs thought to be appropriate for a given syndrome may cause aggravation of seizures in some individuals with that syndrome, even when correctly diagnosed (e.g. lamotrigine in juvenile myoclonic epilepsy).[29]

Although immediate initiation of AED treatment after a single or a few seizures seems unimportant in most, but not all, cases,[14] the actual time taken to achieve full control of seizures may be one factor in determining long-term outcome. The number of seizures over a period of time (seizure density) before initiation of AED treatment has been identified as a prognostic factor for long-term control:[17] it is not known, however, if seizure density after AED initiation has any influence on eventual prognosis in treated cases. Seizures are known to alter gene expression extensively,[30] providing potential pathophysiological mechanisms underpinning the impact of seizure density. In a given individual, one drug may be more likely than another to achieve seizure freedom.

Seizure freedom as an outcome should be the gold standard in the treatment of epilepsy.[31] Only seizure freedom has been proven to improve scores on quality-of-life measures after surgical treatment of refractory epilepsy,[32] for example, and reinstatement of a driving licence in the UK usually depends on seizure freedom (there are some exceptions). Notably, seizure freedom has never been the primary outcome measure in any RCT of AEDs.

The choice of AED, therefore, has important consequences for individual patients in terms of the chances of successful treatment (abolition of seizures), the absence of adverse effects, the speed of achieving control, teratogenicity and risk of seizure exacerbation, even in patients who do respond or who may be destined to do so. Predestination of outcome is strictly unproven, and will be difficult to now establish in mature economies with AED availability, but is likely to be a genuine bioclinical phenomenon.[17]

Pathophysiology and serendipity

For no single epileptic seizure type, disease, pathology or syndrome has a complete or even sufficient mechanistic explanation been elucidated. Consider, by way of example, two conditions: hippocampal sclerosis and periventricular heterotopia (PVH) causing epilepsy.

Hippocampal sclerosis, characterised by the loss of neurons and the presence of gliosis within the hippocampus, is one of the best-studied pathologies underlying the most common type of drug-resistant focal epilepsy syndrome, mesial temporal lobe epilepsy. Even the fact that surgical resection, often curative in this disease, makes available diseased living human brain tissue for detailed scrutiny, at levels from the macromorphological to the genomic, has not generated a mechanistic understanding of the condition: the pathophysiological basis for seizures and epilepsy in mesial temporal lobe epilepsy due to hippocampal sclerosis remains enigmatic.[33] Indeed, while there are known causes of hippocampal sclerosis, such as status epilepticus[34] and exotoxins such as domoic acid from contaminated mussel poisoning,[35] in most cases even the aetiology of this well-recognised and easily demonstrable pathology is unknown.[33]

PVH caused by mutation in the X-linked gene *FLNA*, encoding filamin A, is a rare neurodevelopmental cause of epilepsy. It is now known that deleterious mutations in this gene can underlie some cases of familial or sporadic PVH: in some cases, the PVH goes on to cause epilepsy, which may be drug-resistant, while other patients do not even develop epilepsy.[36] In PVH due to *FLNA* mutation, we do know the ultimate cause of the disease. We have a reasonable understanding of the role of filamin in neurodevelopment.[37] We know much about the pathological anatomy of the periventricular nodules themselves, including the disruptions of neurohistological and immunophenotypic profiles, the abnormal electrical activity that may arise from such nodules, their connectivity with the rest of the brain, and their appearance on imaging. However, we do not know precisely how or why seizures occur (in some patients but not others), nor why epilepsy develops. Therefore, even following a pathological single nucleotide alteration in one gene leading to epilepsy as its primary manifestation, in fact a tangled multilayered raft of changes occurs at several temporal, spatial and functional points, leading eventually to epilepsy.

For most causes of epilepsy, one or more such facets of disease biology, such as identification in vivo, availability of human brain tissue or comparator animal models for study, are unknown or unstudied, let alone understood. Thus, for the vast majority of the epilepsies, there is no rational basis for treatment – agents that are 'successful' are so more by luck than design.

Current clinical practice: evidence base and guidelines

A number of RCTs have been undertaken in epilepsy. The findings of these RCTs have been recently summarised in guideline documents,[2, 38] for the purpose of informing clinical practice. In the context of treating individuals, external validity is evaluated in Chapter 3, but there are certain aspects to evaluating the generalisability of RCTs that are particularly relevant in epilepsy.

Firstly, the published RCTs are overwhelmingly studies of the use of a given drug in cohorts of patients with drug-resistant epilepsy. The patients most commonly have refractory focal epilepsies (rather than refractory idiopathic generalised epilepsies), but nevertheless represent mixed populations of patients with a broad range of underlying subsyndromes (temporal lobe, frontal lobe epilepsies, etc.) and aetiologies (e.g. acquired or inherited causes). Thus the underlying pathophysiology is likely to be varied. These RCTs have examined the effect of a given drug in a spectrum of patients: the studies are thus drug driven, not disease or patient driven. In this sense, the generalisability of the results obtained in the RCTs must be limited: the RCTs are usually designed to satisfy pharmacocentric regulatory requirements rather than pragmatic patient-centred concerns.

Secondly, RCTs are only undertaken for drugs in advanced stages of development or after licensing. In epilepsy, these drugs are almost always selected in the inescapable early stages of development on the basis of their efficacy in a narrow selection of animal seizure models. These models did not emerge from any rational understanding of epilepsy pathophysiology, and have not gained supremacy by design. Thus, most drugs available for the treatment of epilepsy may well not represent good treatments for epilepsy pathophysiologies that are poorly reflected in the models used to filter candidate AEDs.

Thirdly, the natural history of the epilepsies needs to be taken into careful account (see above): many patients with epilepsy go into remission, and the impact of AEDs in general, or any AED in particular, on this prognosis is unknown.[17] A corollary is that almost any syndrome-appropriate AED may appear effective in the majority of patients with newly diagnosed epilepsy. Thus response may not be drug specific.

Lastly, there are few patient-, disease- or syndrome-driven RCTs in epilepsy, bearing in mind the heterogeneity of this condition, and the implications of this heterogeneity, as discussed above. However, individual patients present with a specific cause, type or syndrome of epilepsy, not just with 'epilepsy', even if in a proportion of patients the cause, type or syndrome is not known. Thus, treatment in individuals needs to be determined in the individual context by cause, type or syndrome: RCTs therefore should discriminate or select for these same causes, types or syndromes. There are few such RCTs, but these must be the most useful for generalisability to individuals. RCTs enrolling a wide spectrum of patients may also risk obscuring beneficial effects that drugs may have in a more narrowly defined phenotypic subgroup of patients. Heterogeneous populations necessitate larger sample sizes for the detection of differences.

Some of these issues are recognised in influential documents such as the National Institute for Health and Clinical Excellence (NICE) guidelines on the management of epilepsy in children and adults, which state:

> *The AED treatment strategy should be individualised according to the seizure type, epilepsy syndrome, co-medication and co-morbidity, the individual's lifestyle, and the preferences of the individual and their family and/or carers as appropriate.*[2]

However, the guidelines do not point out that RCT evidence is largely driven by drugs, and much less by 'seizure type, epilepsy syndrome'. Large, inclusive, RCTs are, of course, most likely to provide the most robust evidence base for treatment choices, but in some circumstances subgroup analyses are appropriate. The potential of subgroup analyses, as well as their risks, have been considered in detail.[35] Indeed, for trials in patients with epilepsies, there is arguably an inherent mandate for planned subgroup analyses, given the aetiopathophysiological heterogeneity in the epilepsies.

In the treatment of the majority of individuals with epilepsy, patients and physicians are fortunate that the complex biochemical physiology of the brain can integrate disease (epilepsy, epileptogenesis and seizures) and exogenous chemical agents (AEDs) to produce a comparatively satisfactory outcome with relatively few adverse effects. Within this framework of happenstance, national guidelines provide accessible information for relatively appropriate choices of AEDs. Thus 70% of patients treated with AEDs in mature economies can expect to enter remission,[4] often early after the initiation of small doses of AEDs.

With these provisos in mind, current best practice is well summarised in recent reviews and guidelines,[2, 38, 39] representing a distillation of RCT trial data, large retrospective studies of comparatively well-defined patient groups and expert opinion. Some specific examples are given here. Recommendations supported by RCT data include the preferred use of carbamazepine over valproate as first-line therapy for patients with focal epilepsy.[38] On the other hand, the choice between carbamazepine and lamotrigine (or indeed any other AED) for control of focal seizures is less clear.[39] With respect to teratogenicity, the NICE guidelines state 'Specific caution is advised in the use of sodium valproate because of the risk of harm to the unborn child'.[2] The previous gap in head-to-head comparisons between older and newer AEDs has been partially addressed by the pragmatic SANAD study,[24] although many of the concerns expressed above apply also to this study, despite its size, pragmatism and prospective nature.

The ideal, however, may well be to design clinically meaningful RCTs that are more appropriate for individual diseases within the umbrella label of 'epilepsy': no one would consider designing an RCT for the treatment of 'cancer', or even subgroups such as 'blood cancer'. A very small number of such RCTs do exist for epilepsy. These include a trial of sulthiame for benign childhood epilepsy with centrotemporal spikes (BECTS)[40] and a trial of stiripentol for severe myoclonic epilepsy of infancy (SMEI).[41]

SMEI is a devastating syndrome of childhood epilepsy, due in a proportion (but not all phenotypically defined cases) to a de novo mutation in a gene (*SCN1A*) encoding the alpha subunit of the cerebrally expressed sodium channel. Many (33–100%) patients with SMEI have mutations in *SCN1A*.[42] Characteristically, seizures appear in the first year of life on a background of normal development, and prove refractory to conventional AEDs, and are held responsible for the severe mental retardation that is subsequently observed: it is an epileptic encephalopathy. Although valproate and clobazam do not render such patients seizure free, they are the drugs most commonly used for this syndrome (without an RCT evidence base). The condition is rare, trials in children are difficult and the design of RCTs in this area must meet the concerns of parents and carers as well as regulatory authorities. Despite these limitations, Chiron et al.,[41] in an add-on RCT, were able to demonstrate an absolute reduction in seizure frequency of 69% on stiripentol against an increase of 7% on placebo, with 43% seizure free on stiripentol against none on placebo. For an otherwise devastating and refractory syndrome, this is a remarkable outcome, providing evidence for the use of stiripentol as adjunctive therapy in patients with SMEI, although long-term benefit on neurodevelopment has yet to be shown. Notably: (i) the only other RCT of the use of stiripentol has been published only as an interim report, did not show conclusive evidence of benefit, but did not obviously include children with SMEI;[43] and (ii) the known mechanisms of action of stiripentol (inhibition of cytochrome P450 oxidases and inhibition of synaptosomal reuptake of inhibitory neurotransmitters GABA and glycine) do not obviously target the underlying cause of SMEI where this is known, i.e. *SCN1A* mutation. It would, of course, be interesting to know if the responders in the trial done by Chiron et al.[41] did or did not have *SCN1A* mutation. Thus, even for a relatively phenotypically homogeneous, severe epilepsy syndrome, we may have reasonable evidence for the use of an efficacious drug, but even then we are left with genetic heterogeneity in the causation of the syndrome, and no good biological understanding of disease pathophysiology or drug action.

In summary, although guidelines exist to aid individual AED choice, the evidence base is in fact limited, especially when more detailed patient classification is considered. For the bulk of patients, this may not matter in practice in terms of achieving seizure control, but leaves important issues unaddressed. If syndrome-specific RCTs are to be considered in the epilepsies, multicentre trials will be necessary for adequate power to be obtained.

The future

An understanding of disease biology remains central to progress in rational treatment strategies, whether at the level of the individual patient, syndrome-specific RCTs or giant multicentre broad RCTs. While some epilepsies are monogenic and Mendelian, most are complex traits, resulting from the interplay between environment and individual genetic inheritance and variation. Most individuals with epilepsy are thought to have an oligogenic or polygenic diathesis underlying multiple aspects of disease biology, such as aetiology, susceptibility, clinical manifestation, treatment response, consequences and prognosis. Progress in the genetic contribution to epilepsy susceptibility is proving slow,[44] a parallel to other diseases. On the other hand, progress in disease pharmacogenetics is likely in general to accelerate,[45] although there is no place for complacency in the design and pursuit of pharmacogenetics studies.[46] Genetic heterogeneity for multiple disease aspects, both across and within phenotypic classifications, is a clear reason for subgroup analyses in large RCTs, which by nature recruit broadly across differing types of epilepsy, especially if such analyses are preplanned.[47] It is worth emphasising that genetic heterogeneity in both disease aetiology and drug response might separate such subgroups. The stringency applied to subgroup analyses will need to match that applied to the genetic (association) studies that identify potentially biologically motivated subgroups of patients in the first place.[46]

An example of the potential of pharmacogenetics in individualising treatment decisions based on disease biology comes from the study of the dosing of the two commonly used AEDs, phenytoin and carbamazepine. Both drugs are thought to act at least partly by binding a subunit of the cerebral sodium channel, encoded by the same *SCN1A* gene mutations that cause a variety of epilepsies.[42] The status of a particular single nucleotide polymorphism in *SCN1A* was shown to influence the maximum dose of whichever drug (carbamazepine or phenytoin) patients were exposed to in clinical practice (without knowledge of this genotype).[48] While only a small proportion of the observed numerical variation in dose range across patients could be explained by variation at this *SCN1A* polymorphism, the clinical relevance of the polymorphism could be greater: in addition, it is likely that the rate of dose ramping of either of these two agents tolerable to an individual patient will also be affected by this same *SCN1A* polymorphism. These retrospective findings were not derived from any trial structure, but held across a range of epilepsy phenotypes, and suggest potential for pharmacogenetically driven pragmatic trials of more tailored treatment strategies for licensed AEDs that may provide additional guidance in managing individual patients, allowing better and more rational use of the AEDs already available. Pharmacogenetics might thus help to scale the divide between the bluntness of most RCT data and the needs of the individual.

Complex trait disease susceptibility genetics in epilepsy are less well developed than are the pharmacogenetics, although they have been studied for longer.[45] There are hardly any accepted common genetic variants causing, or associated with, any epilepsy type. An example of one that may turn out to hold true is an association between susceptibility to juvenile myoclonic epilepsy (a type of idiopathic generalised epilepsy) and a common variation in the gene *BRD2*, a neurodevelopmental regulator,[49] although the association may itself not be causal.[50] It is also the case that there is heterogeneity of genetic causation in Mendelian cases of juvenile myoclonic epilepsy,[51, 52] which syndrome is therefore clearly genetically heterogeneous. Thus, analyses of treatment response in any future syndrome-specific RCTs involving patients with the clinical syndrome of juvenile myoclonic epilepsy are very likely to require subgroup analyses, or stratification on entry, potentially driven by genotypic variation. Whether this fundamental principle is applicable in general to other syndromes will depend on the discovery and validation of underlying causal genetic variation for other epilepsy syndromes.

Currently, 'syndrome' is the closest most RCTs (and the epilepsy knowledge base in general) get to 'individual' patients. The most comprehensive classification of an individual's epilepsy is a penta-axial formulation, incorporating ictal phenomenology, seizure type, syndrome and aetiology.[53] Incorporation of additional genetic data in axis 4 may become a necessary part of future efforts to reconcile the need for adequate power with that for external validity of pragmatic RCTs, allowing large numbers of patients to be recruited with limited loss of sensitivity for individual patients.

References

1 Jacoby A, Buck D, Baker G, et al. Uptake and costs of care for epilepsy: findings from a UK regional study. *Epilepsia* 1998; **39:** 776–86.

2 National Institute of Clinical Excellence. *TA76 Epilepsy (Adults) – Newer Drugs: Guidance.* March 2004. Available at: http://www.nice.org.uk/TA076guidance (accessed February 2007).

3 MacDonald BK, Cockerell OC, Sander JW, Shorvon SD. The incidence and lifetime prevalence of neurological disorders in a prospective community-based study in the UK. *Brain* 2000; **123:** 665–76.

4 Sander JW. The epidemiology of epilepsy revisited. *Curr Opin Neurol* 2003; **16:** 165–70.

5 Forsgren L, Beghi E, Oun A, Sillanpaa M. The epidemiology of epilepsy in Europe – a systematic review. *Eur J Neurol* 2005; **12:** 245–53.

6 Heaney DC, MacDonald BK, Everitt A, et al. Socioeconomic variation in incidence of epilepsy: prospective community based study in south east England. *BMJ* 2002; **325:** 1013–16.

7 Sander JW. Infectious agents and epilepsy. In: S Knobler, S O'Connor, SM Lemon, M Najafi M, eds. *The Infectious Etiology of Chronic Diseases: Defining the Relationship, Enhancing the Research and Mitigating the Effects.* Washington, DC: National Academies Press, 2004: 93–99.

8 Sander JW, Bell GS. Reducing mortality: an important aim of epilepsy management. *J Neurol Neurosurg Psychiatry* 2004; **75:** 349–51.

9 MacDonald BK, Johnson AL, Goodridge DM, et al. Factors predicting prognosis of epilepsy after presentation with seizures. *Ann Neurol* 2000; **48:** 833–41.

10 Brodie MJ, Kwan P. Staged approach to epilepsy management. *Neurology* 2002; **58** (suppl 5): S2–S8.

11 Dlugos DJ, Sammel MD, Strom BL, Farrar JT. Response to first drug trial predicts outcome in childhood temporal lobe epilepsy. *Neurology* 2001; **57:** 2259–64.

12 Musicco M, Beghi E, Solari A, Viani F. Treatment of first tonic–clonic seizure does not improve the prognosis of epilepsy. First Seizure Trial Group (FIRST Group). *Neurology* 1997; **49:** 991–98.

13 Temkin NR. Antiepileptogenesis and seizure prevention trials with antiepileptic drugs: meta-analysis of controlled trials. *Epilepsia* 2001; **42:** 515–24.

14 Marson A, Jacoby A, Johnson A, et al., and Medical Research Council MESS Study Group. Immediate versus deferred antiepileptic drug treatment for early epilepsy and single seizures: a randomised controlled trial. *Lancet* 2005; **365:** 2007–13.

15 Berg AT, Shinnar S. Do seizures beget seizures? An assessment of the clinical evidence in humans. *J Clin Neurophysiol* 1997; **14:** 102–10.

16 Semah F, Picot MC, Adam C, et al. Is the underlying cause of epilepsy a major prognostic factor for recurrence? *Neurology* 1998; **51:** 1256–62.

17 Kwan P, Sander JW. The natural history of epilepsy: an epidemiological view. *J Neurol Neurosurg Psychiatry* 2004; **75:** 1376–81.

18 Medical Research Council Antiepileptic Drug Withdrawal Study Group. Randomised study of antiepileptic drug withdrawal in patients in remission. *Lancet* 1991; **337:** 1175–80.

19 Pirmohamed M, James S, Meakin S, et al. Adverse drug reactions as cause of admission to hospital: prospective analysis of 18820 patients. *BMJ* 2004; **329:** 15–19.

20 Prince BS, Goetz CM, Rihn TL, Olsky M. Drug-related emergency department visits and hospital admissions. *Am J Hosp Pharm* 1992; **49:** 1696–700.

21 Kaufman DW, Shapiro S. Epidemiological assessment of drug-induced disease. *Lancet* 2000; **356:** 1339–43.

22 Gilliam F, Carter J, Vahle V. Tolerability of antiseizure medications: implications for health outcomes. *Neurology* 2004; **63** (suppl 4): S9–S12.

23 Adab N, Kini U, Vinten J, et al. The longer term outcome of children born to mothers with epilepsy. *J Neurol Neurosurg Psychiatry* 2004; **75:** 1575–83.

24 Marson AG, Al-Kharusi AM, Alwaidh M, et al., SANAD Study group. The SANAD study of effectiveness of valproate, lamotrigine, or topiramate for generalised and unclassifiable epilepsy: an unblinded randomised controlled trial. *Lancet* 2007; **369:** 1016–26.

25 Berkovic SF. Aggravation of generalized epilepsies. *Epilepsia* 1998; **39** (suppl 3): S11–S14.

26 Perucca E, Gram L, Avanzini G, Dulac O. Antiepileptic drugs as a cause of worsening seizures. *Epilepsia* 1998; **39:** 5–17.

27 Genton P. When antiepileptic drugs aggravate epilepsy. *Brain Dev* 2000; **22:** 75–80.

28 Gelisse P, Genton P, Kuate C, et al. Worsening of seizures by oxcarbazepine in juvenile idiopathic generalized epilepsies. *Epilepsia* 2004; **45:** 1282–86.

29 Biraben A, Allain H, Scarabin JM, et al. Exacerbation of juvenile myoclonic epilepsy with lamotrigine. *Neurology* 2000; **55:** 1758.

30 Becker AJ, Wiestler OD, Blumcke I. Functional genomics in experimental and human temporal lobe epilepsy: powerful new tools to identify molecular disease mechanisms of hippocampal damage. *Prog Brain Res* 2002; **135:** 161–73.

31 Walker MC, Sander JW. Difficulties in extrapolating from clinical trial data to clinical practice: the case of antiepileptic drugs. *Neurology* 1997; **49:** 333–37.

32 Spencer SS, Berg AT, Vickrey BG, et al. Multicenter Study of Epilepsy Surgery. Initial outcomes in the Multicenter Study of Epilepsy Surgery. *Neurology* 2003; **61:** 1680–85.

33 Wieser HG, ILAE Commission on Neurosurgery of Epilepsy. ILAE Commission Report. Mesial temporal lobe epilepsy with hippocampal sclerosis. *Epilepsia* 2004; **45:** 695–714.

34 Wieshmann UC, Woermann FG, Lemieux L, et al. Development of hippocampal atrophy: a serial magnetic resonance imaging study in a patient who developed epilepsy after generalized status epilepticus. *Epilepsia* 1997; **38:** 1238–41.

35 Cendes F, Andermann F, Carpenter S, et al. Temporal lobe epilepsy caused by domoic acid intoxication: evidence for glutamate receptor-mediated excitotoxicity in humans. *Ann Neurol* 1995; **37:** 123–26.

36 Guerrini R, Carrozzo R. Epileptogenic brain malformations: clinical presentation, malformative patterns and indications for genetic testing. *Seizure* 2002; **11** (suppl A): 532–43.

37 Sheen VL, Feng Y, Graham D, et al. Filamin A and Filamin B are co-expressed within neurons during periods of neuronal migration and can physically interact. *Hum Mol Genet* 2002; **11:** 2845–54.

38 Scottish Intercollegiate Guidelines Network. *Diagnosis and Management of Epilepsy in Adults. A National Clinical Guideline.* April 2003. Available at: http://www.sign.ac.uk/pdf/sign70.pdf (accessed February 2007).

39 McCorry D, Chadwick D, Marson A. Current drug treatment of epilepsy in adults. *Lancet Neurol* 2004; **3:** 729–35.

40 Rating D, Wolf C, Bast T. Sulthiame as monotherapy in children with benign childhood epilepsy with centrotemporal spikes: a 6-month randomized, double-blind, placebo-controlled study. Sulthiame Study Group. *Epilepsia* 2000; **41:** 1284–88.

41 Chiron C, Marchard MC, Tran A, et al. Stiripentol in severe myoclonic epilepsy in infancy: a randomised placebo-controlled syndrome-dedicated trial. STICLO study group. *Lancet* 2000; **356:** 1638–42.

42 Mulley JC, Scheffer IE, Petrou S, et al. SCN1A mutations and epilepsy. *Hum Mutat* 2005; **25:** 535–42.

43 Loiseau P, Levy RH, Houin G, et al. Randomized, double-blind, parallel, multicenter trial of stiripentol added to carbamazepine in the treatment of resistant epilepsies. An interim analysis. *Epilepsia* 1990; **31:** 618–19.

44 Tan NC, Mulley JC, Berkovic SF. Genetic association studies in epilepsy: 'the truth is out there'. *Epilepsia* 2004; **45:** 1429–42.

45 Goldstein DB, Tate SK, Sisodiya SM. Pharmacogenetics goes genomic. *Nat Rev Genet.* 2003; **4:** 937–47.

46 Need AC, Motulsky AG, Goldstein DB. Priorities and standards in pharmacogenetic research. *Nat Genet* 2005; **37:** 671–81.

47 Rothwell PM. Treating individuals. 2. Subgroup analysis in randomised controlled trials: importance, indications, and interpretation. *Lancet* 2005; **365:** 176–86.

48 Tate SK, Depondt C, Sisodiya SM, et al. Genetic predictors of the maximum doses patients receive during clinical use of the anti-epileptic drugs carbamazepine and phenytoin. *Proc Natl Acad Sci USA* 2005; **102:** 5507–12.

49 Pal DK, Evgrafov OV, Tabares P, et al. BRD2 (RING3) is a probable major susceptibility gene for common juvenile myoclonic epilepsy. *Am J Hum Genet* 2003; **73:** 261–70.

50 Cavalleri GL, Walley NM, Soranzo N, et al. A multicenter study of *BRD2* as a risk factor for juvenile myoclonic epilepsy. *Epilepsia* 200; **48:** 706–12.

51 Cossett P, Liu L, Brisebois K, et al. Mutation of GABRA1 in an autosomal dominant form of juvenile myoclonic epilepsy. *Nat Genet* 2002; **31:** 184–89.

52 Suzuki T, Delgado-Escueta AV, Aguan K, et al. Mutations in EFHC1 cause juvenile myoclonic epilepsy. *Nat Genet* 2004; **36:** 842–49.

53 Engel J Jr, International League Against Epilepsy (ILAE). A proposed diagnostic scheme for people with epileptic seizures and with epilepsy: report of the ILAE Task Force on Classification and Terminology. *Epilepsia* 2001; **42:** 796–803.

Pharmacogenomic targeting of treatment for cancer

Sharon Marsh and Howard L. McLeod

Introduction

In the UK it has been estimated that approximately 7% of patients are affected by adverse drug reactions (ADRs). Indeed, 1/10 of all National Health Service bed-days are used by patients with ADRs. These ADRs result in the need for the equivalent of 15–20 400-bed hospitals and cost about £380 million a year. ADRs due to cancer chemotherapy are estimated to increase overall hospital costs by 1.9% and drug costs by 15%.[1] Clearly, the current regime of 'one dose fits all' for chemotherapy treatment is not ideal for patients (figure 20.1) and is not cost-effective for the health service. With multiple drug strategies for many cancer types now readily available, pharmacogenetics and pharmacogenomics

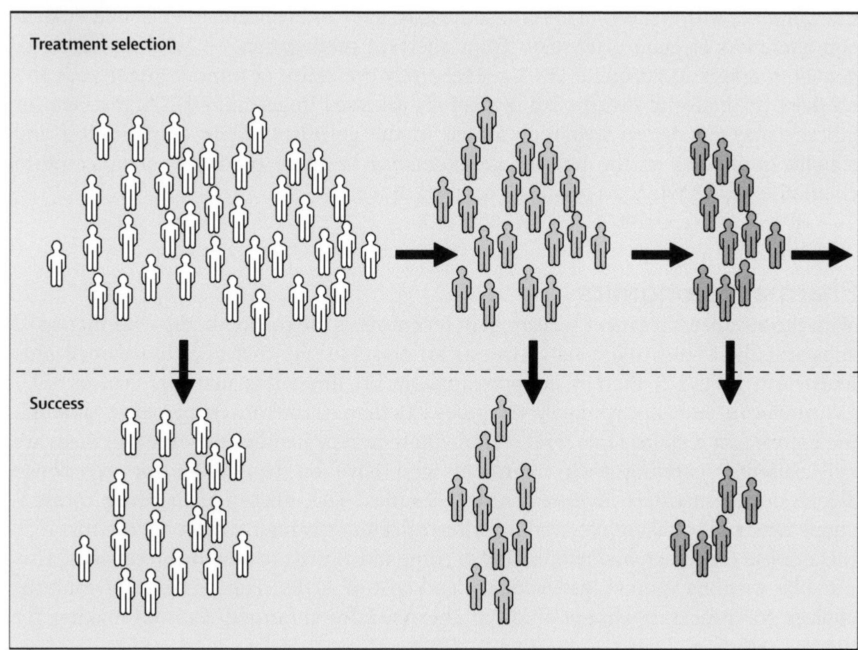

Figure 20.1: **Current drug strategies treat all individuals with the same medication. The fractions that do not have a favourable response are given an alternative drug, and so on. The purpose of pharmacogenetics is to identify the most viable medication for each individual by screening for genetic markers prior to drug selection, thus reducing treatment and monitoring times, improving response rates and reducing toxicity incidence. (Reproduced with permission from the Pharmacogenetics for Every Nation Initiative (http://pgeni.org).)**

encompass the search for answers to the hereditary basis for interindividual differences in drug response,[2, 3] with the ultimate goal of personalised therapy selection.

In addition to environmental influences, as detailed in Chapter 10, variation in the genetic constitution between individuals will have a major impact on drug activity. Single nucleotide polymorphisms (SNPs) account for over 90% of genetic variation in the human genome. The remainder of the variation is caused by insertions and deletions (indels), tandem repeats and microsatellites. With the completion of the human genome project, there has been an explosion in the discovery, characterisation and validation of genetic variation. Over 1.42 million SNPs were initially identified through the human genome project,[4] and a goldmine of SNP information is now readily accessible via publicly available databases.[5] In addition, affordable, high-throughput genotyping technologies are now available, including Taqman, Pyrosequencing, MALDI-TOF and SNP chips/bead arrays, making pretreatment genotyping a real possibility.[6, 7]

Pharmacogenomics includes studies of variations in germline DNA, somatic mutations and variations in RNA expression[8] (figure 20.2). Many studies rely on the availability of DNA and RNA from easily accessible sources, such as blood, buccal smears, etc.[9] In cancer pharmacogenomics, the tumour genome can differ significantly from the germline genome, with regions of chromosome loss, gain and rearrangements, and epigenetic alteration of gene expression from aberrant methylation.[10, 11] Whilst pharmacogenetic markers in germline DNA are relatively predictive of tumour genotype,[12] and markers predictive of toxicity can be usefully assessed in germline DNA, markers for efficacy may not be so well represented in the germline. Gene amplification and somatic mutations in the tumour genome may be more predictive of outcome to chemotherapy agents than germline markers alone.

Pharmacoeconomics

With the advances in cancer treatment in recent years the cost of therapy has increased substantially. Using colorectal cancer as an example, the cost of 5-fluorouracil plus leucovorin (5FU/LV) therapy is approximately 151 times less than the cost of 5FU/LV/irinotecan, and approximately 489 times less than irinotecan/cetuximab.[13] Although the increase in response rate with combination therapy justifies the expense, there are still patients receiving each treatment who have no benefit and/or experience deleterious, sometimes life-threatening, toxicities. The efficacy of the drug combinations needs to be taken into account when selecting treatment; however, the cost may make some combinations inaccessible to some individuals or healthcare services. This must be weighed against the incidence and cost of ADRs. The existence of multiple choices for cancer treatment leads to the need for informed decision-making for therapy selection.

6-Mercaptopurine

6-Mercaptopurine is a commonly used treatment for childhood acute lymphocytic leukaemia. It is regularly used as a daily oral medication for 2–3 years of therapy. Both

6-mercaptopurine and its prodrug, azathioprine, are also used in non-malignant conditions, such as rheumatoid arthritis, inflammatory bowel disease and dermatological syndromes. 6-Mercaptopurine exerts its cytotoxic effect via the incorporation of

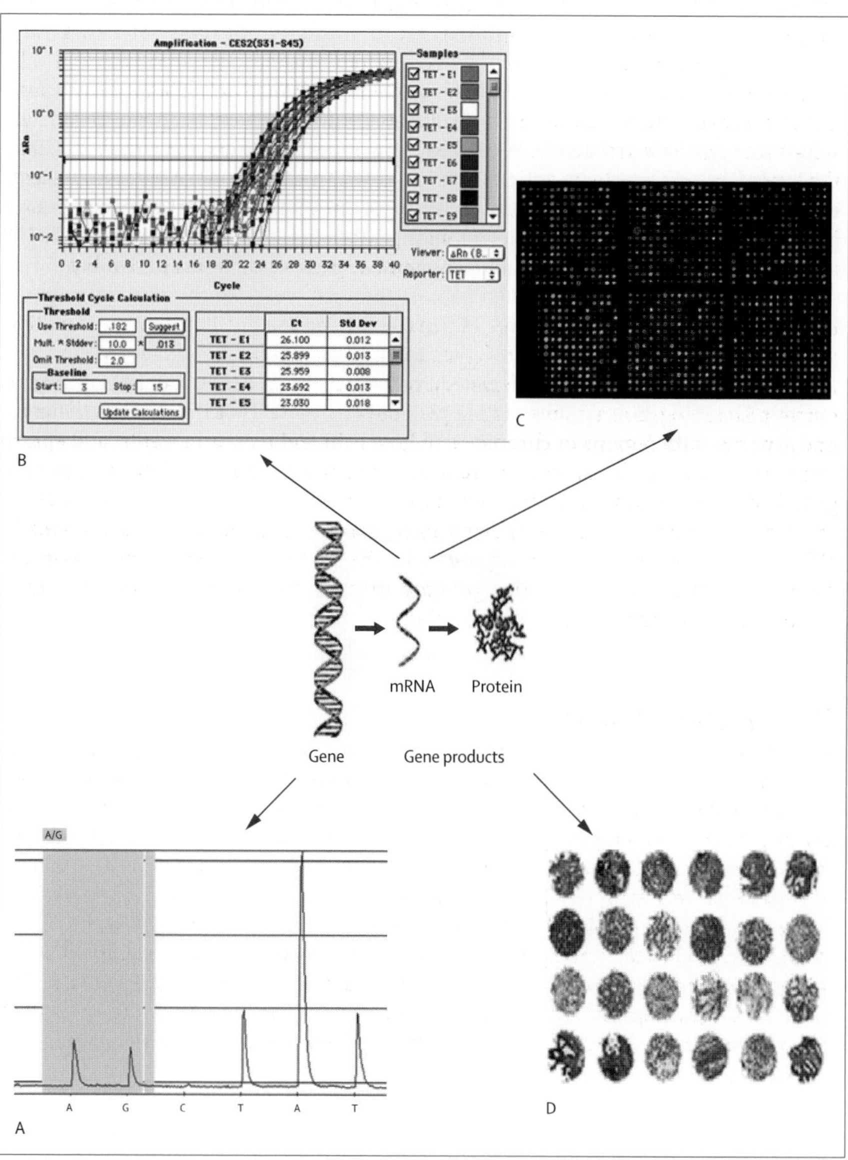

Figure 20.2: **There are many ways to study the genome, including (A) DNA variation at the nucleotide level; (B) RNA expression at the gene level; (C) DNA variation or RNA expression at the whole genome level; and (D) protein expression.**

hioguanine nucleotides into DNA (figure 20.3). 6-Mercaptopurine is also methylated to form methylmercaptopurine by thiopurine methyltransferase (TPMT), and oxidised to thioruic acid via xanthine oxidase (XDH) (see figure 20.3). Underexpression of TPMT leads to increased accumulation of thioguanine nucleotides. This can cause intolerance to mercaptopurine, and lead to severe, life-threatening haematopoietic toxicities.[14, 15]

TPMT

TPMT methylates mercaptopurine, reducing its bioavailability for conversion to thioguanine nucleotides, the cytotoxic form of the drug (see figure 20.3). Approximately 10% of patients have intermediate enzyme activity and 0.3% are deficient for TPMT activity. Intermediate activity patients have a greater incidence of thiopurine toxicity, whereas TPMT-deficient patients have severe or fatal toxicity from mercaptopurine therapy. In 180 children with acute lymphatic leukaemia, patients deficient for TPMT tolerated only 7% of a 2.5-year mercaptopurine treatment regimen. Patients with intermediate TPMT activity tolerated 65% of the total weeks of therapy and patients with normal TPMT activity tolerated 84% of the total weeks.[16]

At least ten variations in the TPMT gene have been associated with low TPMT enzyme activity.[15] Three of these variants (TPMT*2, TPMT*3A and TPMT*3C) account for up to 95% of low TPMT activity phenotypes (figure 20.4). Patients heterozygous for these

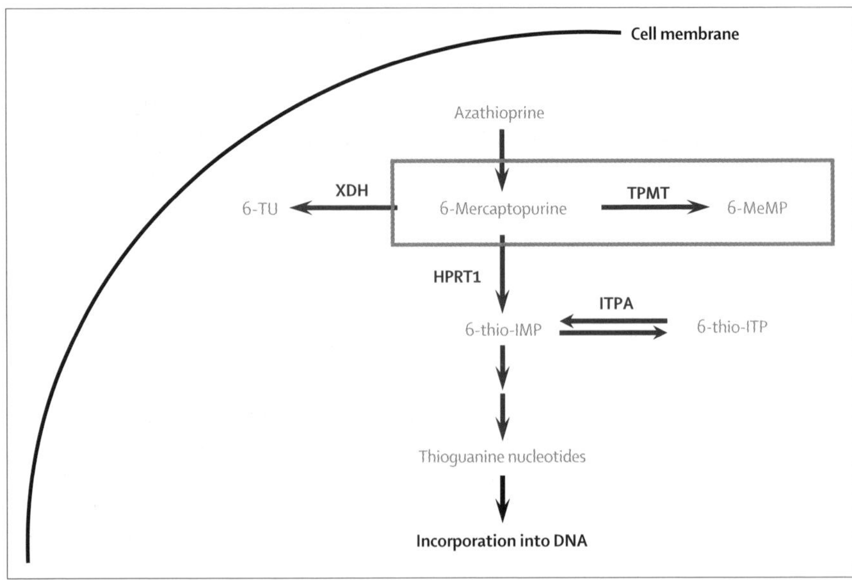

Figure 20.3: **Mercaptopurine pathway, highlighting the role of TPMT in the inactivation of 6-mercaptopurine. Genes (dark green text): XDH, xanthine oxidase; TPMT, thiopurine methyltransferase; HPRT1, hypoxanthine phosphoribosyltransferase; ITPA, inosine triphosphatase. Drug and metabolites (light green text): 6-TU, 6-thiouric acid; 6-MeMP, methylmercaptopurine; 6-thio-IMP, thioinosine monophosphate; 6-thio-ITP, thioinosine triphosphate.**

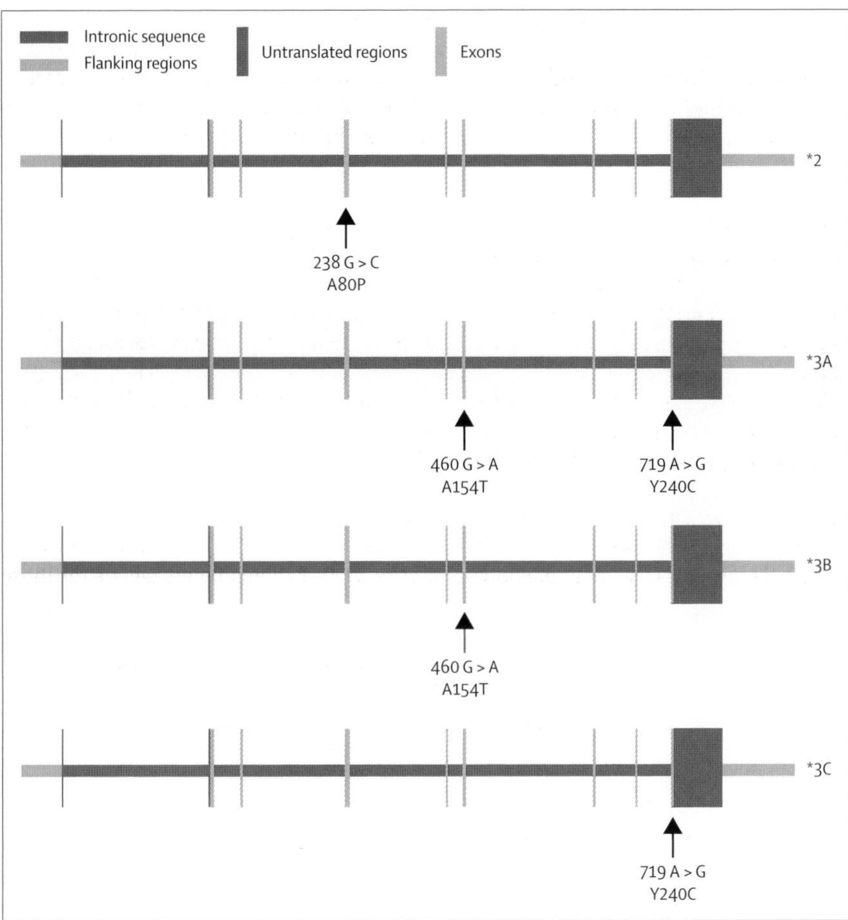

Figure 20.4: **Gene structure of TPMT with the locations of the common clinically relevant alleles TPMT*2, *3A, *3B and *3C. Gene structure courtesy of Derek Van Booven.**

alleles have intermediate TPMT levels, and tolerate approximately 65% of the standard mercaptopurine dosage.[17] Patients homozygous for the variant TPMT alleles are at high risk of severe, sometimes life-threatening, toxicity, requiring significant reductions in drug doses (1/10 to 1/15 of the standard dose). Patients receiving dose reduction because of variant TPMT alleles have similar or superior survival compared to patients with the wild-type allele.[17]

TPMT*3A is the most common allele in Caucasian populations, with a frequency of 3.2–5.7%. TPMT*2 and TPMT*3C alleles are present in 0.2–0.8% of Caucasians. Significant variation in TPMT allele frequencies is seen among different world populations. TPMT*3A is the only variation found in south-western Asians (1%), whereas all variant alleles in African populations are TPMT*3C (5.4–7.6%).[15]

Although currently not a requirement for prescribing mercaptopurine, pretreatment knowledge of a patient's TPMT genotype status is now often used in major centres for dose optimisation, in order prospectively to reduce the likelihood of ADRs in children with acute lymphatic leukaemia.

Irinotecan

Irinotecan (CPT-11; Camptosar) is a camptothecin analogue approved for first-line therapy of advanced colorectal cancer in combination with 5FU/LV.

Irinotecan is a prodrug, which is metabolised into its active form, 7-ethyl-10-hydroxy-camptothecin (SN-38), when inside the cell. Like most drugs, irinotecan activity is not determined by the product of one gene (figure 20.5).[18] Irinotecan can be converted to inactive metabolites via members of the cytochrome P450 3A family (CYP3A4 and CYP3A5), and SN-38 can be inactivated through glucuronidation via the UDP-glucuronosyltransferase enzyme, UGT1A1 (see figure 20.5).[19] Toxicity is a limiting factor for most chemotherapy drugs, including irinotecan. Up to 36% of patients may experience severe, life-threatening diarrhoea and/or neutropenia.[20]

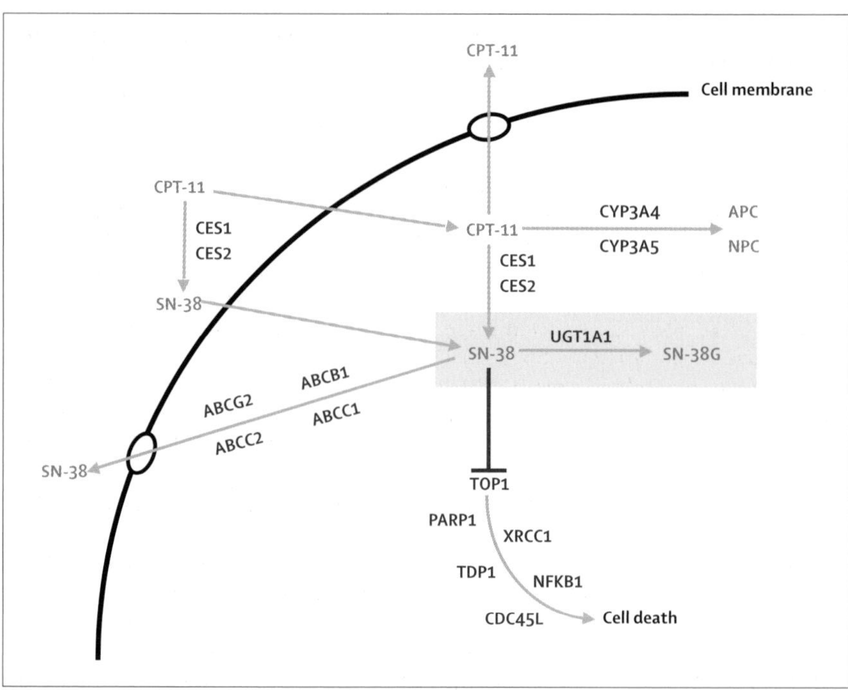

Figure **20.5: Irinotecan pathway, highlighting the role of UGT1A1 in the glucuronidation of the active form of irinotecan, SN-38. Genes are in dark green text, drugs and metabolites are in light green text.**

UGT1A1

The active form of irinotecan, SN-38, can be inactivated through glucuronidation by a member of the UDP-glucuronosyltransferase family, UGT1A1 (see figure 20.5). UGT1A1 is a product of alternative splicing from the UGT1A locus located on chromosome 2q37. At least 13 UGT1A genes are encoded from this locus, including four pseudogenes.[21] UGT1A1 has a unique promoter and a unique exon 1. Exons 2–5 are shared with the UGT1A family of enzymes. The UGT1A1 enzyme is responsible for hepatic bilirubin glucuronidation and is the main UGT1A enzyme involved in SN-38 glucuronidation.

A polymorphic dinucleotide repeat has been identified in the UGT1A1 promoter TATA element (standard nomenclature UGT1A1*28), and consists of five, six, seven or eight copies of a TA repeat [$(TA)_n$TAA], with the $(TA)_6$TAA allele being the most common and $(TA)_7$AA (*28) the most frequently recorded variant allele.[22] The longer the repeat allele, the lower the corresponding UGT1A1 gene expression. Consequently, patients with the 7 and 8 alleles have significantly lower UGT1A1 expression. The frequency of the UGT1A1*28 $(TA)_7$TAA allele has been identified in several world populations, and ranges from approximately 15% in Asian and Amerindian populations, to 45% in sub-Saharan Africans, and is seen in approximately 26–38% of Caucasian, Hispanic and African American populations.[23–25]

As UGT1A1 is responsible for the conversion of SN-38 to the inactive metabolite, SN-38G via glucuronidation, variability in UGT1A1 expression leads to interindividual variation in SN-38G formation.[26, 27] Consequently, the presence of more than six TA repeats in the UGT1A1 promoter region leads to reduced SN-38G formation and the potential for excess SN-38 to be retained in the cell, leading to severe toxicity.

In 2000, Ando et al.[25] published a study of 108 Asian patients treated with irinotecan-containing regimens. Patients with at least one UGT1A1*28 allele encountered severe toxicity compared to patients homozygous for the $(TA)_6$TAA allele ($p < 0.001$).[25] This finding confirmed a report by Iyer et al.,[28] where 20 Caucasian cancer patients treated with irinotecan were assessed for the UGT1A1*28 allele. All patients homozygous for the UGT1A1*28 allele encountered grade 0 or 1 diarrhoea and neutropenia. Patients heterozygous or homozygous for the UGT1A1*28 allele demonstrated a significant trend to lower neutrophil counts ($p < 0.04$). This also correlated with SN-38G production in these patients. A significant trend towards lower SN-38 glucuronidation was seen in patients heterozygous or homozygous for the UGT1A1*28 allele ($p = 0.001$).[28] In a prospective study to confirm these findings of 66 cancer patients receiving irinotecan, UGT1A1*28 was corroborated as a predictive marker for severe neutropenia ($p = 0.02$).[29]

Nine years from the approval to use irinotecan in cancer therapy, the US Food and Drug Administration (US FDA) has requested the inclusion of UGT1A1 genotype information in the drug package insert, with dosing guidelines based on genotype (figure 20.6).[30] One month later, the US FDA approved a clinical test for the UGT1A1*28 allele, which is performed by Third Wave Technologies (Wisconsin, USA; http://www.twt.com), making the integration of pharmacogenetics into clinical practice for cancer treatment a reality.

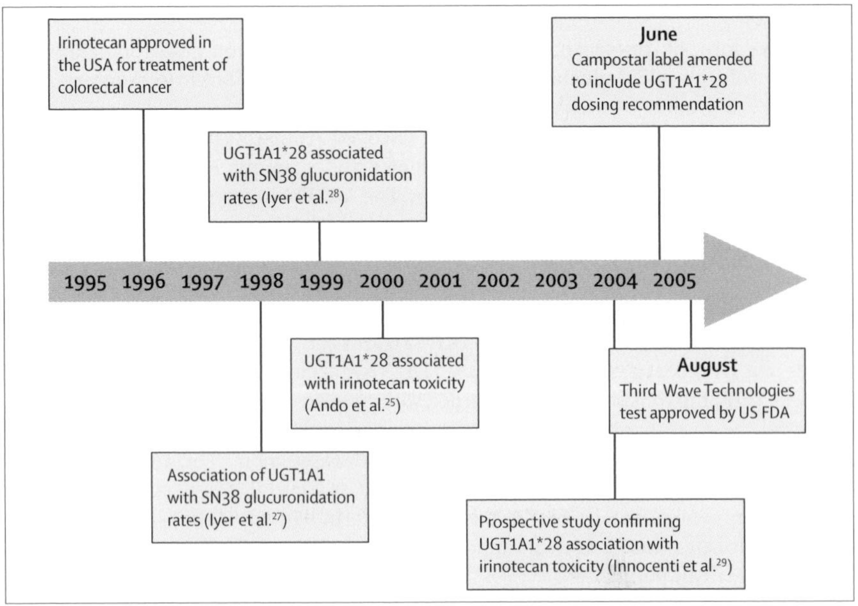

Figure 20.6: **UGT1A1: timeline from irinotecan development to genetic testing.**

Epidermal growth factor receptor inhibitors

Gefitinib (Iressa) and erlotinib (Tarceva) were approved in 2003 and 2004, respectively, by the US FDA as single-agent therapies for patients with metastatic non-small-cell lung cancer (NSCLC) who had previously failed on standard therapies. Gefitinib and erlotinib are inhibitors of the epidermal growth factor receptor (EGFR), specifically inhibiting the EGFR tyrosine kinase domain (figure 20.7). Approximately 10% of patients experience a relative response from these drugs where no other drug has demonstrated efficacy. Response is more frequently seen in females, non-smokers and individuals of Asian descent.[31, 32]

Following the identification of subsets of patients who experienced a response to EGFR inhibitors, efforts were undertaken to determine the underlying mechanism behind the response, or lack of response, by sequencing the EGFR gene from NSCLC tumours. In 2004, Lynch et al.[33] screened the 28 exons of EGFR in nine NSCLC patients who responded favourably to gefitinib, seven patients who did not respond to gefitinib and 25 patients with primary NSCLC who did not receive gefitinib therapy. Of the nine patients who responded to gefitinib therapy, eight had somatic EGFR mutations in the exons corresponding to the tyrosine kinase domain (exons 18–24). Two (of 25) patients who did not receive gefitinib also had EGFR mutations. No mutations were identified in the seven patients who did not respond to gefitinib; in addition, matched normal tissue for patients with mutations were wild-type at all tumour mutation loci.[33] The most common mutations (4/9 patients and 2/25 patients who did not receive gefitinib) were deleted regions in exon 19 of 12–18 nucleotides, all including the deletion of at

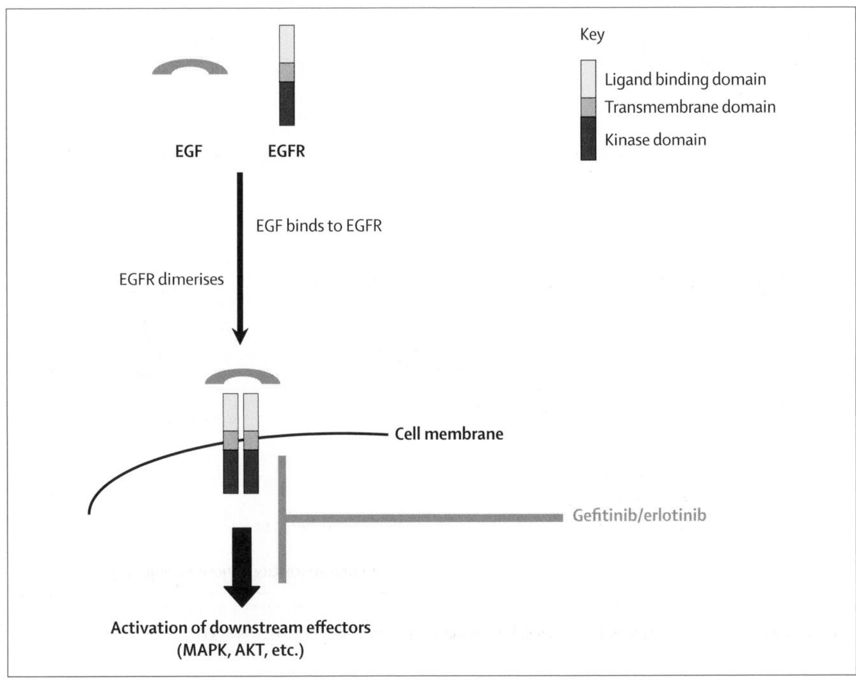

Figure 20.7: **Schematic drawing of the EGFR mechanism. When ligand (e.g. EGF) binding has occurred, EGFR dimerises, causing autophosphorylation of the kinase domain, stimulating tyrosine kinase activity, and subsequently stimulating signalling pathways, including those involved in cell survival and proliferation. Gefitinib and erlotinib inhibit the EGFR tyrosine kinase activity.**

least amino acids 746–750. Non-synonymous mutations leading to amino acid substitutions L858R (2/9 patients), L861Q (1 patient) and G719C (1 patient) were also observed (figure 20.8). No mutations were found in 108 cancer cell lines from diverse cancer types, suggesting these EGFR mutations are lung cancer specific.[33] In a concurrent study, Paez et al.[34] screened tumour DNA from five NSCLC patients who responded to gefitinib and four patients who did not respond. No mutations were identified in the patients who did not respond; however, all five patients who responded had mutations in the EGFR tyrosine kinase domain exons. Three patients had the L858R mutation, three patients had the deleted region in exon 19 corresponding to the loss of amino acids 746–753, and two patients had a mutation causing a G719S amino acid substitution (see figure 20.8).[34] These mutations were confirmed as somatic, as they were not present in matched normal tissue. In 119 unselected NSCLC tumour samples from Japan and the USA, EGFR mutations were more common in the Japanese patients (26%) than the US patients (2%). The highest mutation frequency was seen in Japanese women (57%).[34] These data were confirmed in a later study by Pao et al.,[35] where similar mutations were found in 7/10 patients who responded to gefitinib or erlotinib compared to 0/8 patients who did not respond (see figure 20.8). In addition, Pao et al.[35] identified that 7/15 non-smokers with adenocarcinoma carried EGFR

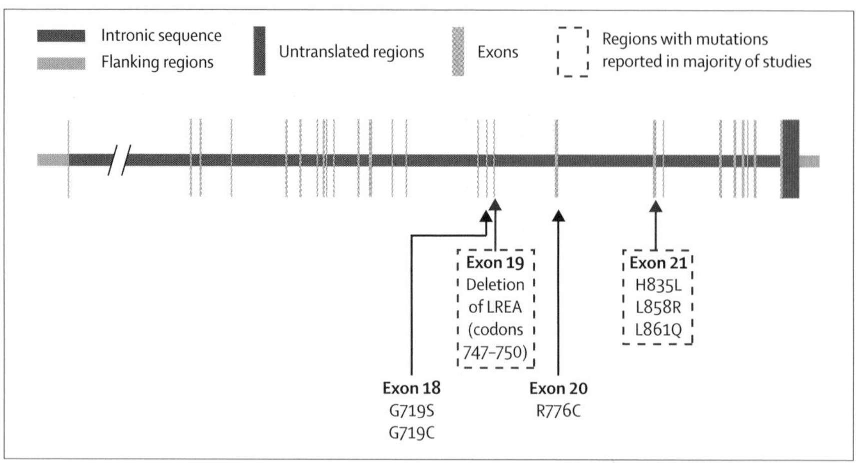

Figure 20.8: **Gene structure of EGFR with the locations of reported mutations in the tyrosine kinase domain.[33–35] (Gene structure courtesy of Derek Van Booven.)**

mutations, whereas only 4/21 former or current smokers with NSCLC carried the mutations ($p = 0.0001$). Collectively, it appears that the highest responder groups are Asian, female, non-smokers, and patients with adeonocarcinomas.[34]

The presence of favourable somatic mutations in EGFR leads to the possibility of screening patients in advance of EGFR inhibitor therapy to select patients likely to respond. As the response rate is low (10%) but dramatic (it occurs in patients who have failed all other therapy), screening tumour tissue should be beneficial for patients who are likely to benefit from gefitinib or erlotinib therapy, and reduce unnecessary administration in patients who would only experience adverse reactions or, at best, no response.

Conclusions

Pharmacogenomic targeting of cancer treatment is rapidly becoming a reality. Approval of genetic testing for UGT1A1*28 in patients prior to irinotecan therapy is an important advance in cancer pharmacogenetics. The identification of somatic mutations responsible for favourable outcome to gefitinib therapy highlights that not all markers for individualised cancer therapy will come from variations identified in germline DNA. Although markers for the toxicity and efficacy of many oncology drugs remain unknown, the examples highlighted here are paving the way for the use of pharmacogeomics for informed decision-making in the clinic.

Acknowledgments

The authors are grateful to Derek Van Booven for his assistance with this chapter. The authors are funded by UO1 GM63340 and R21 CA113491 and R21 CA102461.

References

1 Wiffen P, Gill M, Edwards J, et al. Adverse drug reactions in hospital patients. *Bandolier Extra* 2002. Available at: http://www.jr2.ox.ac.uk/bandolier/Extraforbando/ADRPM.pdf (accessed February 2007).

2 Evans WE, McLeod HL. Pharmacogenomics – drug disposition, drug targets, and side effects. *N Engl J Med* 2003; **348:** 538–49.
3 Marsh S, McLeod HL. Cancer pharmacogenetics. *Br J Cancer* 2004; **90:** 8–11.
4 Sachidanandam R, Weissman D, Schmidt SC, et al. A map of human genome sequence variation containing 1.42 million single nucleotide polymorphisms. *Nature* 2001; **409:** 928–33.
5 Marsh S, Kwok P, McLeod HL. SNP databases and pharmacogenetics: great start, but a long way to go. *Hum Mutat* 2002; **20:** 174–79.
6 Freimuth RR, Ameyaw M-M, Pritchard SC, et al. High-throughput genotyping methods for pharmacogenomic studies. *Curr Pharmacogenom* 2004; **2:** 21–33.
7 Syvanen AC. Toward genome-wide SNP genotyping. *Nat Genet* 2005; **37**(Suppl): S5–S10.
8 Watters JW, McLeod HL. Cancer pharmacogenomics: current and future applications. *Biochim Biophys Acta* 2003; **1603:** 99–111.
9 Lenz HJ. The use and development of germline polymorphisms in clinical oncology. *J Clin Oncol* 2004; **22:** 2519–21.
10 Cheng Q, Yang W, Raimondi SC, et al. Karyotypic abnormalities create discordance of germline genotype and cancer cell phenotypes. *Nat Genet* 2005; **37:** 878–82.
11 McLeod HL, Marsh S. Pharmacogenetics goes 3D. *Nat Genet* 2005; **37:** 794–95.
12 Marsh S, Mallon MA, Goodfellow P, et al. Concordance of pharmacogenetic markers in germline and colorectal tumor DNA. *Pharmacogenomics* 2005; **6:** 873–77.
13 Schrag D. The price tag on progress – chemotherapy for colorectal cancer. *N Engl J Med* 2004; **351:** 317–19.
14 McLeod HL, Relling MV, Liu Q, et al. Polymorphic thiopurine methyltransferase in erythrocytes is indicative of activity in leukemic blasts from children with acute lymphoblastic leukemia. *Blood* 1995; **85:** 1897–902.
15 McLeod HL, Siva C. The thiopurine S-methyltransferase gene locus – implications for clinical pharmacogenomics. Pharmacogenomics 2002; **3:** 89–98.
16 Relling MV, Hancock ML, Boyett JM, et al. Prognostic importance of 6-mercaptopurine dose intensity in acute lymphoblastic leukemia. *Blood* 1999; **93:** 2817–23.
17 Relling MV, Hancock ML, Rivera GK, et al. Mercaptopurine therapy intolerance and heterozygosity at the thiopurine S-methyltransferase gene locus. *J Natl Cancer Inst* 1999; **91:** 2001–08.
18 McLeod HL. Drug pathways: moving beyond single gene pharmacogenetics. *Pharmacogenomics* 2004; **5:** 139–41.
19 Marsh S, McLeod HL. Pharmacogenetics of irinotecan toxicity. *Pharmacogenomics* 2004; **5:** 835–43.
20 Fuchs CS, Moore MR, Harker G, et al. Phase III comparison of two irinotecan dosing regimens in second-line therapy of metastatic colorectal cancer. *J Clin Oncol* 2003; **21:** 807–14.
21 Gong QH, Cho JW, Huang T, et al. Thirteen UDPglucuronosyltransferase genes are encoded at the human UGT1 gene complex locus. *Pharmacogenetics* 2001; **11:** 357–68.
22 Beutler E, Gelbart T, Demina A. Racial variability in the UDP-glucuronosyltransferase 1 (UGT1A1) promoter: a balanced polymorphism for regulation of bilirubin metabolism? *Proc Natl Acad Sci USA* 1998; **95:** 8170–74.
23 Guillemette C, Millikan RC, Newman B, et al. Genetic polymorphisms in uridine diphosphoglucuronosyltransferase 1A1 and association with breast cancer among African Americans. *Cancer Res* 2000; **60:** 950–56.
24 Hall D, Ybazeta G, Destro-Bisol G, et al. Variability at the uridine diphosphate glucuronosyltransferase 1A1 promoter in human populations and primates. *Pharmacogenetics* 1999; **9:** 591–99.
25 Ando Y, Saka H, Ando M, et al. Polymorphisms of UDP-glucuronosyltransferase gene and irinotecan toxicity: a pharmacogenetic analysis. *Cancer Res* 2000; **60:** 6921–26.
26 Innocenti F, Ratain MJ. Irinotecan treatment in cancer patients with UGT1A1 polymorphisms. *Oncology (Huntingt)* 2003; **17:** 52–55.
27 Iyer L, Hall D, Das S, et al. Phenotype-genotype correlation of in vitro SN-38 (active metabolite of irinotecan) and bilirubin glucuronidation in human liver tissue with UGT1A1 promoter polymorphism. *Clin Pharmacol Ther* 1999; **65:** 576–82.
28 Iyer L, Das S, Janisch L, et al. UGT1A1*28 polymorphism as a determinant of irinotecan disposition and toxicity. *Pharmacogenomics J* 2002; **2:** 43–47.
29 Innocenti F, Undevia SD, Iyer L, et al. Genetic variants in the UDP-glucuronosyltransferase 1A1 gene predict the risk of severe neutropenia of irinotecan. *J Clin Oncol* 2004; **22:** 1382–1388.
30 FDA clears Third Wave pharmacogenetic test. *Pharmacogenomics* 2005; **6:** 671–72.
31 Fukuoka M, Yano S, Giaccone G, et al. Multi-institutional randomized phase II trial of gefitinib for previously treated patients with advanced non-small-cell lung cancer (The IDEAL 1 Trial). *J Clin Oncol* 2003; **21:** 2237–46.

32 Cohen MH, Williams GA, Sridhara R, et al. United States Food and Drug Administration Drug Approval summary: Gefitinib (ZD1839; Iressa) tablets. *Clin Cancer Res* 2004; **10:** 1212–18.

33 Lynch TJ, Bell DW, Sordella R, et al. Activating mutations in the epidermal growth factor receptor underlying responsiveness of non-small-cell lung cancer to gefitinib. *N Engl J Med* 2004; **350:** 2129–39.

34 Paez JG, Janne PA, Lee JC, et al. EGFR Mutations in lung cancer: correlation with clinical response to gefitinib therapy. *Science* 2004; **304:** 1497–500.

35 Pao W, Miller V, Zakowski M, et al. EGF receptor gene mutations are common in lung cancers from 'never smokers' and are associated with sensitivity of tumors to gefitinib and erlotinib. *Proc Natl Acad Sci USA* 2004; **101:** 13306–11.

Index

abciximab 184, 191
ABPI 49
absolute cardiovascular risk 247–61
  appropriateness, practical and effectiveness 259–60
  estimation in clinical setting 251–9
  influence of multiple risk factors on 248–9
  influence on treatment benefits 250
absolute risk reduction (ARR) 65, 87, 141, 142, 175, 176, 195
acenocoumarol 158, 159, 164
ACTIVE-A trial 267
ACTIVE-W clinical trial 267
acute coronary syndromes 279–90
acute lymphatic leukaemia 310
acute lymphoblastic leukaemia (ALL) 162
Advanced Ovarian Cancer Trialists' Group 52
adverse drug reactions (ADRs) 151, 307
ageing 97–8
  pharmacology of 99
  predictive equations 105–6
  relevance of outcome measures 99–100
  risk/benefit ratios 98–9
  routine health service data 104–5
  subgroup analysis 102–3
Alzheimer's disease 70, 100, 101, 114
AMADEUS 267
amitriptyline 160
amniotomy 6
amonafide 162
AmpliChip CYP450 165
angina
  prodromal 101
  unstable 14
angioplasty 116
angiotensin converting enzyme (ACE) inhibitors 8, 18, 24, 27, 98, 145–6
angiotensin II receptor blocking drugs 146
animal models 48–9
antiarrhythmic drugs 3, 45, 142, 200
antibiotics 89, 91
anticoagulants 7, 85, 99
anticoagulation 12
anticonvulsants 122
antidepressants 122, 159–61
antiepileptic drugs (AEDs) 17, 297–9, 300–1
antihypertensive drugs 10, 14, 15, 20, 24, 28
antiplatelet therapy 7, 8, 12, 20, 68, 98, 115, 272–3
Antiplatelet Trialists' Collaboration 52
antipsychotic drugs 70, 159–61
antiseizure drugs 297
APACHE-III equation 106
aphasia 114
apolipoprotein E (APOE) gene 159
applicability 61
aprotinin 42
area under the curve (AUC) 221, 227
arylamine 162
aspirin 7–8, 9, 15, 20, 21, 52, 66, 115, 142, 143, 176, 184, 266, 267, 279
asthma 131–4, 239
Asymptomatic Carotid Atherosclerosis Study Group (ACAS) trial 67–8
atenolol 91
ATLANTIS A 293
ATLANTIS B 291, 292
atrial fibrillation 71, 85, 113, 200
  see also atrial fibrillation, stroke prevention and
Atrial Fibrillation Follow-up Investigation of Rhythm Management (AFFIRM) 265–6
Atrial Fibrillation Trial (EAFT) 71, 73
atrial fibrillation, stroke prevention and 265–75
  absolute threshold of benefit 273
  antiplatelet therapy combined with warfarin in elderly patients 272–3
  aspirin in 266
  benefits of blood pressure control 273–4
  cardioversion to sinus rhythm 265–6
  life-long anticoagulation, benefits 270
  obstacles to individualising treatment 274–5
  optimal target intensity of anticoagulation 268–70
  risk of bleeding during anticoagulation 271–2
  warfarin in 266–7
attention deficit hyperactivity disorder 239
azathioprine 162, 164, 309

'Back to Sleep' campaigns 46–8
Bayesian Information Criterion 222
Bayesian statistics 40, 237
BBSRC 49
benefit–harm model 87
benign childhood epilepsy with centrotemporal splices (BECTS) 302
benoxaprofen 99
benzodiazepines 23, 99
beta blockers 19–20, 22, 42–4, 70, 90–1, 105, 146, 171, 188, 279

Index

beta-carotene 27, 28
beta-interferon 195
biological age of individuals 106
biomarkers 105, 164, 165
Birmingham Atrial Fibrillation Trial in the Aged (BAFTA) 266
black box markers 214
blood pressure 4
blood transfusion, perioperative 42
brain ischaemia 112–13
brain, traumatic injury 49
breast cancer 3, 10, 15, 22, 23, 24–5, 28, 39, 64, 84, 144, 178
Brier score 221, 227
bronchiectasis 132
bronchitis, chronic 131
bronchospasm 131
buprenorphine 84
buproprion 160

calcium antagonists 22, 25, 178
Canadian Cooperative Study Group trial 176
cancer
- breast 3, 10, 15, 22, 23, 24–5, 28, 39, 64, 84, 144, 178
- endometrial 17
- lung 105
- non-small-cell lung 45
- oral 18
- ovarian 45, 216

cancer treatment
- 6-mercaptopurine 308–12
- pharmacoeconomics 308

Captopril Prevention Project (CAPPP) trial 6
carbamazepine 122, 298, 301, 303
cardiovascular disease 92
cardiovascular risk 84
cardioversion 265–6
carotid endarterectomy 94, 142, 176–9
- predicting benefit from 200–3
- risk model 197–200

carotid stenosis 14, 67, 142, 205
case–control studies 16, 103
case-crossover analysis 23
causalgia 122
celecoxib 18
central pain 122, 126
cerebral ischaemia 52
cerebrovascular disease 64
cetuximab 308
CHADS 2 scheme awards 270, 273
Chlamydia pneumoniae 144
cholera 18
cholesterol 4
cholinesterase inhibitors 100
chronic inflammatory demyelinating polyradiculoneuropathy 239
chronic obstructive pulmonary disease, pharmaceutical trials 131–4
ciclosporin 151
cisplatinum 122
citalopram 160
clinical credibility. prerequisites for 214
clinical prediction rules 215
clinical trials 3–5
- avoidance of moderate random errors 10–13
- avoidance of moderate systematic errors 5–10
- clinical practice 13–15
- inference based on overall effects on particular outcomes 13–14
- mortality analysis interpretation 14–15
- prespecification of analyses within particular subgroups 14

clofibrate 7
clomipramine 160
clopidogrel 115, 142, 200, 267
clozapine 161
Cochrane Collaboration, The 45, 46
Cochrane Library, The 41, 51
Cochrane Methods Group on Applicability & Recommendations 88
Cochrane Systematic Review 89, 184, 260
codeine 161
cohort studies 16
colon cancer 23, 144
colorectal cancer 18, 23, 24
complex regional pain syndrome type II 122
compliance 7, 62
confounding 18–19
CONSORT 40, 71, 169
contraceptives, oral 23, 84–5
control-rate metaregression 285–6
coronary artery bypass grafting 142, 200
coronary artery catheterisation 22
Coronary Drug Project 7
coronary heart disease 14, 20, 23, 92
corticosteroids 49, 134
- prenatal 45

cost
- of ADRs 307
- of epilepsy 297

Index

of older people 106
Cox regression 217, 220
C-reactive protein 27, 143, 258
c-statistic 221, 227
cumulative meta-analysis 43
cytochrome P450 C19 (CYP2C19) 164
cytochrome P450 2C9 (CYP2C9) 155–9
cytochrome P450 2D6 (CYP2D6) 151, 155, 159–61, 164
and antidepressants 160
and antipsychotics 161
and opioids 161

D statistic 221, 227
DANAMI-2 trial 287–9
data-dependent emphasis 7–9
dementia 15, 18
desipramine 160
detection bias 19, 22
dexfenfluramine 17
dextromethorphan 161
diabetes 83, 126, 239
diabetic coma 3
diabetic neuropathies 121, 123, 124, 125, 126
diethylstilboestrol 17
Digitalis Investigation Group (DIG) 24
digoxin 24, 99
dihydrocodeine 161
dihydropyrimidine dehydrogenase (DPD) 162
diltiazem 146
dipyridamole 52, 75, 115
diuretics 22, 146
divalproex sodium 164
doctor–patient relationship 62, 140
domoic acid 299
double dummy placebo technique 86
doxepine 160

Early Breast Cancer Trialists' Collaborative Group 52
ECASS II 293
elderly patients
atrial fibrillation, stroke prevention 268–70, 272–3
'*n*-of-1' trial 103–4, 241
neglect of 106
selection into trials 100–2
subgroup analysis 102–3
see also ageing
emphysema 131
endarterectomy 142, 176, 178, 191
endometrial cancer 17
enoxaparin 142, 200, 289
epidermal growth factor receptor inhibitors 314–16
epilepsy 75, 101, 143, 239
choice of AED 297, 298–9
choice of agent in 297–304
cost 297
evidence base and guidelines 300–2
future 302–4
incidence 297
pathophysiology and serendipity 299–300
escitalopram 160
ESPRIT trial 52
ethics 40–1
'*n*-of-1' trial 237, 241
ethylmorphine 161
etifibatide 184
European Carotid Surgery Trial (ECST) 64, 66, 71, 173, 176, 177, 200–1, 203, 204
European System for Cardiac Operative Risk Evaluation (EuroSCORE) 222–4
events per variable (EPV) 216
evidence-based medicine 111
extensive metabolisers (EM) 155
external validity of randomised controlled trials 61–77
adverse effects of treatment 76–7
characteristics of randomised patients 71–3
composite outcome measures 75–6
intervention, control treatment and pre-trial or non-trial management 72–3
length of treatment and follow-up 76
outcome measures and follow-up 74–6
patient-centred outcomes 75
scales 74
selection of patients 68–71
by eligibility criteria 68–70
enrichment strategies 70
prior to consideration of eligibility 68
reporting 71
run-in periods 70
selection beyond the eligibility criteria 70
setting 64–8
country 64–7
healthcare system 64
participating centres and clinicians 67–8
surrogate outcomes 74
extrapolation to primary care 87–8
false-negative results 10–11

Index

false-positive results 12–13
fenfluramine 17
fibrinogen 27
fibrinolytic therapy 8, 10, 11, 13, 14, 102
fibromyalgia 239
5-fluorouracil 162, 308
fluoxetine 160
fluvoxamine 160
forest plot 43
Framingham Heart Study 251, 258

gabapentin 122, 123, 125
Galt formula 99
gefitinib (Iressa) 163, 315
generalisability 61, 214
genetic polymorphisms 154
gentamycin 99
Global Initiative for Asthma (GINA) 132
Global Initiative for Chronic Obstructive Disease (GOLD) workshop guideline 132
GRACE model 289, 290
Gruppo Italiano per lo Studio della Streptochinasi nell'Infarcto Miocardico (GISSI) randomised trial 8, 10, 70
GUSTO trial 184, 281–5

H_2-receptor antagonists 93
hazard ratios 221
Heart Protection Study 146
hemianopia 14
heparin 15, 66, 142, 184
hexamethonium 41
hippocampal sclerosis 299
HIV/AIDS 3, 144, 145, 162
homocysteine 27
homeopathy 64
hormone replacement therapy (HRT) 17, 18, 23, 28, 46, 53, 144
Hosmer–Lemeshow test 221
hydrazine 162
hydrocodone 161
hypercholesterolaemia 84
hypertension 239
Hypertension Detection Follow-up Program 250

idraparineux 267
imatinib (Gleevec) 163
imipramine 160
imputation 217
indirect estimation of effect 87–8
induction of labour 6
instrumental variable estimation 22
intention-to-treat analysis 7
interindividual variation in drug response 152–65
  causes 152
  CYP2C9, VKORC1 and warfarin 155–9
  CYP2D6, antidepressants, antipsychotics and opioids 159–61
  individuality of genomes 153–4
  mercaptopurine, irinotecan and trastuzumab 162–3
  monogenic causes or polymorphisms of drug response 154–5
  N-acetyltransferase and isoniazid 161–2
intermediate metabolisers (IM) 155
international normalised ratio (INR) 155, 268
International Study of Infarct Survival
  First (ISIS-1) 49
  Second (ISIS-2) 7, 10, 176
intracranial haemorrhage (ICH) 71
intrauterine growth retardation 12
inverse care law 105
irinotecan (CPT-II) 162–3, 308, 312–13, 316
isoniazid 161–2
itraconazole 22
IV-ACS 184

juvenile myoclonic epilepsy 298, 303

labour, induction of 6
lamifiban 184
lamotrigine 122, 298, 301
Lancet, The 42, 49, 51–2, 53
leucovorin 308
leukaemia
  acute lymphatic 310
  acute lymphoblastic (ALL) 162
levorphanol 122
logistic regression 220
lorcainide 38
lumpectomy 10, 64
lung cancer 105

magnesium 15
magnetic resonance imaging (MRI) 272
MALDI-TOF 308
maprotiline 160
mastectomy 10, 64
mastoiditis 91

MCA disease 115–16, 117
Medical Research Council (MRC) 49, 50–1, 100, 141, 174
Medline 41
mega-trial 10, 11, 53
melanoma, malignant 17, 23
meningococcal disease 84, 93
mercaptopurine 162–3, 164
meta-analysis 5, 8–9, 17–18, 39, 52, 114, 183–91
  conventional 184–5
  individual patient data 188–90
  of randomised trials 42
  of subgroup differences 187–8
meta-regression 185–7, 285–6
methadone 122
mianserin 160
migraine 239
mirtazepine 160
miscarriages of treatment 142
model to predict survival among patients with end-stage liver disease (MELD) 213
morphine 122
motor neuron disease 101
multidimensional subgroup analyses 199
multidrug resistant 1 (MDR1 gene) 159
multiple imputation 217
multiple sclerosis 75, 121, 126, 195
myasthenia gravis 101
myocardial infarction 14, 19, 22, 38, 42–5, 101–3, 171, 200
  acute (AMI) 7–8, 13, 70, 176, 224, 279

N-acetyltransferase 161–2
National Institute for Health and Clinical Excellence (NICE) 184, 301
National Institutes of Health (US) 45, 70, 71
National Service Framework (UK) 259
neuropathic pain, pharmaceutical trials 121–34
  adverse effects 124
  clinical characteristics 123
  outcome measures and follow-up 123–4
  recommendations for future trials 127–8
  selection of patients 123
  setting 122–3
  trial protocol versus routing practice 123
NHS Research and Development Programme 49
nicotine gum 83
nimodipine 48
NINDS trial 290, 293
'*n*-of-1' trials 37, 83, 85–7, 94, 183, 231–42
  analysis 235–7
  Bayesian statistics 237
  clinical examples 241
  definition 232
  design 233
  double-blind treatment allocation 233–4
  drug-induced adverse effects 241
  elderly patients 103–4, 241
  ethics 237, 241
  follow-up and outcome evaluation 234–5
  informed consent 232
  interventions 232
  limitations 238
  outcome measures (treatment targets) 234
  preliminary, unblinded, run-in period of active treatment 232–3
  qualitative evaluation 235
  quantitative evaluation 235
  readiness of patient to change behaviour 232
  replication 235
  research examples 242
  setting 232
  sign test 236
  strengths 237–8
  Student's paired *t*-test 236–7
  subject 232
  treatment effectiveness 242
  treatment intervals 234
  treatment periods (cycles) 234
  value to clinicians and researchers 238–41
    clinician 241
    disease 239
    patient 239
    support services241
    treatment 240
    trial design 240–1
  visual assessment 235–6
non-Q-wave infarction 184
non-randomised assessment of treatment 16–28
non-small-cell lung cancer 45
non-valvular fibrillation 142
North American Symptomatic Carotid Artery Endarterectomy Trial (NASCET) 20, 201
nortriptyline 160
NSAIDs 18, 68, 73, 74, 86, 99
number needed to harm (NNH) 122, 124, 126
number needed to quit (NNQ) 122, 124, 126
number needed to treat (NNT) 15, 84, 122, 124, 126, 141–2, 195, 197
observational studies 4, 15–28

Index

absolute effects of treatment 27–8
assessment of adverse effects of treatment 16–18
assessment of beneficial effects of treatment 18
control of biases 22–3
estimation of potential effects of treatment 25–8
limitations 16
relative effects of treatment 25–7
results from randomised trials 24–5
small random errors in 23–4
sources of bias 18–22
bias due to differential detection of outcomes 22
differential recall of treatment exposure 21
factors associated with treatment and outcome 18–21
oestrogen 23
oestrogen receptor alpha 144
oestrogen replacement therapy *see* hormone replacement therapy
olanzepine 161
older people 97–107
costs 106
neglect 106
selection into trials 100–2
well-being of 97–8
omeprazole 93
opiate addiction 84
opioids 122, 159–61
oral cancer 18
osteoarthritis 86, 239
otitis media 87, 89, 91
ovarian cancer 45, 216
overfitted models 217
oxcarbazepine 298
Oxford Record Linkage Study (ORLS) 104–5
oxycodone 122, 161
oxytocin 6

painful diabetic neuropathy 122, 124–5, 126
paracetamol 86
PARAGON-B 184
Parkinson's disease 100, 239
paroxetine 160
patient preference 62, 140
penicillin 18, 84
prehospital 93
peptic ulcer 85, 113
peripheral neuropathic pain 126
periventricular heterotopia (PVH) 299
perphenazine 161
phantom limb pain 121, 122, 126
pharmacodynamics 99
pharmacogenetics 153, 190
clinical potential of 164–5
therapeutic lessons from 163–4
pharmacogenomics 152, 153, 162–3
clinical potential of 164–5
therapeutic lessons from 163–4
pharmacokinetics 99
phenoprocoumon 158, 159
phentermine 17
phenytoin 298, 303
PICO mnemonic 90, 91, 93
placebo effect 62, 140, 232
plagiarism 40
platelet glycoprotein IIb/IIIa inhibitors (PGIs) 184
poliomyelitis 6
polypill 260
poor metabolisers (PM) 155
post-randomisation characteristics 9–10
post-stroke pain 121, 126
postherpetic neuralgia 121, 122, 124, 126
postsurgical nerve injury pain 126
pravastatin 144
pre-eclampsia 12, 15
pregabalin 122, 123, 125
prehospital penicillin 93
prevention paradox 205
primary care
application of evidence to individual patient 91–3
benefits and harms, different, in 90–1
benefits and harms, types 89–90
transferability of evidence to 88–91
versus other settings 83–5
PRISM trial 184
PRISM-PLUS 184
probability models 213
procainamide 162
progestin 23
prognostic models 213–27
PROGRESS trial 273
progressive supranuclear palsy 101
propafenone 160
Prospective Cardiovascular Munster (PROCAM) study 258
proton pump inhibitors 93

Index

PSEP 221, 224, 227
publication bias 38
PURSUIT model 184, 289, 290
pyrosequencing 308

quality-adjusted life years (QALYs) 106
quality-of-life assessment 100
quinidine 160
quitiazepine 161

R^2 measures 221, 227
random errors 4
  minimising 5–16
  moderate 10–13
randomisation, proper 5–7
randomised controlled trials (RCTs) 5–16, 20, 131, 139, 173, 195, 199, 231
  in neuropathic pain 121–8
  see also external validity of randomised controlled trials
ranitidine 93
recall bias 19, 21
recombinant factor X 164
referral rates from primary care 84
relative risk reduction (RRR) 88, 144, 175
research misconduct 40
reserpine 24
responses to treatment, clinically important 139–46
  arguments against attempts to target treatment 140
  biological heterogeneity 144
  comorbidity 145–6
  genetic heterogeneity 144
  heterogeneity related to risk 141–2
  multiple underlying pathologies 143
  pathophysiological heterogeneity 143–4
  severity or stage of disease 144–5
  situations where differences are expected 140–6
  timing of treatment 145
  underuse of treatment 146
rheumatoid arthritis 74, 76
rifampicin 161
risk models
  accessibility of results 203–4
  carotid endarterectomy 197–200
  case studies 222–5
    lessons from 225–6
    predicting 4-year mortality in older adults 222
    predicting death from acute myocardial infarction 224
    predicting operative mortality of patients undergoing cardiac surgery 222–4
  comparing predictions with observations 221
  developing a useful prognostic model 214–15
  external validation 220
  individual variation in absolute risk 195–7
  internal validation 220
  measuring intrinsic prognostic information 220–1
  need to validate a prognostic model 215–18
  predicting benefit from carotid endarterectomy 200–3
  prespecifying adequate performance 221
  quantifying performance 226–7
  study design 219–20
  temporal validation 220
  using individual risk to target treatment 204–9
  validation of prognostic model 218–21
risperidone 161
road-traffic accidents 23, 104
rofecoxib 18
roxithromycin 144

salazosulfapyridine 162
Salk polio vaccine studies 6
schizophrenia 74, 76
SCORE Project 258
scurvy 49
seizure type, epilepsy syndrome 301
selective serotonin reuptake inhibitors (SSRIs) 160
senile dementia 101
sertraline 160
severe myoclonic epilepsy of infancy (SMEI) 302
single nucleotide polymorphisms (SNPs) 153–4, 308
smoking clinics 83
SNP chips/head arrays 308
sodium valproate 301
somatotropin 164
spinal cord injury 126
spinal cord injury pain 121
stage-of-change model 232

Index

Standard and New Antiepileptic Drugs (SANAD) trial 301
statins 10, 14, 18, 90, 98, 205
status epilepticus 299
Stevens–Johnson syndrome 17
STOP trial 141, 142
streptokinase 8, 281–5
stroke 7, 14, 15, 20, 21, 28, 68, 105, 113–14, 290–3
  acute 191
  acute ischaemic 48
  atrial fibrillation and 265–75
  risk of 197
Stroke Prevention in Atrial Fibrillation (SPAF) III risk stratification 270
Stroke Prevention in Reversible Ischaemia Trial (SPIRIT) 71, 73
Student's paired *t*-test 236–7
subgroups, treatment in 169–80
  interpretation 176–8
  multidimensional subgroup analysis 179
  statistical analysis and reporting 171–6
  trial design 169–73
syringomyelia 121
systematic reviews 37–54, 114, 139
systemic errors 4
  minimising 5–16
  moderate 5–10
systolic blood pressure 143

tacrine 70
tamoxifen 15, 178
Taqman 308
tetracyclic compounds 160
TGN1412 39
thalidomide 17, 21
thiazide 146
thiopurine methyltransferase (TPMT) 162, 310–12
thioridazine 161, 164
thrombolytic predictive instrument (TPI) 280
thrombolytic therapy 44, 103
  versus primary coronary intervention (PCI) 285–9
ticlopidine 115
time-to-event data 217
TIMI model 289, 290
timolol 98
tirofiban 184
tissue plasminogen activator (tPA) 281–5
toxic epidermal necrolysis 17
tramadol 122
transient global amnesia 101
transient ischaemic attacks (TIAs) 8, 26, 76, 94, 112, 115, 116, 143, 179, 196, 205
trastuzumab 162–3
trials, limitations of 112–14
tricyclic antidepressants 160
trigeminal neuralgia 122
troponin 189
tuberculosis 66, 132, 162
tyrosine kinases 163

UGT1A1 164, 313
UK Prospective Diabetes Study 28
ulcer
  leg 15
  peptic 85, 113
ultrarapid metabolisers (UM) 155
Uniform Requirements for Manuscripts Submitted to Biomedical Journals 71
unstable angina 184
unstable angina/non-ST-segment-elevation myocardial infarction (UA/NSTEMI) 289–90

validity 214
valproic acid 151, 164
vascular disease 101
venlafaxine 160
vesnarinone 15
vitamin E 27
VKORC1 155–9
volunteer effects 101

warfarin 71, 76, 85, 88, 113, 115, 151, 155–9, 164, 266–7
  in elderly atrial fibrillation patients 272–3, 274
Warfarin–Aspirin Recurrent Stroke (WARS) study 115
WASID trial 115
Wellcome Trust 49
Wellcome Trust Witness Seminar 46
willingness to please bias 232
Women's health initiative 23
wrongful treatment 142

xanthine oxidase (XDH) 310
ximelagatran 267

zidovudine 3
ziprasidone 161